ADVANCES IN EMBRYO TRANSFER

Edited by **Bin Wu**

Advances in Embryo Transfer
Edited by Bin Wu

Published by InTech
Janeza Trdine 9, 51000 Rijeka, Croatia

Publishing Process Manager Iva Simcic

Technical Editor Teodora Smiljanic

Cover Designer InTech Design Team

Additional hard copies can be obtained from orders@intechopen.com

Advances in Embryo Transfer, Edited by Bin Wu
p. cm.
ISBN 978-953-51-0318-9

For EU product safety concerns:
IN TECH d.o.o., Prolaz Marije Krucifikse Kozulić 3, 51000 Rijeka, Croatia,
info@intechopen.com or visit our website at intechopen.com.

Meet the editor

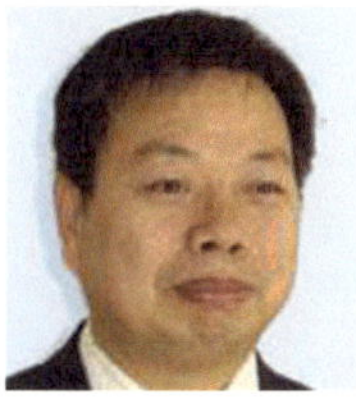

Bin Wu, Ph.D., HCLD is currently a scientific laboratory director at Arizona Center for Reproductive Endocrinology and Infertility, USA. He received his training in genetics and reproductive biology at the Northwest Agricultural University in China and Cornell University, New York and post-doctor training at University of Guelph, Canada. He was promoted as a professor at the Northwest Agricultural University. As an embryologist, he later joined in the Center for Human Reproduction in Chicago. Dr. Wu has membership for many professional associations, such as American Society for Reproductive Medicine; International Embryo Transfer Society; Society for the Study of Reproduction; American Association of Bioanalysts and European Society of Human Reproduction and Embryology. Also, he has obtained some significant research awards from these professional associations.

Contents

Preface

Embryo transfer technology has become one of the prominent high businesses worldwide in human and animal reproduction. As human in vitro fertilization (IVF) technique rapidly develops in infertility treatment, not only animal IVF has offered a very valuable tool to study mammalian fertilization and early embryo development as treatment, but also its commercial applications have being increased quickly. So far, this technology has gone through three major changes, that is, (1) traditional embryo transfer (in vivo embryo production by donor superovulation) in animals, especially in cow, (2) in vitro embryo production by ovum pick up with in vitro fertilization (OPU-IVF) in human and animals and (3) notably current cloning technique by somatic cell nuclear transfer and transgenic animal production. Embryo transfer technology has widely been used in animal industry to improve animal breeds. In human, many IVF clinic centers have been set up for infertility couple treatment over the whole world.

As embryo transfer techniques have accumulated over long period, many kinds of books about embryo transfer on human and various animals have been published. Most of books have described embryo transfer procedures and manipulation protocols. The purpose of this book does not concentrate on the detail description of basic embryo transfer techniques and procedures, while we will update and review some new developed theories and technologies and focus on discussing some encountered problems during embryo transfer and give some examples how to improve pregnancy rate by innovated techniques so that readers, especially embryologists and physicians for human IVF programs, may acquire some new and usable information as well as some key practice techniques.

This book contains four parts with 16 chapters. Firstly, an optimal stimulation scheme for ovaries, particularly natural and minimal stimulation of ovaries, has been discussed in the first part. Then, one paper analyzed that how many oocytes per retrieval will be the best for human IVF practice. If one stimulation scheme produces too many eggs, it often results in hyperstimulation syndrome. Thus, a chapter reviewed hyperstimulation syndrome diagnosis, prevention and treatment. In the second part, some advanced technologies in insemination have been listed. After introduction of normal sperm physiology, sperm meiotic chromosome abnormalities and DNA fragmentation infertile patients are analyzed. Then, newly developed intracytoplasmic sperm injection (ICSI) techniques, such as intracytoplasmic morphologically-selected sperm injection (IMSI) and selection of hyaluronan bound sperm for use in ICSI (PICSI), have been reviewed. Finally, we introduced some new techniques and methods which can make azoospermic men realize their dream to have children. In the third part, it will mainly discuss how to increase pregnancy rate by improving embryo transfer procedures including optimal embryo transfer skills, blastocyst selection and single embryo transfer, and the relationship of intercourse and pregnancy success rate. In the last part, endometrial receptivity and embryo implantation are discussed, interestingly, more than 20 biomarkers have been found in uterus to determine embryo implantation window and pregnancy failure. Thus, this book will greatly add some new information for embryologists and IVF physicians to improve human IVF pregnancy rate.

Great thanks go to all authors who gladly contributed their time and expertise to prepare these outstanding chapters included in this book.

Bin Wu, Ph.D., HCLD (ABB)
Arizona Center for Reproductive Endocrinology and Infertility
Tucson, Arizona
USA

Part 1

Introductory Chapter

1

Advances in Embryo Transfer

Bin Wu
Arizona Center for Reproductive Endocrinology and Infertility, Tucson, Arizona USA

1. Introduction

Embryo transfer refers to a step in the process of assisted reproduction in which one or several embryos are placed into the uterus of a female with the intent to establish a pregnancy. Currently this biotechnology has become one of the prominent high businesses worldwide. This technique, which is often used in connection with *in vitro* fertilization (IVF), has widely been used in animals or human, in which situations the goals may vary. In animal husbandry, embryo transfer has become the most powerful tool for animal scientists and breeders to improve genetic construction of their animal herds and increase quickly elite animal numbers which have recently gained considerable popularity with seedstock dairy and beef producers. In human, embryo transfer technique has mainly been used for the treatment of infertile couples to realize their dream to have their children. The history of the embryo transfer procedure goes back considerably farther, but the most modern applicable embryo transfer technology was developed in the 1970s (Steptoe and Edwards, 1978). In the last three decades, embryo transfer has developed into a specific advanced biotechnology which has gone through three major changes, "three generations"---the first with embryo derived from donors (*in vivo*) by superovulation, non-surgical recovery and transfer, especially in cattle embryos, the second with *in vitro* embryo production by ovum pick up with *in vitro* fertilization (OPU-IVF) and the third including further *in vitro* developed techniques, especially innovated embryo micromanipulation technique, which can promote us to perform embryo cloning involved somatic cells and embryonic stem cells, preimplantation genetic diagnosis (PGD), transgenic animal production etc. At the same time, commercial animal embryo transfer has become a large international business (Betteridge, 2006), while human embryo transfer has spread all over the world for infertility treatment. Just only in the United States of America there are 442 assisted reproductive technology (ART) centers with IVF programs in 2009 report of the Centers for Disease Control and Prevention. Embryo transfer, besides male sperm, involves entire all process from female ovarian stimulation (start) to uterine receptivity (end). During this entire process, many new bio-techniques have been developed (Figure 1). These techniques include optimal ovarian stimulation scheme, oocyte picking up (OPU) or oocyte retrieval, *in vitro* maturation (IVM) of immature oocytes, *in vitro* fertilization (IVF) and intracytoplasmic sperm injection (ICSI), preimplantation genetic diagnosis (PGD), blastocyst embryo culture technology, identification of optimal uterine environment etc. Here, we will review some key newly developed biotechnologies on human embryo transfer.

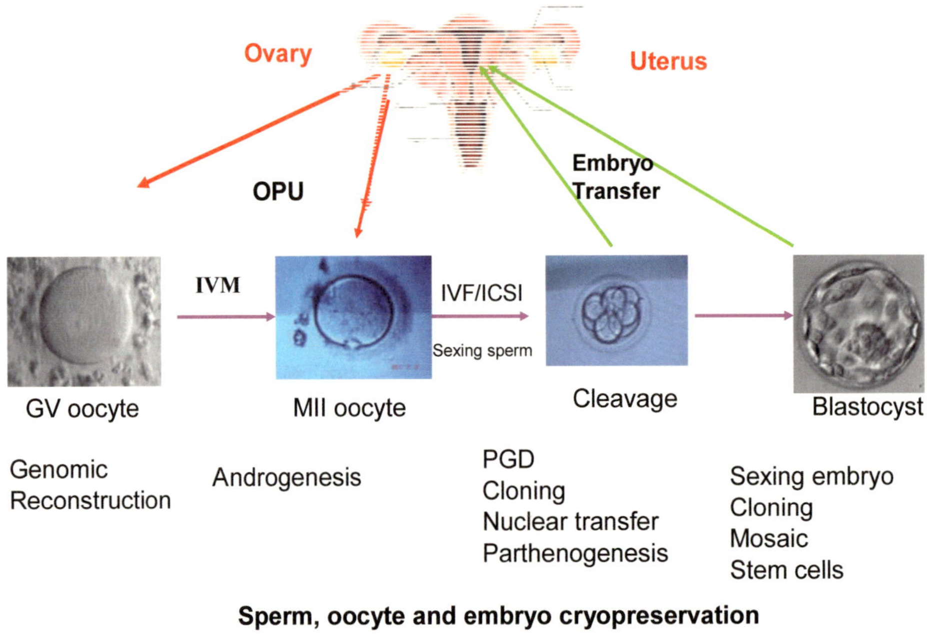

Fig. 1. Schematic representation of main embryo biotechnologies which can involve from ovary to uterus.

2. Ovarian stimulation technique

So far we have known that female ovary at birth has about 2 million primordial follicles with primary oocytes and at puberty ovary has 300,000 to 400,000 oocytes. From puberty, oocytes start frequently to grow, mature and ovulate from ovaries under endocrine hormone stimulation, such as follicle stimulating hormone (FSH), luteinizing hormone (LH) and estradiol, but normal fertile woman usually ovulate only an oocyte per menstrual cycle. This will ensure women to be able to have a normal single baby pregnancy. However, in an attempt to compensate for inefficiencies in IVF procedures, patients need to undergo ovarian stimulation using high doses of exogenous gonadotrophins to allow retrieval of multiple oocytes in a single cycle. Current IVF stimulation protocols in the United State generally involve the use of 3 types of drugs: 1) a medication to suppress the LH surge and ovulation until the developing eggs are ready, GnRH-agonist (gonadotropin releasing hormone agonist) such as Lupron and GnRH-antagonist such as Ganirelix or Cetrotide; 2) FSH product (follicle stimulating hormone) to stimulate development of multiple eggs such as Gonal-F, Follistim, Bravelle, Menopur; 3) HCG (human chorionic gonadotropin) to cause final maturation of the eggs. The use of such ovarian stimulation protocols enables the selection of one or more embryos for transfer, while supernumerary embryos can be cryopreserved for transfer in a later cycle (Macklon et al. 2006). Currently the standard regimen procedures for ovarian stimulation have been set up in all IVF centers (Santos, et al., 2010) in which almost centers use exogenous gonadotrophins as routine procedure to stimulate patients' ovaries to obtain multiple eggs. This technique works very well in most patients. Thus, this leads to setting up many drug companies to produce all kind of stimulation drugs for human assisted reproductive technology (ART). However, evidences of recent several year studies have showed that ovarian stimulation may itself have detrimental effects on oogenesis, embryo quality, uterus endometrial receptivity and perhaps perinatal outcomes. The retrieval oocyte number is also considered to be an important prognostic variable in our routine IVF practice (see Chapter 3 in this book). Also, if this stimulation scheme produces too many eggs, it often results in hyperstimulation syndrome. Standard IVF requires the administration of higher dosages of injectable medications to stimulate the growth of multiple eggs. These medications are expensive and are associated with certain potential health risks. Careful monitoring must be performed to ensure safety and efficacy. While these factors lead to increased costs and time commitment for the patient, the result is an increased number of embryos available for transfer. Additionally, in standard or traditional IVF, cryopreservation of surplus embryos for transfer in a non-stimulated cycle may be available. The overall expected take-home baby rate with standard IVF varies considerably, based primarily upon the patient's age. Recently some IVF centers have begun to use natural or minimal stimulation on IVF and obtained good results.

The recent popularity of Mini-IVF (minimal stimulation IVF), Micro-IVF, natural cycle for IVF, oocyte *in vitro* maturation (IVM) has attested to the changes taking place in the practice of advanced reproductive technologies (Edward, 2007). This technique has some advantage and has good future use. A common feature all of these procedures share is the use of less infertility medications. The reduction in medication use compared to a normal IVF cycle ranges from a 50% to a 100% reduction. If the less medication is used, the less monitoring is required (blood test and ultrasounds). The amount of reduction in monitoring depends on the procedure being done and the philosophy of the practice. For most of these approaches, fewer eggs are involved, which may mean there is less work for the laboratory to do. Some programs will discount their routine laboratory charges compared to regular IVF and patients may pay less expense (see Chapter 2). Also, the most significant risk of routine IVF, severe ovarian hyperstimulation syndrome, could be decreased in all of these procedures or completely eliminated in some pure natural IVF cycles and programmed IVM cycles (Tang-Pedersen et al., 2012). This can be very important for some women with severe polycystic ovary syndrome (PCOS) who are at increased risk for significant discomfort or even (rarely) hospitalization with routine IVF approaches. However, this technique needs more times of oocyte retrieval and results in a lower pregnancy rate per egg retrieval cycle because only one or a very few eggs may be retrieved per cycle. Thus, this technique may be used in some specific woman populations, such as younger women less than 30 years old or aged women over 40 years old. In this book, the impact of ovarian stimulation and underlying mechanisms will be reviewed and some strategies for reducing the impact of ovarian stimulation on IVF outcomes are also addressed. (Please further read Chapter 2 in this book).

As describing above, ovarian hyperstimulation syndrome (OHSS) usually occurs as a result of taking hormonal medications that stimulate oocyte development in woman's ovaries. In OHSS, the ovaries become swollen and painful and its symptoms can range from mild to severe. About one-fourth of women who take injectible fertility drugs get a mild OHSS form, which goes away after about a week. If woman becomes pregnant after taking one of these fertility drugs, her OHSS may last several weeks. A small proportion of women taking fertility drugs develop a more severe OHSS form, which can cause rapid weight gain, abdominal pain, vomiting and shortness of breath. In order to prevent OHSS occur, some effective steps should be taken. If the OHSS has happened, specific treatment should be guided by the severity of OHSS. The aim of the treatment is to help relieving symptoms and prevent complications. Chapter 4 of this book has given a detail review about OHSS diagnosis, prevention and treatment.

3. Advances in insemination and *in vitro* fertilization technology

Embryo development begins with fertilization. Prior to fertilization, both the oocytes and the sperm must undergo a series of maturational events to acquire their capacity to achieve fertilization. Much research in this area has been geared toward improving reproductive efficiencies of farm animals and preserving endangered species. An important milestone of embryo transfer is *in vitro* fertilization (IVF). In animals, IVF has offered a very valuable tool to study mammalian fertilization and early embryo development. *in vitro* fertilization is a process by which retrieval oocytes fertilized by sperm outside the body, *in vitro*. IVF is a major treatment in infertility when other methods of assisted reproductive technology have failed. This technique has become a routine procedure and widely been used in human infertile treatment all over the world. IVF was initially created to help those women whose fallopian tubes were blocked not allowing for fertilization to occur. Over the years through, this technique has become very efficient in achieving pregnancies for several other situations including unexplained infertility. So far many infertile couples may obtain their dreamed children by IVF technique. However, IVF isn't just for issues relating to women. Male sperm amount and quality has a determined effect on egg fertilization. Sperm dysfunction is associated with the inability of sperm to bind and penetrate the oocyte zona pellucida. During last two decades, micromanipulation techniques have undergone some major developments which include partial zona dissection (PZD), subzonal sperm injection (SUZI) and intracytoplasmic sperm injection (ICSI). These methods greatly improve oocyte fertilization rate. More importance is that ICSI technique can solve sever male infertility problem including 1) complete absence of sperm (azoospermia); 2) low sperm count (oligozoospermia); 3) abnormal sperm shape (teratozoospermia); 4) problems with sperm movement (asthenozoospermia); 5) completely immobile sperm (necrozoospermia). To further review the development of these technologies, four chapters about sperm treatment have been listed in this book.

Firstly, some basic knowledge of sperm physiology has been described and evaluation of male infertility has been discussed (Chapter 5). Secondly, the sperm chromosomal abnormality has a significant effect on embryo quality and pregnancy rate. Even so it may result in a lot of miscarriage after pregnancy. Currently there are many researches about sperm abnormality including sperm chromosomal examination, sperm DNA fragmentation analysis. Thus, a chapter about meiotic chromosome abnormalities and spermatic FISH in infertile patients with normal karyotype has listed (Chapter 6). This chapter indicates that the incidence of spermatic aneuploid in the infertile population is as three times as in the fertile population and using FISH technique may diagnosis testicular sperm meiosis. This is a very interesting result. Thirdly, in the recent years, ICSI technique has experienced a great development to intracytoplasmic morphologically-selected sperm injection (IMSI) and a method for selection of hyaluronan bound sperm for use in ICSI (PICSI) (Parmegiani et al., 2010a,b; Said & Land 2011; Berger et al., 2011). These innovations have significantly increased egg fertilization and pregnancy rates in many IVF clinics. The major aim of these techniques is to select a normal good spermatozoon without any dysfunction for ICSI to obtain a good quality embryo for transfer. Oligozoospermic men often carry seminal populations demonstrating increased chromosomal aberrations and compromised DNA integrity. Therefore, the *in vitro* selection of sperm for ICSI is critical and directly influences the paternal contribution to preimplantation embryogenesis. Hyaluronan (H), a major constituent of the cumulus matrix, may play a critical role in the selection of functionally competent sperm during *in vivo* fertilization (Parmegiani et al., 2010a). Hyaluronan bound sperm (HBS) exhibit decreased levels of cytoplasmic inclusions and residual histones, an increased expression of the HspA2 chaperone protein and a marked reduction in the incidence of chromosomal aneuploidy. The relationship between HBS and enhanced levels of developmental competence led to the current clinical trial (Worrilow et al., 2010). Thus, as a HBS test, a PCISI technique, a method for selection of hyaluronan bound sperm for use in ICSI, has been developed to treat oligozoospermic and asthenozoospermic man infertility problem (Parmegiani et al., 2010b). Additionally, recent advanced intracytoplasmic morphologically-selected sperm injection (IMSI) technique has been used to treat sperm morphology problem (teratozoospermia). These techniques have begun to be used in some IVF centers. Thus, some detail technologies for sperm selection have been reviewed in chapter 7.

Finally, the most sever cases of male infertility are those presenting with no sperm in the ejaculate (azoospermia). Some men have a condition where their reproductive ducts may be absent or blocked (obstructive azoospermia or OA), where others may have no sperm production with normal reproductive anatomy (non-obstructive azoospermia or NOA). Azoospermia is found in 10% of male infertility cases. Patients with OA due to congenital bilateral absence of the vas deferens or those in whom reconstructive surgery fails have historically been considered infertile. Men who can not produce sperm in their testes with apparent absence of spermatogenesis diagnosed by testicle biopsy are classified as NOA. Once testicular and epidiymal function can be verified, surgery is justified to correct or remove the blockage. Current optimal method for treatment of azoospermic men is to acquire sperm from testicles or epididymides by means of surgery or non-surgery (Wu et al., 2005). However, in some situations, no any mature spermatozoon can be obtained from either semen or surgical testicular biopsy tissues. Thus immature haploid spermatids or diploid spermatocytes or spermatogonia, or even somatic cells like Sertoli cell nuclei or Leydig cells may also be considered as a sperm to transfer paternal DNA into maternal oocyte to form embryo for transfer. In the chapter of advances in fertility options of azoospermic men (Chapter 8), the optimal applications of testicular biopsy sperm, round or elongated spermatids from azoospermic men to human IVF have been discussed and some new technologies to produce artificial sperm from stem cells and somatic cells as well as sperm cloning have been designed. Application of these technologies will make no sperm men realize their dream to have a child.

4. Procedure for embryo transfer

The procedure of embryo transfer is very crucial and great attention and time should be given to this step. The embryo transfer procedure is the last one of the *in vitro* fertilization process and it is a critically important procedure. No matter how good the IVF laboratory culture environment is, the physician can ruin everything with a carelessly performed embryo transfer. The entire IVF cycle depends on delicate placement of the embryos at the proper location near the middle of the endometrial cavity with minimal trauma and manipulation. The ultimate goal of a successful embryo transfer is to deliver the embryos atraumatically to the uterine fundus in a location where implantation is maximized.

The transfer of embryos can be accomplished in several different fashions including transfallopian (ZIFT), transmyometrial and transcervical ways. Today the majority of embryo transfers are performed via the cervical canal into the uterine cavity by a specific catheter. In order to optimize the embryo transfer technique, although Mansour and Aboulghar (2002) had a good review paper about embryo transfer procedure, two chapters of this book indicated that several precautions should be taken (Chapter 9 and 10). The first and most important is to avoid the initiation of uterine contractility. This can be achieved by the use of soft catheters, gentle manipulation and by avoiding touching the fundus. Secondly, proper evaluation of the uterine cavity and utero-cervical angulation is very important, and this can be achieved by performing dummy embryo transfer and by ultrasound evaluation of the utero-cervical angulation and uterine cavity length. Another important step is the removal of cervical mucus so that it does not stick to the catheter and inadvertently remove the embryo during catheter withdrawal. Finally, one has to be absolutely sure that the embryo transfer catheter has passed the internal cervical os and that the embryos are delivered gently inside the uterine cavity.

Embryo stage for transfer also has an important influence on IVF pregnancy outcome. As we know, the time and number of transfer embryos have an obvious effect on pregnancy. Current IVF technique may make many infertility couple to realize their dream to have children, but many treated patients by IVF program have multiple pregnancy problems which present a serious perinatal risk for mother and child. This is mainly due to the transfer of three or four early cleavage stage embryos. In order to reduce multiple pregnancies, the best way is to transfer single embryo. However, this will greatly decrease pregnancy rate. Many studies have showed that good quality embryo on morphology will have a high chance for implantation, especially good blastocyst stage embryo for transfer. Thus, prolonged cultivation of embryos to the blastocyst stage has become a routine practice in the human *in vitro* fertilization program (IVF) since the first commercial sequential media were developed in 1999. The advantage of blastocyst culture is able to select the activated genome embryos (Braude et al., 1988) which have higher predictive values for implantation on the basis of their morphological appearance as compared with earlier embryos (Gardner and Schoolcraft, 1999; Kovačič et al., 2004) and in a reduction in the number of transferred embryos without compromising pregnancy rate (Gardner et al., 2000). Also transfer of blastocyst stage embryos is matching better synchronized with endometrial receptivity for embryo implantation. Interestingly, Kovačič et al's studies (see chapter 11) have showed that single or double blastocyst transfer results in similar pregnancy rates in young patient groups, but the twin rate remains unacceptably high after the transfer of two blastocysts, especially if at least one of them is morphologically optimal. Thus, based on evaluation of blastocyst embryo morphology, single embryo transfer is feasible for young couple patients so as to prevent multiple pregnancies in IVF program.

Also, frozen/thawed embryo transfer (FET) has become a routine procedure in all IVF centers throughout the world. This treatment involves implanting embryos that were retrieved from the patient during a previous IVF cycle and held safely in a frozen state. However, FET often results in lower pregnancy rate than fresh embryo transfers. This is because freezing and thawing may damage the morphological characteristics of embryos and survival rate of embryo blastomeres resulting into lower implantation rates. Thus, the evaluation after embryo thawing and transferring one or several real alive embryos will greatly improve pregnancy rate. In chapter 12, a simple research report has showed a pregnancy comparison following transfer of cultured versus non cultured frozen thawed human embryos. This study provides a feasible method to determine embryo alive after embryo thawing by overnight embryo culture to select the embryos with blastomere cleavage for transfer. Transferring cleaving embryos after embryo frozen and thawing will significantly increase pregnancy rate (Joshi et al., 2010).

So far, there is still a contradictory whether intercourse is encouraged or not after embryo transfer. A large of randomized control trials suggest that intercourse around the time of embryo transfer improve embryo implantation rates and increase pregnancy rate, but some studies showed no significant difference. Chapter 13 examines the available evidences suggesting why intercourse is beneficial or harmful to assisted reproductive technique outcome.

5. Embryo implantation and endometrial receptivity

After transfer procedure, embryo will continue growing and finally hatching out from zona pellucida to start implantation in the uterus. Thus, implantation is the final frontier to embryogenesis and successful pregnancy. Over the past three decades, tremendous advances have made in the understanding of human embryo development and its implantation in the uterus. Implantation is a process requiring the delicate interaction between the embryo and a receptive endometrium. This interactive process is a complex series of events that can be divided into three distinct steps: apposition, attachment and invasion (Chapter 15, Norwitz et al., 2001). This intricate interaction requires a harmonized dialogue between embryonic and maternal tissue. Thus, implantation represents the remarkable synchronization between the development of the embryo and the differentiation of the endometrium. As long as these events remain unexplained, it is very difficult to improve the success of IVF treatment. In last few years, many researches have focused on both enhancing the quality of the embryos and understanding the highly dynamic tissue of the endometrial wall (Horne et al., 2000) because there is a close relationship between endometrial receptivity and embryo implantation. Not only does woman pregnancy depend on embryo quality, but also it depends on uterine receptivity because uterine endometrium must undergo a serious changes leading to a short time for embryo implantation called the "implantation window". Outside of this time the uterus is resistant to embryo attachment. How to determine this window time is very important for obtaining a high pregnancy rate. Determining molecular mechanisms of human embryo implantation is an extremely challenging task due to the limitation of materials and significant differences underlying this process among mammalian species. Recently some papers have reviewed some adhesion molecules in endometrial epithelium during tissue integrity and embryo implantation (Singh and Aplin, 2009) and the trophinin has been identified as a unique apical cell adhesion molecule potentially involved in the initial adhesion of trophectoderm of the human blastocyst to endometrial surface epithelia (Fukuda, 2008). In the mouse, the binding between ErbB4 on the blastocyst and heparin-binding epidermal growth factor-like growth factor on the endometrial surface enables the initial step of the blastocyst implantation. L-selectin and its ligand carbohydrate have been proposed as a system that mediates initial adhesion of human blastocysts to the uterine epithelia. The evidence suggests that L-selectin and trophinin are included in human embryo implantation and their relevant to the functions and these cell adhesion mechanisms in human embryo implantation have been described (Fukuda, 2008). Interestingly, some important biomarkers including essential expression of proteins, cytokines and peptides can be detected in the uterine endometrium during embryo implantation (Aghajanova et al., 2008). Also, human cumulus cells may be used as biomarkers for embryo and pregnancy outcomes (Assou et al., 2010). Thus, this book selected two very interesting papers about mechanism of embryo implantation (Chapter 14, and 15). These two articles have explored the mystery of the mechanisms controlling the receptivity of the human endometrium. About 20 biomarkers have been described and studied to distinguish embryo implantation window time as days 20-24 of menstrual cycle. This is very interesting to determine embryo transfer time and to improve pregnancy rate. Additionally, screening for receptivity markers and testing patients accordingly may allow for increasing use a single embryo transfer.

From a clinical point of view, the repeated implantation failure is one the least understood causes of failure of IVF. The causes for repeated implantation failure may be because of reduced endometrial receptivity, embryonic defects or multifactorial causes. Various uterine pathologies, such as thin endometrium, altered expression of adhesive molecules and immunological factors, may decrease endometrial receptivity, whereas genetic abnormalities of the male or female, sperm defects, embryonic aneuploidy or zona hardening are among the embryonic reasons for failure of implantation. Endometriosis and hydrosalpinges may adversely influence both. Recent advances into the molecular processes have delineated possible explanations why the embryos fail to implant. Our selected chapters also have a detail description about embryo implantation failure and some feasible treatment methods have been recommended.

6. Fertility cryopreservation

Fertility cryopreservation is a vital branch of reproductive science and involves the preservation of gametes (sperm and oocytes), embryos, and reproductive tissues (ovarian and testicular tissues) for use in assisted reproduction techniques. The cryopreservation of reproductive cells is the process of freezing, storage, and thawing of spermatozoa or oocytes. It involves an initial exposure to cryoprotectants, cooling to subzero temperature, storage, thawing, and finally, dilution and removal of the cryoprotectants, when used, with a return to a physiological environment that will allow subsequent development. Proper management of the osmotic pressure to avoid damage due to intracellular ice formation is crucial for successful freezing and thawing procedure. So far there are two major techniques for reproductive cell or tissue cryopreservation: slow program frozen-thawing processes and vitrification method. Slow program has widely used in many IVF programs for a long time and it has been proved to be a feasible practice for human and other animal sperm and embryo freezing. In the last decade, many scientists and embryologists are more interested in vitrification method because this technique may freeze oocytes and embryos with an ultra-fast speed to avoid ice formation within cell during cryopreservation. Thus, it may save freezing time and obtain a higher survival rate. In order to understand and apply these two methods to human and other animal IVF program, a detail review on reproductive cell cryopreservation including sperm, oocyte, embryo and testicular/ovarian biopsy tissues has been included in this book (Chapter 16).

7. Future use of newly developed embryo transfer technologies

As our description in introduction section, embryo transfer has experienced three major changes, "three generations." In the human, major application of these techniques focus on the second stage where *in vitro* embryo production is performed by ovum pick up with *in vitro* fertilization (OPU-IVF) for infertile couple treatment. However, the third stage including further developed techniques, especially innovated embryo micromanipulation techniques, can promote us to perform various embryo manipulation including cloning involved somatic cells and embryonic stem cells, preimplantation genetic diagnosis (PGD), transgenic animal production etc. As Figure 1 showed, early oocytes may be obtained by current *in vitro* culture of ovarian tissue and primordial germ cells (PGCs), because female PGCs may become oogonia, which are mitotically divided several times in the ovaries and enter the prophase of first meiosis (Eppig et al., 1989). In the germinal vesicle stage (GV), oocyte reconstruction may be conducted by the nuclear transfer technique (Takeuchi et al., 1999). In higher organisms including humans, both nucleus and mitochondria contain DNA. Mitochondrion is located outside the nucleus in the cytoplasm and is an organelle responsible for energy synthesis. Oocyte contains rich mitochondria in a large amount of cytoplasm (Spikings et al., 2006). In normal sexual reproduction, offspring inherit their mitochondrial DNA from the mother. This type of inheritance pattern is generally known as maternal inheritance. When the mother passes defective mitochondria to the child, fatal heart, liver, brain or muscular disorders can result. In order to prevent this genetic disease, getting rid of mother defective mitochondrial DNA, mother nuclear DNA may be transferred into a normal enucleated ovum provided a third donor (Figure 2). The purpose of the donation of an enucleated cell is to provide the child with non-defective mitochondria, from a woman other than the mother. This results in a three-parent embryo. Its nucleus is formed by the fusion of sperm and mother's oocyte nucleus, and its cytoplasm is provided by the enucleated donor cell. Thus, this child has the inheritance of DNA from three different sources, the nuclear DNA is from his father and mother, and his mitochondrial DNA is mainly through the donor (Zhang et al., 1999).

Also, some aged women can not produce normal fertilization eggs and well-development embryos. The major problem is that the aged egg lacks synthesizing some components of maturation promoter factors, such as cyclin B, *c-Mos* proto-onco protein, cytostatic factor (Wu et al., 1997a, b). Thus, the new developed technique of oocyte (egg) reconstruction including nuclear transfer and cytoplasm replace may increase age woman pregnancy opportunity. Nuclear transfer is to transfer an age woman nucleus into young woman enucleated egg so that aged woman nucleus may complete a normal meiosis (Figure 2). The cytoplasm nuclear transfer (Figure 3) may replace partly aged oocyte cytoplasm with younger oocyte cytoplasm by transferring part of one woman's egg into another's (Cohen, 1998). In this case, the healthy portion of a donor egg (the cytoplasm) may supplement the defective portion of the infertile recipient's egg and to help it survive, hence making one good egg. Thus, the infertile woman's genetic legacy is preserved because the nucleus of this egg is made available from the infertile woman and the donor cytoplasm (which simply contains mitochondrial DNA that gives the egg energy to survive) contributes only one percent of the embryo's genetic makeup. Once the egg is fertilized, the embryo is implanted in the infertile woman's uterus. Unfortunately, after many babies were born in the U.S. using human cytoplasmic transfer (HCT), ethical and medical complications spurred the

U.S. government to curtail the procedure in 2001. Today, fertility scientists must file an investigational clinical trial application to continue research in this area, and the New Hope Fertility Center in New York intends to obtain approvals and continue our research. It is likely that with continued research this technique may prove its efficacy and safety in the future. It should be understood that the methods of the present invention are applicable to non-human species and, where the law permits, to humans.

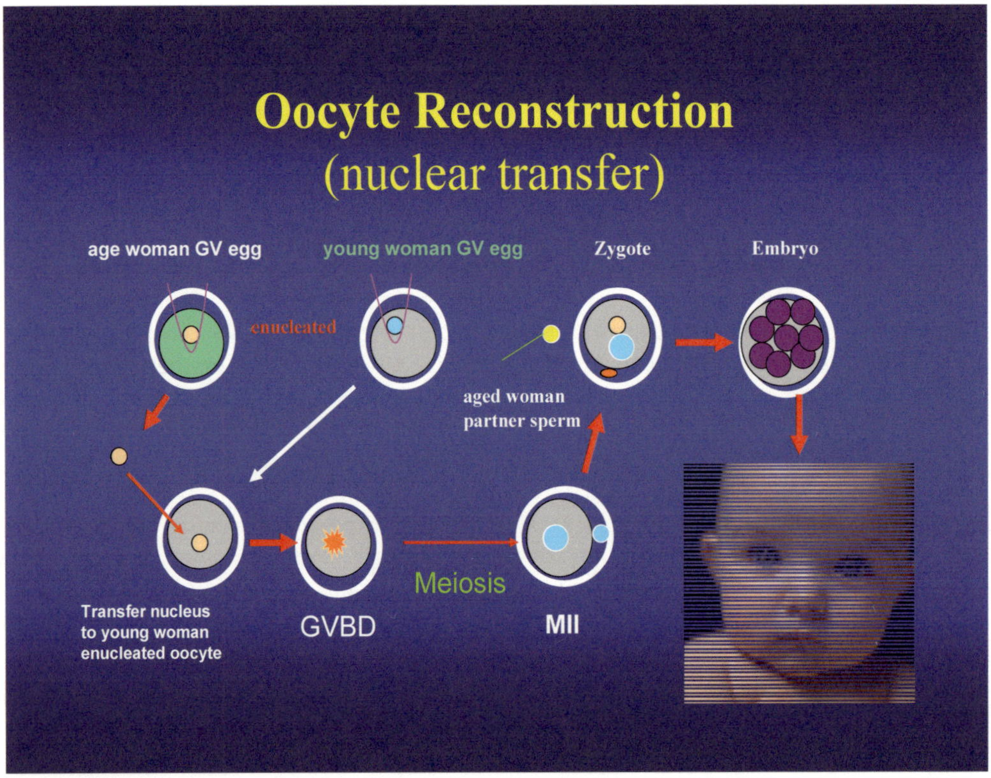

Fig. 2. Scenario for oocyte reconstruction by nuclear transfer technique. An aged woman oocyte nucleus is transferred into a young woman enucleated oocyte so that young woman immature oocyte will induce aged woman nucleus to complete meiosis during oocyte maturation. Then the aged woman husband sperm will be injected into this reconstructed oocyte to form a normal embryo for transfer.

Further, during oocyte *in vitro* maturation (IVM) and *in vitro* fertilization (IVF), some techniques such as sperm sexing, oocyte activation, parthenogenesis have been developed and applied in animal researches and human infertility treatment. Sex selection is the attempt to control the sex of the offspring to achieve a desired sex animal. It can be accomplished in several ways, including sperm sex selection and preimplantation embryo sex selection. A number of reviews have addressed the use of sexed semen in cattle (Seidel and Garner, 2002; Seidel, 2003). The current successful method for separating semen into X- or Y-bearing chromosome sperm is to use flow cytometry to sort sperm for artificial insemination or IVF (DeJarnette et al. 2007, Blondin et al., 2009). However, in human treatment, sex selection seems to have ethical problem. Thus, sperm sexing may be used in

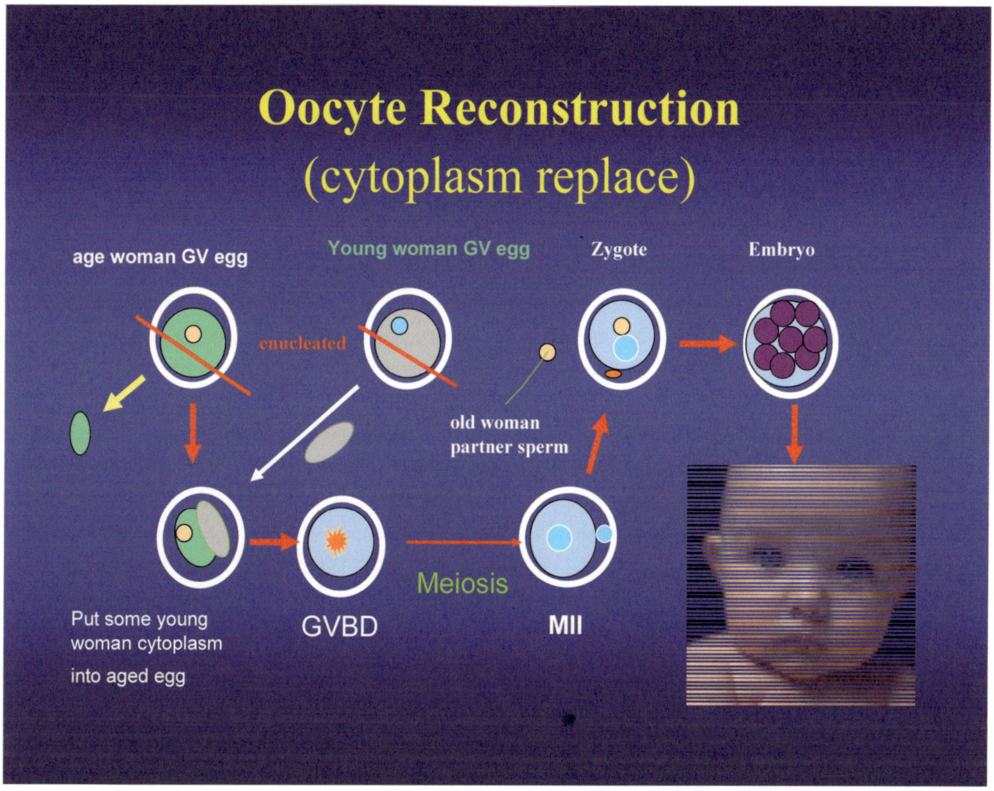

Fig. 3. Scenario for oocyte reconstruction by partly cytoplasm replace technique. Firstly small amount cytoplasm of aged woman oocyte is removed out and partly young woman oocyte cytoplasm will be transferred into this oocyte so that young woman oocyte cytoplasm will induce aged woman nucleus to complete meiosis during oocyte maturation. Then the aged woman husband sperm will be injected into this reconstructed oocyte to form a normal embryo for transfer.

related x-chromosome disease inherit treatment. One major limitation of sperm sexing is low efficient for low sperm motility. Oocyte activation may increase oocyte fertilization or result in parthenogenesis. Combining with reliable nuclear transfer method, this oocyte activation may produce pathenogenetic bimatermal embryos (Kawahara et al., 2008) or andrenogenetic bipaternal embryos (Wu and Zan, 2011, Tesarik 2002). In the chapter 9 of this book, the scenario for using immature oocyte to induce male somatic cell complete meiosis has been described. The nucleus of immature oocyte is removed and a male diploid cell was injected to this enucleated oocyte. After completing meiotic division, the induced haploid nucleus was transferred into normal female mature oocyte to form a biparental embryo for transfer. Also, a scenario for sperm genome cloning technique is displayed in this chapter. A single sperm is injected into enucleated oocyte and this oocyte goes through a parthenogenesis process to become a 4-8 cell haploid embryo. A single blastomere is transferred into a normal mature oocyte to form a zygote. The developed embryos are transferred to recipient mice to deliver offspring. Also, nuclear transfer studies have shown that nuclei from not growing oocytes have already been competent to mature into MII stage when transferred into fully grown germinal vesicle-stage oocytes. However, the resultant oocytes lack developmental competence, and nuclei from oocytes more than 65 µm in diameter first become competent to support term development after fertilization *in vitro* (Niwa et al., 2004).

After the fertilization, the zygote will be formed and two obvious pronuclei could be observed at this stage. The genetic manipulation of the prenuclear stage embryo has resulted in two fundamental discoveries in reproductive biology (Wilmut et al., 1991). By pronuclear removal and exchanges, the principle of genetic imprinting has been convincingly demonstrated. By injecting foreign DNA into one of the two pronuclei of the zygote, the resulting offspring may contain a functional foreign gene in the genome, known as transgenesis. Production of transgenic animals has great application in agriculture and medicine (Niemann and Kues 2003). In agricultural animals, the transgenic technology may be applied to develop lines of animals for faster growth, higher quality beef products or disease resistance (Greger 2010). Transgenic practices of last decade have proved that by inserting a single growth regulating gene into an animal of agricultural value, animal growth rate and feed efficiency could be greatly increased and fat deposition could be obviously reduced. This technique has been transforming the entire meat animal industry (Wheeler, 2007). In human, it is possible to target genetic sequences into predetermined sites in the host DNA, to transfer a given gene for some genetic disease therapy.

Animal cloning may involve embryo cloning and adult somatic cell cloning. During early development before 8-cell stage, embryonic cells may be dis-aggregated into individual blastomeres. Each blastomere has a totipotency which is able to potentially to develop into a viable embryo following nuclear transfer and to regenerate whole new individuals, this is, cloning. Also, embryo division is a kind of cloning and it may produce identical twin. In the human IVF, one blastomere often is removed from embryo for genetic diagnosis to examine some genetic disease and sex determination by fluorescent *in situ* hybridization (FISH) technique or polymerase chain reaction (PCR). The biopsied embryo could develop normal fetus and deliver health babies. Also, the process of freezing and thawing can be fairly harsh on the embryos and often not all of the cells or embryos survive. After freezing and thawing, one or several lysed blastomeres often occur in some embryos and these damaged cells are thought to either disrupt the development of the embryo or produce negative factors as they degenerate to affect survival blastomere growth. Recently new technique attempts to remove these lysed cells from embryo by making a small hole in the zona pellucida with acid or laser. The removal of lysed cells will restore the embryo's developmental potential. Cell number and morphology was also significantly improved compared with embryos without lysed cell removal (Elliott et al., 2007). This method has been shown to dramatically increase the implantation potential of human embryos and pregnancy rate (Nagy et al., 2005).

Also, many data showed a significant negative correlation between the degree of embryo fragmentation and rate of blastocyst development (Eftekhari-Yazdi et al., 2006). As above method, this fragmentation of embryo also may be removed. Some studies have indicated that the removal of fragmentation from fresh embryo on day 3 may increase the rate of blastocyst development (Alikani et al., 1999; Eftekhari-Yazdi et 2006).

At the blastocyst stage, two distinct cell lines in the embryos may be observed, the inner cell mass (ICM) and the trophectoderm (TE) cells. Inner cell mass cells are totipotent stem cells which will give rise to all different tissues in the fetus. By *in vitro* culturing ICM cells, the lines of embryonic stem (ES) cells have been developed. ES cells have the ability to remain undifferentiated and proliferate indefinitely *in vitro* while maintaining the potential to differentiate into derivatives of all three embryonic germ layers. Thus, combining cloning and nuclear transfer technique, the specific stem cells may be produced from ICM of embryos. Recent achievement showed that completely differentiated cells (both fetal and adult) may be reprogrammed to return to multipotential embryonic cells, that is the induced pluripotent stem cells (iPSCs) with qualities remarkably similar to embryonic stem cells-like state by being forced to express genes and factors important for maintaining the defining properties of embryonic stem cells (Takahashi and Yamanaka 2006;Yu et al., 2007).This discovery has created a valuable new source of pluripotent cells for drug discovery, cell therapy, and basic research.

For more than a decade, preimplantation genetic screening (PGS) and PGD have been used to assist in the identification of aneuploid embryos on Day 3. However, current strategies, based upon cell biopsy followed by FISH, allow less than half of the chromosomes to be screened. Currently, the FISH technique has gradually been replaced by the competitive genomic hybridization (CGH) or microarray analysis (Wells, et al., 2008). This analysis can evaluate all chromosomes by the trophectoderm biopsies of blastocyst embryos, which may significantly reduce embryo harm than Day 3 embryo. Trophectoderm biopsy involves removing some cells from the trophectoderm component of an IVF blastocyst embryo. The removed cells can be tested for chromosome normality, or for a specific gene defect using PGD or preimplantation genetic screening test. Some microarray platforms also offer the advantage of embryo fingerprinting and the potential for combined aneuploidy and single gene disorder diagnosis. However, more data concerning accuracy and further reductions in the price of tests will be necessary before microarrays can be widely applied.

8. Conclusions

Not only has embryo transfer already been one of the prominent high businesses worldwide for animal breed genetic improvement and creating new animal breeds, but also it has become a major tool for the treatment of infertile couples to realize their dream to have their children. The new developed embryo biotechnology has been able to make no sperm (azoospermia) men realize their dream to have a child. In the meantime, the innovation of various technologies, such as ovarian optimal stimulation scheme, new developed ICSI techniques, ultra-sound guide embryo transfer, embryo selection, seeking uterus biomarkers, have greatly improved transfer embryo pregnancy rates. As new embryo culture method improved and PGD, PGS, CGH and microarray analysis techniques developed, a single good quality embryo may be chosen for transfer and multiply pregnancies may significantly be reduced. Also, embryo cryopreservation technique, especially vitrification, has greatly increased embryo survival after thawing and made a single egg retrieval have more opportunity for pregnancy. Newly developed technologies such as embryo cloning, nuclear transfer, transgenic animals, stem cells etc. have demonstrated great promises for application in agricultural and biomedical sciences. Currently, these technologies have been being or will be used in human infertility treatment. In the next decade, these technologies will not only greatly promote animal genetic improvement and create new animal breeds, but also significantly improve human reproductive health.

9. References

Aghajanova L, Hamilton AE, and Giudice LC(2008) Uterine Receptivity to Human Embryonic Implantation: Histology, Biomarkers, and Transcriptomics. *Semin Cell Dev Biol* 19(2): 204–211

Alikani M, Cohen J, Tomkin G, Garrisi GJ, Mack C, Scott RT (1999) Embryo fragmentation and fragmentation removal in IVF. *Fertility and Sterility* 71(5):836-842

Assou S, Haouzi D, De Vos J, Hamamah S (2010) Human cumulus cells as biomarkers for embryo and pregnancy outcomes. *Mol Hum Reprod* 16 (8): 531-538

Berger DS, AbdelHafez F, Russell H, Goldfarb J, Desai N (2011) Severe teratozoospermia and its influence on pronuclear morphology, embryonic cleavage and compaction. *Reprod Biol Endocrinol* 9: 37

Betteridge KJ, 2006: Farm animal embryo technologies: Achievements and perspectives. *Theriogenology* 65: 905-913.

Blondin P, Beaulieu M, Fournier V, Morin N, Crawford L, Madan P, King WA (2009) Analysis of bovine sexed sperm for IVF from sorting to the embryo. *Theriogenology* 71: 30-38.

Braude, P. Bolton, V & Moore, S. (1988). Human gene expression first occurs between the four- and eight-cell stages of preimplantation development. *Nature* 332(6163):459-461.

Cohen J, Scott R, Alikani M, Schimmel T, Munné S, Levron J, Wu L, Brenner C, Warner C, Willadsen S (1998) Ooplasmic transfer in mature human oocytes. *Mol Hum Reprod* 4(3): 269-280

DeJarnette JM, Nebel RL, Marshall CE, Moreno JF, McCleary CR, Lenz RW (2007) Effect of sex-sorted sperm dosage on conception rates in Holstein heifers and lactating cows. *J Dairy Sci* 91:1778-1785.

Edwards, RG (2007) IVF, IVM, natural cycle IVF, minimal stimulation IVF - time for a rethink. *Reprod Biomed Online* 15(1):106-19.

Eftekhari-Yazdi P, Valojerdi MR, Ashtiani SK, Eslaminejad MB, Karimian L (2006)

Effect of fragment removal on blastocyst formation and quality of human embryos. *Reprod Biomed Online* 13(6):823-32.

Elliott TA, Colturato LFA, Taylor TH, Wright G, Kort HI, Nagy ZP (2007) Lysed cell removal promotes frozen–thawed embryo development. *Fertil Steril* 87(6): 1444-1449.

Eppig JJ, Schroeder AC(1989) Capacity of mouse oocytes from preantral follicles to undergo embryogenesis and development to live young after growth, maturation, and fertilization in vitro. *Biol Reprod* 41:268-276

Fukuda MN (2008) An integrated view of L-selectin and trophinin function in human embryo implantation. *J Obs Gyn Res* 34(2) 129-136.

Gardner, DK & Schoolcraft, WB (1999) *in vitro* culture of human blastocysts. In: Jansen R, Mortimer D (eds) Toward reproductive certainty: fertility and genetics beyond. Parthenon Publishing, Carnforth, UK. pp. 378-388.

Gardner DK, Lane M, Stevens J, Schlenker T and Schoolcraft WB (2000) Blastocyst score affects implantation and pregnancy outcome: towards a single blastocyst transfer. *Fertil Steril 73, 1155–1158.*

Greger M (2010) Transgenesis in Animal Agriculture: Addressing Animal Health and Welfare Concerns. *J Agric Environ Ethics* DOI 10.1007/s10806-010-9261-7

Guerif F, Bidault R, Cadoret V, Couet ML, Lansac J, Royerel D (2002) Parameters guiding selection of best embryos for transfer after cryopreservation: a reappraisal. *Hum Reprod* 17 (5): 1321-1326.

Horne AW, White JO, Lalani EL-N (2000) The endometrium and embryo implantation: A receptive endometrium depends on more than hormonal influences. *BMJ* 321(7272): 1301–1302.

Joshi BV, Banker MR, Parel PM, Shah PB (2010) Transfer of human frozen-thawed embryos with further cleavage during culture increases pregnancy rates. *J Hum Reprod Sci* 3(2): 76-79.

Kawahara M, Obata Y, Sotomaru Y, Shimozawa N, Bao S, Tsukadaira T, Fukuda A, Kono T (2008) Protocol for the production of viable bimaternal mouse embryos *Nature Protocols* 3: 197-209

Kovacic B, Vlaisavljevic V, Reljic M, Cizek-Sajko M (2004) Developmental capacity of different morphological types of day 5 human morulae and blastocysts. *Reprod Biomed Online* 8, 687-694

Macklon NS, Stouffer RL, Giudice LC & Fauser BC (2006) The science behind 25 years of ovarian stimulation for *in vitro* fertilization. *Endocrine Reviews* 27:170–207.

Mansour RT, Aboulghar MA (2002) Optimizing the embryo transfer technique. *Hum. Reprod.* 17(5): 1149-1153.

Margalioth EJ, Ben-Chetrit A, Gal M, Eldar-Geva T (2006) Investigation and treatment of repeated implantation failure following IVF-ET. *Hum Reprod* 21(12): 3036-3043.

Nagy ZP, Taylor T, Elliott T, Massey JB, Kort HI, Shapiro DB (2005) Removal of lysed blastomeres from frozen-thawed embryos improves implantation and pregnancy rates in frozen embryo transfer cycles. *Fertil Steril* 84:1606–12.

Niemann H and Kues WA (2003) Application of transgenesis in livestock for agriculture and biomedicine. *Animal Reprod Sci* 79: 291–317.

Niwa K, Takano R, Obata Y, Hiura H, Komiyama J, Ogawa H, Kono T (2004) Nuclei of Oocytes Derived from Mouse Parthenogenetic Embryos Are Competent to Support Development to Term. *Bio Reprod* 71(5):1560-1567

Norwitz ER, Schust DJ and Fisher SJ (2001) Implantation and the survival of early pregnancy. *N Engl J Med* 345:1400–1408.

Parmegiani L, Cognigni GE, Bernardi S, Troilo E, Ciampaglia W, Filicori M (2010a) "Physiologic ICSI": Hyaluronic acid (HA) favors selection of spermatozoa without DNA fragmentation and with normal nucleus, resulting in improvement of embryo quality. *Fertil Steril* 93:598-604

Parmegiani L, Cognigni GE, Ciampaglia W, Pocognoli P, Marchi F, Filicori M (2010b) Efficiency of hyaluronic acid (HA) sperm selection. *J Assist Reprod Genet* 27(1):13-6

Said TM, Land JA (2011) Effects of advanced selection methods on sperm quality and ART outcome: a systematic review. *Hum Reprod Update* doi: 10.1093/humupd/dmr032 First published online: August 25, 2011

Santos MA, Kuijk EW, Macklon NS (2010) The impact of ovarian stimulation for IVF on the developing embryo. *Reproduction* 139:23-34.

Seidal GE.Jr, Garner DL (2002) Current statue of sexing mammalian spermatozoa. *Reproduction* 124:733-743.

Seidel GE Jr (2003) Economic of selecting for sex: the most important genetic trait. *Theriogeneology* 59:585-598.

Singh H, Aplin JD (2009) Adhesion molecules in endometrial epithelium: tissue integrity and embryo implantation. *J Anatomy* 215 (1) 3-13.

Spikings ED, Alderson J, John JCSt (2006) Transmission of mitochondrial DNA following assisted reproduction and nuclear transfer *Hum Reprod Update* 12 (4): 401-415.

Steptoe PC, Edwards RG(1978) Birth after the preimplantation of a human embryo. *Lancet* 2:366.

Takahashi K,Yamanaka S (2006) Induction of pluripotent stem cells from mouse embryonic and adult fibroblast cultures by defined factors. *Cell* 126(4) 663-676.

Takeuchi T, Ergun B, Huang TH, Rosenwaks Z, Palermo GD(1999) A reliable technique of nuclear transplantation for immature mammalian oocytes. *Hum Reprod* 14 (5): 1312-1317.

Tang-Pedersen M, Westergaard LG, Erb K, Mikkelsen AL (2012), Combination of IVF and IVM in naturally cycling women. *Reprod BioMed Online* 24(1) 47-53.

Tesarik J (2002) Reproductive semi-cloning respecting biparental embryo origin: Embryos from syngamy between a gamete and a haploidized somatic cell. *Hum Reprod* 17 (8):1933-1937.

Wells D, Alfarawati S, Fragouli E (2008) Use of comprehensive chromosomal screening for embryo assessment: microarrays and CGH. *Mol Hum Reprod* 14(12):703–710

Wheeler MB(2007) Agricultural applications for transgenic livestock. *Trends in Biotechnology* 25(5): 204-210.

Wilmut I, Hooper ML and Simons JP(1991) Genetic manipulation of mammals and its application in reproductive biology. *J Reprod Fert* 92:245-279.

Worrilow KC, Eid S, Matthews J, Pelts E, Khoury C, Liebermann J (2010) Multi-site clinical trial evaluating PICSI®, a method for selection of hyaluronan bound sperm (HBS) for use in ICSI: improved clinical outcomes. *Human Reprod* 25(suppl 1): 6-9.

Wu B, Ignotz G, Currie WB, Yang X (1997a) Dynamics of maturation-promoting factor and its constituent proteins during *in vitro* maturation of bovine oocytes. *Bio Reprod* 56: 253-259.

Wu B, Ignotz G, Currie WB, Yang X (1997b) Expression of Mos proto-oncoprotein in bovine oocytes during maturation *in vitro*. *Biol Reprod* 56:260-265.

Wu B, Wong D, Lu S, Dickstein S, Silver M, Gelety T (2005) Optimal use of fresh and frozen-thawed testicular sperm for intracytoplasmic sperm injection in azoospermic patients. *J Assist Reprod Genet* 22: 389-394.

Wu B, Zan LS (2011) Enhance beef improvement by embryo biotechnologies. *Reprod Domestic Animals* (in press)

Yu J, Vodyanik MA, Smuga-Otto K, Antosiewicz-Bourget J, Frane JL, Tian S, Nie J, Jonsdottir GA, Ruotti, V, Stewart R, Slukvin II, Thomson JA (2007) Induced pluripotent stem cell lines derived from human somatic cells. *Science* 318:1917-1920.

Zhang J, Wang CW, Krey L, Liu H, Meng L, Blaszczyk A, Adler A and Grifo J (1999) *in vitro* maturation of human preovulatory oocytes reconstructed by germinal vesicle transfer. *Fertil Steril* 71:726–731.

Part 2

Optimal Stimulation for Ovaries

2

Minimal and Natural Stimulations for IVF

Jerome H. Check
Cooper Medical School of Rowan University, Department of Obstetrics and Gynecology, Division of Reproductive Endocrinology & Infertility, Camden, New Jersey USA

1. Introduction

In vitro fertilization-embryo transfer (IVF-ET) procedures have widely been used in most reproductive centers for many years. The protocol aim is to create a maximum number of oocytes to allow selection of the best embryos and provide extra embryos for future embryo transfers without undergoing ovarian hyperstimulation. So far, most IVF centers enjoy very good pregnancy rates using these conventional stimulation protocols. However, the conventional stimulation requires higher dosages of FSH injections, which are very expensive. Sometimes, the process of ovarian hyperstimulation creates health risks especially the dreadful ovarian hyperstimulation syndrome (OHSS). There has been a recent interest in using a much lower dosage of FSH to use for controlled ovarian hyperstimulation (COH) protocols for IVF. The multiple variations of IVF lower dosage include starting on day 5 instead of day 3 with FSH dosages 50% lower so called minimal (min) stimulation IVF, even lower dosages of FSH starting the gonadotropins even later allowing apoptosis of "less quality" follicles with dosage of FSH 1/4 to 1/3 of conventional dosages (micro IVF) or natural cycle IVF which can be completely natural or used with a gonadotropin releasing hormone antagonist and a mild dosage of FSH to allow better timing of oocyte retrieval. Other options - mild stimulation can also utilize other drugs that either block estrogen receptors on the pituitary or inhibit estradiol production by inhibiting the aromatase enzyme that recruits less follicles, e.g., clomiphene citrate or letrazole either alone or followed by low dose FSH stimulation. In some instances dosages of FSH above conventional levels are used especially women with diminished oocyte reserve in an effect to stimulate more follicles. This is referenced to as high dosage FSH stimulation.

For years the attitude of IVF centers has been "the more eggs the merrier." This chapter will discuss the benefits and risks of these various ovarian stimulation protocols. Also there will be a description as to the advantages and disadvantages of conventional vs. mild stimulation vs. high dosage FSH stimulation according to the degree of ovarian oocyte reserve.

2. Basic theory of ovarian stimulation

2.1 Oogenesis and hormone function on ovarian

A necessary factor for the development of antral follicles into dominant follicles is a hormone called the follicle stimulating hormone (FSH). In those normal ovulating women, a complex interaction occurs between the FSH and granulosa theca cells of these follicles which are associated with up and down regulation of FSH receptors on these granulosa-theca cells. This process of FSH receptor up and down regulation is possibly related to the pulsatility of the gonadotropin releasing hormone (GnRH) which causes pulsatile release of FSH and luteinizing hormone (LH), leading to the progressive increase in estradiol (E2). The rise in E2, in turn, suppresses FSH release from gonadotropin cells leading to the usual recruitment and the development of only one dominant follicle each cycle from the multiple antral follicles. Though over simplified, basically the follicle developing the most FSH receptors in the granulosa cells is the one that can continue to develop into a dominant follicle despite the progressive drop in serum FSH from the early follicular phase to mid-cycle. Theoretically, but not proven, this process leads to the selection of at least one of the best quality antral follicles in the group to develop one mature oocyte each month. Follicles that have not developed adequate FSH receptors will undergo atresia in the presence of decreasing serum FSH (1).

With the advent of follicle maturing drugs, e.g., clomiphene citrate or gonadotropins, it was realized that raising serum FSH by using drugs that cause endogenous or using exogenous gonadotropins can allow the recruitment and development of multiple antral follicles to the dominant follicle stage. Follicles with less development of FSH receptors can respond to a higher FSH stimulus.

Because of multiple follicles the rising serum E2 levels can sometimes induce the luteinizing hormone (LH) surge before any one follicle has attained full maturity with a metaphase II oocyte. Thus most of these conventional IVF COH protocols using 225 to 300 units of FSH from day 2 or 3 of the menstrual cycle will also add either a gonadotropin releasing hormone (GnRH) agonist from mid-luteal phase until the human chorionic gonadotropin trigger in the late follicular phase of the next cycle or a GnRH agonist from early follicular phase or a GnRH antagonist from the mid to late follicular phase to prevent premature luteinization and cancellation of the oocyte retrieval.

2.2 Types of ovarian reserve and serum FSH and LH pattern

One of the ways to determine the oocyte reserve is to measure the number of antral sized follicles in the early follicular phase which is known as the antral follicle count. Two main hormones suppress the secretion of FSH by the pituitary - E2 and inhibin B. Since antral follicles make very little estrogen but do secrete inhibin B, women with less antral follicles will generally have an elevated serum FSH on day 2 or 3 because less inhibin B is secreted from less follicles (1).

Women with normal oocyte reserve will generally demonstrate on day 3 a serum FSH greater than LH but the FSH will be ≤11 mIU/mL. Women with supra-normal antral follicles, produce an increased amount of total estrogens related to conversion of androstenedione to estrogen. The positive feedback effect of estrogen on LH release from the pituitary but negative effect on the FSH secretion, frequently is manifested with an LH/FSH ratio greater than 1.8 to 1.

In the natural cycle the endogenous FSH advances the antral follicles and with the rise in serum E2, serum FSH gradually declines allowing monofollicular ovulation from the one dominant follicle that acquired the most FSH receptors. The challenge for natural oocyte retrieval is to retrieve the oocyte at the appropriate time interval from the LH surge to allow advancement of the oocyte to the meta-phase II stage.

So far although the germinal vesicle stage or metaphase I oocyte may be in vitro cultured to the metaphase II stage and further fertilized and cryopreserved for the subsequent embryo transfer, live deliveries have been reported with a lower expected pregnancy rate (2).

3. Types of FSH stimulation for follicular development

3.1 Mild stimulation protocols

There are a spectrum of mild stimulation protocols varying from no exogenous FSH at all to 150 units FSH from days 3-5 with a possible increase to 225 U of FSH if a GnRH antagonist is added or the serum E2 fails to rise sufficiently.

It seems logical and there is some supporting evidence that it is not a coincidence which of the antral follicles develops into the dominant follicle, and thus it may be the best follicle with the "best" oocyte. It seems reasonable that the first follicles to undergo atresia have the least quality oocytes. The ones progressing past the mid-follicular phase may have better quality related to better FSH receptors in the granulosa theca cells. If one does not intervene at this point by a small dosage of exogenous FSH the continued drop in FSH from rising serum E2 will cause atresia of these "better follicles" also except the one dominant follicle.

The problem with a completely natural cycle is that one cannot predict when the spontaneous LH surge will occur. Thus, we may face the risk that the oocyte could release before oocyte retrieval. Even though a bolus injection of human chorionic gonadotropin (hCG) is used before the spontaneous LH rise, it must be done without compromising the maturity of the follicle and the oocyte within.

In order to overcome this problem, some IVF centers trying to attain the one best dominant follicle will wait until the dominant follicle approaches a 14mm size and boost with 75 IU FSH with or without a GnRH antagonist. A natural cycle with a boost of FSH protocol can also be used with a mild GnRH agonist protocol to prevent premature luteinization. One method is to use a GnRH agonist for only 3 days, e.g., day 2-4 to prevent a premature LH surge in the late follicular phase (3,4). Actually, the GnRH agonist mildly stimulates the follicles and this stimulation is maintained by a low dosage of FSH starting around day 5 or later. Another method is to use a diluted dosage of the GnRH agonist and a low dosage FSH from the early follicular phase known as the microdose flare (5).

A mild stimulation protocol sometimes uses an anti-estrogen drug which recruits less of the antral follicles followed by a low dosage of FSH (or LH and FSH combined). For example, 100mg clomiphene citrate may be given from days 3-7 or 5-9 with 75-150 IU of FSH started on the last day of clomiphene (6-8). Another selective estrogen modulator, e.g., tamoxifen or an aromatase inhibitor, e.g., letrozole can be substituted for the clomiphene (9,10). Mild stimulation could employ 75-150 IU FSH or human menopausal gonadotropin from days 3-5 of the menstrual cycle. This can be used by any of the GnRH antagonist or agonist regimens that were previously mentioned. It should be noted that frequently when starting a GnRH antagonist, e.g., cetrorelix or ganirelix, one raises the FSH dosage by 75 IU.

3.2 Conventional stimulation protocols

There are several variations of conventional COH regimens. They usually either employ a GnRH agonist from mid luteal phase or sometimes the GnRH agonist from day 2, so called short flare protocol trying to take advantage of the initial "agonistic" effects of GnRH agonist before the negative effect on gonadotropin release occurs later in the follicular phase. Some cases use a GnRH antagonist from the late follicular phase sometimes when the leading follicle reaches 14mm. Most conventional COH protocols start with 225-300 IU FSH frequently, but not always, with the addition of 75-150 IU LH. Many IVF centers will try to induce multiple follicles with 225-300 IU FSH, then decrease by 75-150 IU in an effort to continue the stimulation of the advancing follicles but not stimulate much smaller follicles. Usually, hCG is given when the two leading follicles reach 18-20mm. Sometimes a GnRH agonist is used in 1 or 2 injections to stimulate endogenous gonadotropin release instead of hCG to reduce the risk of OHSS (11).

3.3 High dose FSH protocols

The high dosage FSH protocols are those that start with greater than 300 U of FSH. They are frequently used by IVF-ET centers to try to increase the follicular response in previous poor responders.

4. Theoretical advantages of various stimulation schemes – Normal oocyte reserve

4.1 Conventional FSH stimulation over mild stimulation

Conventional COH produces more oocytes and thus more embryos. Theoretically this procedure will obtain more top quality embryos for transfer, especially considering a blastocyst transfer. With more embryos there will be a greater opportunity for subsequent frozen embryo transfer. A frozen embryo transfer does not create a risk of OHSS and is usually much less expensive than fresh IVF cycle. Furthermore there is no cost for expensive gonadotropins and GnRH agonists or antagonists and no charge for anesthesia. The most important aim of IVF program is to obtain a live delivered pregnancy from a given oocyte harvest whatever a fresh or frozen embryo transfer is performed (12). Thus, the more embryos obtained, the greater the chance of achieving a pregnancy per oocyte harvest (12).

4.2 Mild dosage FSH stimulation over conventional stimulation

One main advantage of mild FSH stimulation is low cost of medication. Also, the price of the IVF-ET cycle can be greatly reduced because of less work in the embryology laboratory. Our IVF center has reduced the price by 50% when the mild stimulation method is used. Also, using less FSH markedly reduces the risk of OHSS.

Interestingly, one of the arguments in favor of conventional stimulation is that the more embryos developed the better chance of chromosomally normal embryos. Proponents of mild stimulation consider that oocytes with meiotic errors identified in the natural ovulatory process are more likely to undergo apoptosis and can not advance to a dominant follicle stage. A randomized controlled trial comparison of mild vs. conventional COH on rates of aneuploidy found that both regimens created the same number of chromosomally normal embryos, i.e., an average of 1.8 per cycle (13). Thus no higher number of chromosomally normal embryos is produced by conventional higher FSH dosage regimens than mild stimulation according to this study (13).

Also, some IVF programs favor transferring chromosomally normal embryos by pre-implantation genetic diagnosis (PGD). Completing this procedure requires more oocytes and embryos. Current PGD fluorescent in situ hybridization (FISH) technique has been replaced by the competitive genomic hybridization or microarray analysis which can evaluate all chromosomes. The trophectoderm biopsies of blastocyst embryos may significantly reduce embryo harm than day 3 embryo biopsy (14). However, these procedures add extra expense and need for higher FSH dosage stimulation. The mild stimulation could allow natural selection of the best oocytes. Thus the best embryo may be obtained at a much lower price.

4.3 Relationship of stimulation scheme with embryo cryopreservation

Another way to avoid severe OHSS is to freeze all embryos and defer transfer, but this places the burden on an IVF center of having a good success rate with their frozen embryo transfers. One advantage of mild stimulation is if the cryopreservation program is not superb they do not have to fear a lower chance of pregnancy if fresh embryos are transferred. In fact, when evaluating a given center's pregnancy rate per transfer, one should not ignore the concept of pregnancy rate per oocyte harvest. Pregnancy should be evaluated based on fresh or frozen embryo transfer together or at a minimum the pregnancy rate of the first transfer irrespective if it is fresh or frozen (12).

One theoretical advantage of mild stimulation is that it allows "mother nature" to recruit the best follicles. It is possible that all multiple embryos produced by conventional stimulation have morphologically similar quality, but they may have poor likelihood of implantation. The oocytes with chromosome abnormalities are more likely to undergo atresia. If there is a good cryopreservation program, all embryos will eventually be transferred. However, those IVF centers that do not excel in embryo freezing programs may not transfer the "best ones" on fresh transfer but the odds of transferring the better embryos fresh may be greater with mild stimulation.

5. Controlled ovarian stimulation – Effects on the post-ovulatory endometrium

By comparing pregnancy rates from infertile oocyte donors sharing half their oocytes with recipients, a very significant adverse effect of COH has been suggested based on a much higher pregnancy rate in recipients vs. donors (15). However it became clear that a good portion of the differential was related to the failure to realize that salpingectomy should be performed for hydrosalpinges (16-18). There still does appear to be a mild adverse effect of conventional COH on embryo implantation in some women as evidenced by comparing pregnancy rates in infertile donors and their recipients in the era of salpingectomy for hydrosalpinges (19).

Sometimes one case can vividly establish an interesting concept that controlled studies can not so firmly establish. One woman with amenorrhea from polycystic ovarian syndrome was promoted to ovulate every cycle with clomiphene citrate or gonadotropins plus progesterone in the luteal phase for 6 years. All known infertility factors were corrected but she failed to conceive. This woman had 10 IVF-ET cycles with 92 embryos for fresh transfer in three top IVF centers without pregnancy, but in her 11th IVF cycle, all embryos were purposely cryopreserved. Finally she conceived and delivered a healthy baby on her first frozen embryo transfer (20). After that, this woman started naturally to ovulate and spontaneously conceived by natural intercourse and finally a healthy baby was born with luteal phase progesterone supplementation (21).

Kerin et al showed that the aspiration of only preovulatory graafian follicle for purpose of IVF-ET following spontaneous ovulation did not cause a luteal phase defect (22). Yet as far back as 1980, Edwards, Steptoe and Purdy suggested that the luteal phase of all stimulated cycles is abnormal (23). When Edwards et al published their data, the use of GnRH agonists and antagonists were not used as part of the COH protocol. Thus the luteal phase defects had to be related to the use of follicle stimulating drugs (23). With the advent of GnRH agonists various theories developed suggesting that they were responsible for luteal phase defects related to a delay in pituitary recovery from suppression by the GnRH agonists. However a subsequent study showed that despite rapid recovery of pituitary function when GnRH antagonists were used luteal phase deficiency still persists and pregnancy rates greatly suffer unless supplemental progesterone or hCG injections are given (24).

Thus the prevalent theory today for the etiology of luteal phase deficiency following COH and IVF-ET is related to the supra-physiological concentration of steroids secreted by multiple corpora lutea during the early luteal phase which directly inhibit LH release by negative feedback to the pituitary and hypothalamus.

Bourgain and Devroey summarized the adverse effects of FSH stimulation on the post-ovulatory endometrium (25). Compared to natural cycle, FSH stimulation cycles showed 1) premature secretory changes in the post-ovulatory and early luteal phase of IVF cycles followed by a large population of dyssynchronous glandular and stromal differentiation in the mid-luteal phase; 2) a modified endometrial steroid receptor regulation; 3) a profound anti-proliferative effect in IVF cycles and 4) support was provided for the theory of the implantation window with premature expression of various endometrial products including pinopodes, integrins and leukemia inhibitory factor (25). Some studies demonstrated that an immunomodulatory protein known as the progesterone induced blocking factor (PIBF) may be much earlier detected in the early luteal phase following COH. The PIBF is expressed by gamma/delta T cells at the maternal fetal interface which in turn inhibits local natural killer cell activity. This factor supports premature trophoblast invasion as a cause of failure of embryo implantation in some circumstances since the production of PIBF requires trophoblastic invasion to allow this allogeneic stimulus to induce P receptors on gamma/delta T cells (26). These data suggest premature trophoblast invasion may account for failure for successful implantation (26). It is clear that periovulatory maturation exceeding 3 days results in extremely poor (possibly zero) pregnancy rates (25).

It is suspicious that the aforementioned woman who experienced 6 years of ovulation induction and 10 IVF-ET cycles with 92 embryos for transfer and finally got pregnancy with frozen ET cycle and a natural cycle conception might have the advancement of the periovulatory window and premature trophoblast invasion to explain these findings (20, 21). However, some evidence indicates that luteal phase inadequacy can be corrected by adding supplemental progesterone or hCG in the luteal phase so as to increase pregnancy rates per transfer in the modern IVF era (27-33), but some studies thought that the luteal phase support does not increase the delivery rate (34).

6. Author's experience with conventional vs. mild FSH stimulation

The ideal study to determine the proper therapeutic recommendation could be based on a large prospective randomized controlled trial (RCT), but very few studies have been conducted. Meta-analysis of prospective studies can increase the power but frequently there are journal reviewer and author biases in the publication of multiple studies. Clinically important conclusions can be reached from large retrospective studies comparing two therapeutic options if there are no apparent biases or inadvertent confounding variables. It is impossible to compare conventional vs. mild FSH stimulation with a large prospective RCT since there is little motivation for a pharmaceutical company to fund such a study.

When comparing conventional vs. mild COH protocols it is essential that the concept of pregnancy rate per harvest is taken into consideration. Thus a credible large retrospective study must come from an IVF center with a good pregnancy rate following frozen embryo transfer. Our IVF center developed a modified slow-cool embryo cryopreservation technique that allows equal pregnancy rates with the transfer of fresh or frozen thawed embryos (35-37). Thus our center data would qualify to evaluate pregnancy rate per first transfer, i.e., fresh or frozen, in case all embryos needed to be cryopreserved because of the risk of OHSS. Similarly our center could evaluate the pregnancy rate per harvest before requiring the need for another COH IVF-ET cycle with consideration of transfer of all frozen embryos (12).

We summarize data on the decision for using conventional vs. mild FSH stimulation in women with normal ovarian reserve from a large retrospective study over a 10 year time period (data was presented at the 2011 World Congress of IVF in Tokyo, Japan). These data were based strictly on financial reasons with 50% less charge for IVF-ET plus reduction on at least 50% of the cost of FSH drugs. No significant differences were found in two stimulation schemes (Table 1 and 2). If one looks for a trend for higher pregnancy rate it would favor mild FSH stimulation for first transfers irrespective of fresh or frozen embryos.

	High stim cycle			Low stim cycle		
Age at retrieval	Totals	≤35	36-39	Totals	≤35	36-39
# of Retrievals	859	536	323	396	265	131
# of Transfers	678	418	260	288	194	94
% Clinical pregnancy/transfer	44.5	50.2	35.4	43.8	51.0	28.7
% Ongoing/transfer	39.8	46.4	29.2	41.3	47.9	27.7
% Delivered/transfer	36.1	41.9	26.9	38.5	44.8	25.5
Implantation rate (%)	27.0	32.1	19.7	30.0	34.6	20.1

Table 1. Pregnancy rates of the first retrieval with fresh embryo transfer cycles

	High stim cycle			Low stim cycle		
Age at retrieval	Totals	≤35	36-39	Totals	≤35	36-39
# of Transfers	790	498	292	342	238	104
% Clinical pregnancy/transfer	43.5	49.2	33.9	44.4	49.6	32.7
% Ongoing/transfer	39.4	45.8	28.4	41.8	46.6	30.8
% Delivered/transfer	35.7	41.2	26.4	39.2	43.7	28.8
Implantation rate (%)	26.0	31.0	18.6	29.8	33.0	22.2

Table 2. Pregnancy rates for the first transfer - fresh or frozen Ets

Also, no significant differences were found in pregnancy rate per oocyte harvest (Table 3) in the younger groups, a higher pregnancy rate trend with conventional stimulation was observed. The only significant difference was that women aged 36-39 had a higher pregnancy rate with conventional stimulation than mild stimulation (32.5% vs. 26.7%, $p<0.05$).

	High stim cycle			Low stim cycle		
Age at retrieval	Totals	≤35	36-39	Totals	≤35	36-39
% Clinical pregnancy/transfer	55.9	64.4	41.8	48.2	57.0	30.5
% Ongoing/transfer	49.2	58.0	34.7	44.4	52.5	28.2
% Delivered/transfer	45.3	53.0	32.5	41.9	49.4	26.7

Table 3. Pregnancy rates per oocyte oocyte harvest

7. Diminished oocyte reserve and infertility

It is well known that as age advances, the antral follicles in the early follicular phase become less and less (38). With the less antral follicles, the less inhibin B is secreted, which leads to a higher day 3 FSH level as long as it is not being falsely lowered by a higher serum E2 level from a more advanced follicle. The oocytes of women with advanced reproductive age are much more prone to meiosis errors which result in a very high percentage of embryos with aneuploidy. Even if they have normal serum FSH, the women over age 45 rarely achieve pregnancies (39).

One explanation to the phenomena associated with poor pregnancy rates and high miscarriage rates is that the oocytes with the best mitochondria are more likely to advance to a secondary oocyte and eventually develop into antral follicles because there is a natural selection of the best follicles with oocytes with the best mitochondria. By natural selection, older women have "de-selected" follicles. Less than adequate mitochondria lead to a greater risk of meiosis errors which cause poor pregnancy rates and higher miscarriage rates.

Another alternate hypothesis is that the selection of follicles is simply positional but age itself leads to aging of the mitochondria in the follicles and further leads to meiosis errors. Several 1980s studies found very poor pregnancy rates even in younger women with diminished oocyte reserve as manifested by elevated day 3 serum FSH levels (40-43). Even in the modern IVF era some of the top IVF centers still claim extremely poor (or even zero) live delivery rate in younger women despite the transfer of several normal morphologic embryos especially if day 3 FSH exceeded 15 mIU/mL (44,45). Based on these data the conclusion favored by many reproductive endocrinologists (but not this author) is that the poor pregnancy rates are related to poor quality oocytes allegedly with quality more akin to women of advanced reproductive age (46).

8. Author's experience with diminished oocyte reserve

If remaining oocytes in women with marked diminished oocyte reserve were of the same poor quality as their 52 year old "FSH" peers where pregnancy rate is almost zero, it is difficult to explain how a group of women with hypergonadotropic amenorrhea and estrogen deficiency for a minimum of one year achieved a pregnancy rate of 28% (19/68) in those who ovulated and a live rate of 11.7% per ovulation cycle without any assisted reproductive procedure (47). The techniques used to induce ovulation involve gonadotropin suppression with ethinyl estradiol plus restoration of down-regulated FSH receptors followed by low dose gonadtoropin therapy in some but not all cases (47). A study of euestrogenic women age ≤39 with a mean serum 18.9 mIU/mL FSH and without assisted reproductive technology achieved a clinical and ongoing 6 month pregnancy rate of 46.1% and 34.6%, respectively (48). Successful pregnancies could be achieved without ART not only in menstruating women with serum FSH levels >100 pg/mL (49), but also in a woman in apparent menopause with serum FSH levels of 164 mIU/mL (50), and even women in apparent menopause with ovaries appearing as streaked gonads (51,52). A successful pregnancy was even achieved by merely lowering the elevated FSH and restoring sensitivity to endogenous FSH in a 40 year old woman in apparent menopause with several years of amenorrhea and estrogen deficiency with a documented serum FSH of 124 mIU/mL (but a claimed level of 180 mIU/mL) who failed to conceive despite 4 previous transfers of fresh embryos derived from donor oocytes (53). At the 2011 American Society for Reproductive Medicine we presented data on natural cycle conception in women aged ≤37 with day 3 serum FSH >15 mIU/mL using natural cycles or mild FSH stimulation plus progesterone support in the luteal phase. The clinical and live delivered pregnancy rates after 3 treatment cycles were 41.6% (n=24) and 33.3% respectively vs. 70.8% and 62.5% respectively for matched controlled women with normal (≤8 mIU/mL) day 3 serum FSH.

Successful pregnancies have been recorded in apparent menopausal women with tubal factor by ovulation induction following restoring sensitivity of some of the few remaining follicles and by lowering the elevated serum FSH levels (54, 55). One menstruating woman with an elevated day 3 serum FSH achieved 3 live deliveries out of 4 IVF-ET cycles with ICSI over an 8 year time span (56). Roberts et al.'s study showed that any age women who ever once had a serum FSH more than 15mIU/mL can not achieve a live pregnancy even if they stimulate adequately and have morphologically normal embryos (45). Their hypothesis suggested that high serum FSH results in a loss of best oocytes and the remaining ones have poor quality similar to ≥45 year old woman (45), but the fact that live delivered babies have been achieved despite the extreme of oocyte depletion suggests Roberts et al's hypothesis is incorrect (45,46,57).

Recently, a study evaluated the relative effect of blastomere number and fragmentation indices of day 3 embryos on pregnancy and implantation rates by undergoing IVF women with a markedly decreased egg reserve and >15 mIU/mL serum FSH levels (57). The study consisted of only women having a single embryo transfer. Transferring embryos with over 6 blastomeres (which represented 65% of the transfers) showed 40% clinical pregnancy rate per transfer and 31.7% live birth rate, while transferring only 4 and 5 cell embryos had just 3.8% and 9.5% pregnancy rates (57).

Many controlled ovarian hyperstimulation regimens for women with normal egg reserve begin on day 2 or 3 with at least 225mIU/mL FSH and frequently 300mIU/mL. When attempting to stimulate a woman with diminished egg reserve, most IVF centers will increase the starting dosage of FSH hoping to get more follicles. Women with the least egg reserve will usually fail to respond to high dosage gonadotrophins, thus, their cycles are cancelled. However, the reports are generally only in those women with greater egg reserve and response sufficient to obtain possibly a minimum of 5 oocytes and very poor pregnancy rates when conventional or high FSH COH protocols are used (40-45).

9. Hypothesis to explain the discrepancy in results with the aforementioned studies with negative outcome vs. the author's positive experience

The principal of trying to establish ovulation in an apparent menopausal woman is based on the assumption that some antral follicles are still present but they have acquired a resistance to exogenous and endogenous gonadotropins because the chronically high level of serum FSH causes down regulation of the FSH receptor (58). The theory implies that lowering the serum FSH by exogenous estrogen can allow restoration of the down-regulated FSH receptors leading to the development of a dominant follicle by stimulation with endogenous and/or exogenous gonadotropins (59). One could argue that the estrogen may directly improve the sensitivity of the follicles to FSH without the need to suppress endogenous FSH. However, the fact against this theory is that ovulation induction in hypergonadotropic amenorrhea can also be achieved by lowering the serum FSH with either gonadotropin releasing hormone (GnRH) agonists or antagonists (47, 59, 60).

At the cellular level an adverse effect of an excessive exposure to hormonal stimulation is frequently regulated by receptor down regulation. This would explain the frequent observation of a high dose FSH failing to stimulate any or just a few follicles whereas mild dosage FSH allows a better response. A vivid example was an iatrogenic menopausal woman caused by raising her endogenous FSH levels with clomiphene citrate. By simply stopping the clomiphene therapy, she was able to restore ovulation by stimulating 3 dominant follicles with a serum E2 >800pg/mL in a natural cycle (61). Thus the probable explanation for such diverse success results is the use of mild vs. conventional or supra-conventional dosages of exogenous FSH to try to stimulate more dominant follicles. Otherwise there were no differences in methodology used for IVF in this population.

Though it is not known for sure why high dosage FSH stimulation results in such poor outcome in these women, the adverse effect seems to affect the embryo rather than the endometrium (author's unpublished experience on cryopreservation). Deferring fresh transfer does not overcome the adverse effect in women with diminished oocyte reserve. Two possible mechanisms of the high dosage FSH leading to poor pregnancy rates could be that the increase of FSH in the follicular phase causes higher meiosis errors which results in aneuploidal embryos or the high FSH down-regulates the receptors leading to the production of implantation factors attached to the embryo itself.

10. The author's mild stimulation protocol for women with diminished oocyte reserve

The basic principle of using mild FSH stimulation for women with diminished oocyte reserve is try to avoid adding exogenous FSH while the endogenous serum FSH is already elevated. It is important to restore FSH receptors in granulosa-theca cells by lowering the serum FSH in women who appear to be in menopause (62, 63). The author's preference is to use compounded ethinyl estradiol to lower the high serum FSH since it is inexpensive and helpful to create adequate endometrial thickness and good cervical mucus so that in case the oocyte is released before retrieval, it is possible for conception with intercourse. In contrast to other estrogen preparations, such as serum 17-beta estradiol assay, ethinyl estradiol allows detection of a recruited follicle and determination of maturity (64). Also, ethinyl estradiol allows the lengthening of the follicular phase to give more exposure time of the endometrium to estrogen so that endometrial progesterone receptors obtain proper development (65, 66).

Sometimes in this scenario of reversing menopause the FSH remains elevated while a single follicle grows and the serum E2 rises. In this case the better way may be to allow completely natural development of the follicle without the addition of exogenous FSH (55). If the FSH is only mildly elevated but the follicular maturation is not rapidly progressing enough, a boost of low dosage (75-150 IU) FSH may be used at that point. Similarly, if there are only 1-2 antral follicles and the high serum FSH decreased to the normal range, the low dosage gonadotropins (FSH or LH/FSH combination) may be used at this point.

In the aforementioned study of women with very high FSH and single embryo transfer there were 92 initiated cycles in women doing completely natural cycles (57). Sixty of them lead to oocyte retrieval. The data are analyzed according to cycles initiated but excluding some cancellation cases because of very little expense for medication, the cancellation for not reaching a mature follicle or release of oocyte before retrieval does not have the same negative impact as cancellation of stimulation with conventional or high dosage FSH. Only 19 of the 60 (33%) retrievals led to an embryo transfer and 21% clinical pregnancy and 16% live delivery.

The group "good enough" to allow a boost of gonadotropins had a somewhat better outcome in that about 70% (80/116) proceeded to oocyte retrieval leading to about a 75% transfer rate. The clinical and live delivered rate per transfer for this group was 29% and 24% respectively (57). With just diminished ovarian reserve as evidenced by a 3 day serum FSH >12 mIU/mL but where frequently (but not always) the woman is euestrogenic, one common technique is to allow natural follicular maturation to proceed until the endogenously rising E2 decreases the serum FSH in the follicular phase when either 75-150 IU FSH is added. This group will frequently have more than one embryo to transfer.

If the day 3 FSH is only mildly elevated or top normal mild stimulation consists of 75-150 IU FSH initially around day 5, and a GnRH antagonist is added later. This less severe group can perform a lot better. Almost all of these initiated cycles go to retrieval and most retrievals lead to embryo transfers. Our data showed that miscarriage rates are directly proportional to age but not the FSH level (presented at the 2011 Pacific Coast Reproductive Society). Comparing relative pregnancy rates based on age and rising FSH levels in younger women ≤age 39 was listed in Table 4 and older women aged 40-44 in Table 5. It is clear that until age 43 the FSH level does not negatively affect the live delivered rates when the mild stimulation are used. Actually since these data were obtained to evaluate aneuploidy as evidenced by miscarriage rates, all IVF cycles were included. Thus there may have been some bias with the normal FSH group since our IVF center attracts some difficult cases who failed several previous IVF cycles in other centers, while the high FSH group may never have any previous IVF cycles being rejected because of their high day 3 FSH levels.

Age at time of retrieval	≤35				36-39			
Baseline FSH levels (mIU/mL)	≤11	12-14	15-17	>17	≤11	12-14	15-17	>17
# transfers	2120	111	37	88	1313	120	47	93
% live delivered preg/transfer	45.1	42.3	48.6	45.5	33.4	35.0	29.8	36.6
% SAB/clin. pregnancy	11.9	13.9	13.3	12.8	17.2	11.4	7.1	22.9

Table 4. Pregnancy rates by age and FSH levels - younger group

Age at time of retrieval	40-42				43-44			
Baseline FSH levels (mIU/mL)	≤11	12-14	15-17	>17	≤11	12-14	15-17	>17
# transfers	737	103	30	65	121	30	18	25
% live delivered preg/transfer	23.1	20.4	30.0	27.7	24.0	10.0	0.0	8.0
% SAB/clin. pregnancy	27.3	32.3	36.4	30.4	34.4	75.0	100.0	75.0

Table 5. Pregnancy rates by age and FSH levels - older group

11. Other studies using mild stimulation for diminished oocyte reserve

Not all studies agree that mild stimulation is the key for achieving a reasonable pregnancy rate in "poor responders". Kolibianakis et al did not achieve any live pregnancies in 78 modified natural cycles although they started 100 unit FSH and ganirelix when the follicle reached ≥16mm but no hormonal studies were obtained (44). Possibly they did not wait long enough for full maturation of the follicle before administering hCG injection (44). Kim et al found a 13.5% live delivered pregnancy rate with low dose FSH but not higher than the 16.7% live birth rate from a multidose FSH dosage (67). Thus this study does not support the idea of poor outcome in other studies related to the high dose FSH regimen. However, it should be noted that the dosage of 225 IU FSH daily is a lower dosage than most centers treat women with diminished oocyte reserve where frequently higher dose FSH regimens are used.

Another retrospective study compared the implantation rates according to natural vs. various types of regimens using conventional and high dosage FSH IVF dosages in women whose response was so poor that only one embryo to transfer. Authors reported a 20% rate (6/30) with natural vs. 8.3% (23/274) with high dose FSH (68). Though these studies used "lower dosage" FSH stimulation, they did not adhere to the tenets of the author's specific regimen. These differences in protocol could explain somewhat lower pregnancy rates in this other study (69).

12. Conclusions

Women with normal oocyte reserve seem to have a similar chance of live deliveries following IVF-ET whether they use mild or conventional FSH stimulation protocols. Considering the risk of OHSS and the increased cost from conventional FSH stimulation, it is logical to use milder FSH stimulation for women with normal oocyte reserve. Perhaps for women of advancing reproductive age, i.e., >age 35, it is better to choose the conventional FSH dosage stimulation. If the cryopreservation techniques are used, frozen extra embryos for women at this age will provide the hope for infertile couples to have another child in the future.

A lot of data supports the use of low dose FSH protocols for women with diminished oocyte reserve. It seems logical that the very poor pregnancy rate in women with diminished oocyte reserve recorded by some of the finest IVF-ET centers was not related to poor quality oocytes, rather than a direct adverse effect of the conventional or high dosage of FSH used. The main principle for those women is not to further increase FSH level but to wait for endogenous or exogenous estrogen to lower the FSH closer to normal levels before instituting any FSH stimulation.

13. References

[1] Check JH: Understanding the physiology of folliculogenesis serves as the foundation for perfecting diagnosis and treatment of ovulatory defects. Clin Exp Obst Gyn, in press.
[2] Check ML, Brittingham D, Check JH, Choe JK: Pregnancy following transfer of cryopreserved-thawed embryos that had been a result of fertilization of all vitro matured metaphase, or germinal stage oocytes: Case report. Clin Exp Obst Gyn 28:69-70, 2001.
[3] Howles CM, Macnamee MC, Edwards RG: Short term use of an LHRH agonist to treat poor responders entering an in vitro fertilization programme. Hum Reprod 1987;2:655-656.
[4] Check JH, Nowroozi K, Chase JS: Comparison of short versus long-term leuprolide acetate-human menopausal gonadotropin hyperstimulation in in vitro fertilization patients. Hum Reprod 7:31-34, 1992.
[5] Sharara FI, McClamrock HD: Use of Microdose GnRH agonist protocol in women with low ovarian volumes undergoing IVF. Hum Reprod 2001;16:500-503.
[6] Shanis B, Check JH, O'Shaughnessy A, Summers D: Improved pregnancy rates (PRs) in older patients or those with elevated baseline FSH levels with short flare or clomiphene-hMG hyperstimulation protocols. In: IX World Congress on In Vitro Fertilization and Assisted Reproduction, International Proceedings Division. eds: Aburumieh A, Bernat E, Dohr G, Feichtinger W, Fischl, Huber J, Muller E, Szalay S, Urdl W, Zech H. Monduzzi Editore. pgs. 279-283, 1995.
[7] Check JH, Davies E, Adelson H: A randomized prospective study comparing pregnancy rates following clomiphene citrate and human menopausal gonadotropins therapy. Hum Reprod 1992;7:801-805.
[8] Trounson AO, Leeton JF, Wood C, Webb J, Wood J: Pregnancies in human by fertilization in vitro and embryo transfer in controlled ovulatory cycle. Science 1981;212:681-682.
[9] Garcia-Velasco JA, Moreno L, Pacheco A, Guillen A, Duque L, Requena A, Pellicer A: The aromatase inhibitor letrozole increases the concentration of intraovarian androges and improves in vitro fertilization outcome in low responder patients: a pilot study. Fertil Steril 2005;84:82-87.

[10] Mitwally MF, Caster RF: Use of an aromatase inhibitor for induction of ovulation in patients with an inadequate response to clomiphene citrate. Fertil Steril 2001;75:305-309.

[11] Check JH, Nazari A, Barnea ER, Weiss W, Vetter BH: The efficacy of short-term gonadotrophin-releasing hormone agonists versus human chorionic gonadotrophin to enable oocyte release in gonadotrophin stimulated cycles. Hum Reprod 8:568-571, 1993.

[12] Katsoff B, Check JH, Choe JK, Wilson C: Editorial article: A novel method to evaluate pregnancy rates following in vitro fertilization to enable a better understanding of the true efficacy of the procedure. Clin Exp Obst Gyn 2005;32:213-216.

[13] Baart EB, Martini E, Elkemans MJ, Van Opstal D, Beckers N, Verhoeff A, Macklon NS, Fauser B: Milder ovarian stimulation for in-vitro fertilization reduces aneuploidy in the human pre-implantation embryos: a controlled trial. Hum Reprod 2007;22:980-988.

[14] Schoolcraft WB, Treff NR, Stevens JM, Ferry K, Katz-Jaffe M, Scott RT Jr: Live birth outcome with trophectoderm biopsy, blastocyst vitrification, and single-nucleotide polymorphism microarray-based comprehensive chromosome screening in infertile patients. Fertil Steril 2011;96:638-640.

[15] Check JH, Choe JK, Katsoff D, Summers-Chase D, Wilson C: Controlled ovarian hyperstimulation adversely affects implantation following in vitro fertilization-embryo transfer. J Assist Reprod Genet, 16:416-420, 1999.

[16] Strandell A, Waldenstrom U, Nilsson L, Hamberger L: Hydrosalpinx reduces in vitro fertilization/embryo transfer pregnancy rate. Hum Reprod 1994;9:861-863.

[17] Shelton KE, Butier L, Toner JP: Salpingectomy improves the pregnancy rate in in vitro fertilization patients with hydrosalpinx. Hum Reprod 1996;11:523-525.

[18] Choe J, Check JH: Salpingectomy for unilateral hydrosalpinx may improve in vivo fecundity. Gynecol Obstet Invest 48:285-287, 1999.

[19] Check JH, Choe JK, Nazari A, Fox F, Swenson K: Fresh embryo transfer is more effective than frozen ET for donor oocyte recipients but not for donors. Hum Reprod, 16:1403-1408, 2001.

[20] Check JH, Choe JK, Nazari A, Summers-Chase D: Ovarian hyperstimulation can reduce uterine receptivity. A case report. Clin Exp Obst Gyn 27(2):89-91, 2000.

[21] Check JH, Check ML: A case report demonstrating that follicle maturing drugs may create an adverse uterine environment even when not used for controlled ovarian hyperstimulation. Clin Exp Obst Gyn 28:217-218, 2001.

[22] Kerin JF, Broom TJ, Ralph MM, et al: Human luteal phase function following oocyte cycles. Br J Obstet Gynecol 1981;88:1021-8.

[23] Edwards RG, Steptoe PC, Purdy JM: Establishing full-term human pregnancies using cleaving embryos grown in vitro. Br J Obstet Gynecol 1980;87:737-756.

[24] Albano C, Grimbizis G, Smitz J, Riethmuller-Winzen H, Reissmann T, Van Steirteghem A, Devroey P: The luteal phase of nonsupplemented cycles after ovarian superovulation with human menopausal gonadotropin and the gonadotropin-releasing hormone antagonist Cetrorelix. Fertil Steril 1998;70:357-9.

[25] Bourgain C, Devroey P: the endometrium in stimulated cycles for IVF. Hum Reprod Update 2003;9:515-522.

[26] Check JH, Check ML: Evidence that failure to conceive despite apparent correction of ovulatory defects by follicle-maturing drugs may be related to premature trophoblast invasion. Med Hypoth 2002 Oct;59(4):385-8.

[27] Check JH: Luteal phase support in assisted reproductive technology treatment: focus on Endometrin® (progesteorne) vaginal insert. Ther Clinic Risk Manag 2009;5:403-7.

[28] Doody KJ, Schnell VL, Foulk RA, et al. Endometrin for luteal phase support in a randomized, controlled, open-label, prospective in-vitro fertilization trial using a combination of Menopur and Bravelle for controlled ovarian hyperstimulation. Fertil Steril, 2009;91:1012-7.

[29] Fatemi HM, Popovic-Todorovic B, Papanikolaou E, et al: An update of luteal phase support in stimulated IVF cycles. Hum Reprod Update 2007;13:581-90.

[30] Chakravarty BN, Shirazee HH, Dam P, Goswami SK, Chatterjee R, Ghosh S: Oral dydrogesterone versus intravaginal micronised progesterone as luteal phase support in assisted reproductive technology (ART) cycles: results of a randomized study. J Steroid Biochem Mol Biol 2005;97:416-20.

[31] Nosarka S, Kruger T, Siebert I, et al: Luteal phase support in in vitro fertilization: meta-analysis of randomized trials. Gynecol Obstet Invest 2005;60:67-74.

[32] Araujo E Jr, Bernardini L, Frederick JL, et al: Prospective randomized comparison of human chorionic gonadotropins versus intramuscular progesterone for luteal phase support in assisted reproduction. J Assist Reprod Genet 1994;11:74-8.

[33] Ludwig M, Finas A, Katalinic A, et al: Prospective, randomized study to evaluate the success rates using HCG, vaginal progesterone or a combination of both for luteal phase support. Acta Obstet Gynecol Scand 2001;80:574-582.

[34] Nyboe AA, Popovic-Todorovic B, Schmidt KT, Loft A, Lindhard A, Hojgaard A, Ziebe S, Hald F, Hauge B, Toft B: Progesterone supplementation during early gestations after IVF or ICSI has no effect on the delivery rates: a randomized controlled trial. Hum Reprod 2002;17:357-61.

[35] Baker AF, Check JH, Hourani CL: Survival and pregnancy rates of pronuclear stage human embryos cryopreserved and thawed using a single step addition and removal of cryoprotectants. Hum Reprod Update May 1996;2:271 (CD-ROM), Item 12.

[36] Check JH, Summers-Chase D, Swenson K, Choe JK, Yuan W, Lurie D: Transfer success of frozen-thawed embryos at different cell stages at cryopreservation. Reprod Technol 10:201-205, 2000.

[37] Check JH, Katsoff B, Choe JK: Embryos from women who hyperrespond to controlled ovarian hyperstimulation do not have lower implantation potential as determined by results of frozen embryo transfer. In: International Proceedings of the 13th World Congress on In Vitro Fertilization and Assisted Reproduction and Genetics, Monduzzi Editore, Pgs. 109-113, 2005.

[38] Goldenberg RL, Grodin J, Rodbard D, Ross GT: Gonadotropins in women with amenorrhea: the use of follicle stimulating hormone to differentiate women with and without ovarian failure. Am J Obstet Gynecol 1973:11:1003.

[39] Manken J, Trussel J, Larsen U: Age and infertility. Science 1986;233:1389.

[40] Muasher SJ, Eohninger S, Simonetti S, Matta J, Ellis LM, Liu H-C, et al: The value of basal and/or stimulated serum gonadotropin levels in prediction of stimulation response and in vitro fertilization outcome. Fertil Steril 1988;50:298.

[41] Fenichel P, Grimaldi M, Olivero J-F, Donzeau M, Gillet J-Y, Harter M: Predictive value of hormonal profiles before stimulation for in vitro fertilization. Fertil Steril 1989;51:845.

[42] Scott RT, Toner JP, Muasher SJ, Oehninger S, Robinson S, Rosenwaks Z: Follicle-stimulating hormone levels on cycle day 3 are predictive of in vitro fertilization outcome. Fertil Steril 1989;51:651.

[43] Tanbo T, Dale PO, Abyholm T, Stokke KT: Follicle-stimulating hormone as a prognostic indicator in clomiphene citrate/human menopausal gonadotropin-stimulated cycles for in vitro fertilization. Hum Reprod 1989;4:647.

[44] Kolibianakis E, Zikopoulos K, Camus M, Tounaye H, Van Steirteghem A, Devroey P: Modified natural cycles for IVF does not offer a realistic chance of parenthood in poor responders with high day 3 FSH levels as a last resort prior to oocyte donation. Hum Reprod 2004;19:2545.

[45] Roberts JE, Spandorfer S, Fasouliotis SJ, Kashyap S, Rosenwaks Z: Taking a basal follicle-stimulating hormone history is essential before initiating in vitro fertilization. Fertil Steril 2005;83:37.

[46] Nassari A, Mukherjee T, Grifo JA, Noyes N, Krey L, Copperman AB: Elevated day 3 serum follicle stimulating hormone and/or estradiol may predict fetal aneuploidy. Fertil Steril 1999;71:715.

[47] Check JH, Nowroozi K, Chase JS, Nazari A, Shapse D, Vaze M: Ovulation induction and pregnancies in 100 consecutive women with hypergonadotropic amenorrhea. Fertil Steril 53(5):811-816, 1990.

[48] Check JH, Peymer M, Lurie D: Effect of age on pregnancy outcome without assisted reproductive technology in women with elevated early follicular phase serum follicle-stimulating hormone levels. Gynecol Obstet Invest 45:217-220, 1998.

[49] Check JH, Check ML, Katsoff D: Three pregnancies despite elevated serum FSH and advanced age: Case report. Hum Reprod 15(8):1709-1712, 2000.

[50] Check ML, Check JH, Kaplan H: Pregnancy despite imminent ovarian failure and extremely high endogenous gonadotropins and therapeutic strategies: Case report and review. Clin Exp Obst Gyn 2004;31:299-301.

[51] Check JH, Chase JS, Wu CH, Adelson HG: Ovulation induction and pregnancy with an estrogen-gonadotropin stimulation technique in a menopausal woman with marked hypoplastic ovaries. Am J Obstet Gynecol 1989;160:405-406.

[52] Shanis BS, Check JH: Spontaneous ovulation and successful pregnancy despite bilateral streaked ovaries. Infertility 15:70-77, 1992.

[53] Check JH, Katsoff B: Successful pregnancy with spontaneous ovulation in a woman with apparent premature ovarian failure who failed to conceive despite four

transfers of embryos derived from donated oocytes. Clin Exp Obst Gyn 2006;33:13-15.
[54] Check JH, Summers D, Nazari A, Choe J: Successful pregnancy following in vitro fertilization-embryo transfer despite imminent ovarian failure. Clin Exp Obst Gyn, 27(2):97-99, 2000.
[55] Check ML, Check JH, Choe JK, Berger GS: Successful pregnancy in a 42-year-old woman with imminent ovarian failure following ovulation induction with ethinyl estradiol without gonadotropins and in vitro fertilization. Clin Exp Obst Gyn 2002;29:11-14.
[56] Check JH, Katsoff B: Three successful pregnancies with in vitro fertilization embryo transfer over an eight year time span despite elevated basal serum follicle stimulating hormone levels - Case report. Clin Exp Obst Gyn 2005;32:217-221.
[57] Check JH, Summers-Chase D, Yuan W, Horwath D, Wilson C: Effect of embryo quality on pregnancy outcome following single embryo transfer in women with a diminished egg reserve. Fertil Steril 2007 Apr;87(4): 749-56.
[58] Check JH: Pharmacological options in resistant ovary syndrome and premature ovarian failure. Clin Exp Obst Gyn 2006;33:71-77.
[59] Check JH: The concept and treatment methodology for inducing ovulation in women in apparent premature menopause. Clin Exp Obst Gyn 2009;36:70-73.
[60] Check JH, Katsoff B: Ovulation induction and pregnancy in a woman with premature menopause following gonadotropin suppression with the gonadotropin releasing hormone antagonist, cetrorelix - a case report. Clin Exp Obstet Gynecol 2008;35(1):10-12.
[61] Check JH: Multiple follicles in an unstimulated cycle despite elevated gonadotropins in a perimenopausal female. Gynecol Obstet Invest, 33:190-192, 1992.
[62] Check JH, Chase J: Ovulation induction in hypergonadotropic amenorrhea with estrogen and human menopausal gonadotropin therapy. Fertil Steril 42: 919-922, 1984.
[63] Check JH, Wu CH, Check M: The effect of leuprolide acetate in aiding induction of ovulation in hypergonadotropic hypogonadism: A case report. Fertil Steril 49(3):542-543, 1988.
[64] Check JH: The multiple uses of ethinyl estradiol for treating infertility. Clin Exp Obst Gyn 2010;37:249-251.
[65] Katsoff B, Check MD: Successful pregnancy in a 45-year-old woman with elevated day 3 serum follicle stimulating hormone and a short follicular phase. Clin Exp Obstet Gynecol 2005;32:97-98.
[66] Check JH, Adelson H, Lurie D, Jamison T: The effect of the short follicular phase on subsequent conception. Gynecologic and Obstetric Investigation. 34:180-183, 1992.
[67] Kim C-H, Kim SR, Cheon YP, Kim SH, Cahe AD, Kang BM: Minimal stimulation using gonadotropin releasing hormone (GnRH) antagonist and recombinant human follicle stimulating hormone vs. GnRH antagonist multi-dose protocol in low responders undergoing in vitro fertilization/intracytoplasmic sperm injection. Fertil Steril 2009;92:2082-2084.

[68] Ata B, Yakin K, Balaban B, Urman B: Embryo implantation rates in natural and stimulated assisted reproduction treatment cycles in poor responders. Reprod Biomed Med Online 2008;77:207-212.

[69] Verberg MFG, Macklon NS, Nargund G, Frydman R, Devroey P, Broekmans FJ, Fauser BCJM: Mild ovarian stimulation for IVF. Hum Reprod Update 2009;15:13-29.

3

Does the Number of Retrieved Oocytes Influence Pregnancy Rate After Day 3 and Day 5 Embryo Transfer?

Veljko Vlaisavljević, Jure Knez and Borut Kovačič
Department of Reproductive Medicine, University Medical Centre Maribor
Slovenija

1. Introduction

Decisions associated to ovarian stimulation approach are an essential component of medically assisted reproduction (MAR). Considerable amount of research in this field has enhanced our understanding of certain biological phenomena taking place in the process and also brought along novel means of ovarian stimulation. Nevertheless, there is still not enough evidence to suggest the optimal number of oocytes collected at retrieval in order to predict the occurrence of successful pregnancy and most importantly, birth of a live baby. First, this chapter will describe certain historical developments in MAR. Next, current ovarian stimulation protocols and desired aims of modern era ovarian stimulation, embryo culture and embryo transfer outcome will be discussed. A single-centre MAR results analysis was performed in a ten year span in order to help resolve one of the ultimate questions: what is the optimal number of oocytes needed to achieve clinical pregnancy after embryo transfer?

2. Milestones in evolution of ovarian stimulation and embryo transfer

Ever since the beginnings of MAR, increasing the chance of a live birth has been the most important aim of researchers' efforts. The first successful embryo transfers (ETs) resulting in pregnancy by Edwards and Steptoe in the early 1970s were carried out in natural cycles. This means that only one oocyte was harvested at follicle aspiration (which was at the time performed laparoscopically). Hundred-and-one ETs were attempted before the first successful delivery of the world's first IVF (in vitro fertilization) baby Louise Brown in 1978 (Edwards & Steptoe, 1980). In these first attempts that paved the way for future extensive worldwide MAR success, Edwards and Steptoe described 65 natural cycles that yielded 45 oocytes from 44 patients and resulted in 3 successful deliveries. Thus, pregnancy rate was 9.1% and delivery rate 6.8% per oocyte retrieval.

Since then, research has brought along many improvements to MAR. In the early 1980s, one of the most important steps was the introduction of human menopausal gonadotrophin (HMG), which allowed for controlled ovarian hyperstimulation (COH) and multiple follicular growth. This enabled the retrieval of multiple oocytes at pick-up and thus substantially increased the likelihood of successful embryo replacement and subsequent pregnancy. This finding has ignited further research and development that has improved gonadotrophin formulation and efficiency, but detailed illustration of this process is beyond the scope of this chapter.

3. Current challenges in ovarian stimulation

3.1 Ovarian hyperstimulation syndrome

The development and implementation of gonadotrophins that allowed for controlled ovarian hyperstimulation (COH) in MAR has brought along a possibility of potentially life-threatening complication, namely ovarian hyperstimulation syndrome (OHSS) (Brinsden et al., 1995). It has been established that the risk of OHSS increases proportionally with an increase in ovarian response to stimulation as measured by the number of ovarian follicles, number of retrieved oocytes and serum estradiol concentration on the day of human chorionic gonadotrophin (hCG) administration (Asch et al., 1991). In our previous research, it has been demonstrated that the risk of OHSS increases with rising number of harvested oocytes and the risk is significantly higher in patients with more than ten collected oocytes (Reljič et al., 1999). Severe OHSS is a serious and potentially life-threatening complication of MAR treatment and has a mean incidence of 1-3% in MAR programmes involving standard ovarian stimulation protocols (Fauser et al., 1999). However, to date, there are no reliable predictors of its occurrence. Owing to these facts, many investigations in recent decade have been aimed towards less aggressive, milder forms of ovarian stimulation and to procedures that could eliminate the risk of OHSS (Revelli et al., 2011).

3.2 Ovarian stimulation strategies

Ovarian stimulation is the crucial component in medically assisted reproduction. In current practice, long acting gonadotrophin-releasing hormone (GnRH) agonist pituitary suppression combined with recombinant or purified urinary exogenous follicle stimulating hormone (FSH) is the most frequently used stimulation protocol (Macklon et al., 2006). However, in light of making MAR more "patient friendly", there is a recent trend toward milder stimulation protocols in order to reduce the chances of complications and not lastly, to lower the costs of MAR treatment (Fauser et al., 1999). With the availability of GnRH antagonists in ovarian stimulation protocols, administration of FSH can be delayed to mid-follicular phase, thus reducing the amount of gonadotrophins used for stimulation and minimizing exogenous hormonal interferences that are present in conventional hormonal stimulation (Fauser & van Heusden, 1997). On the other hand, regarding reduction of OHSS, conventional stimulation protocols employing GnRH antagonists allow for substitution of human chorionic gonadotrophin (hCG) with GnRH agonist for ovulation triggering. Using this procedure, OHSS can be eliminated almost completely even in high responding patients with high numbers of retrieved oocytes (Humaidan et al., 2011).

Despite the novel approaches to ovarian stimulation, the number of retrieved oocytes is still considered to be an important prognostic variable in everyday MAR practice. However, the relation between the number of oocytes and MAR outcome is poorly understood as studies performed on this subject present with conflicting results (Hamoda et al., 2010; Letterie et al., 2005; Meniru et al., 1997; Sunkara et al., 2011; Yoldemir et al., 2010). Moreover, as IVF procedures are performed in increasing extent globally, new, restrictive legislation policies in certain countries limit the amount of oocytes per cycle that can be used in MAR procedures. Due to the lack of reliable data, experts' opinions of such legislation effects on treatment success are too often contradictory. Thus, further research is needed to establish the role of number of harvested oocytes in MAR outcome prediction.

3.3 Embryo cultivation and transfer strategies

In the scenario of transfer of more than one embryo, multiple gestations are the most common complication of pregnancies achieved through MAR. Thus, in recent times, scientific societies have propagated the idea that the goal of medically assisted procreation must be the achievement of a singleton pregnancy (European Society of Human Reproduction and Embryology [ESHRE] Task Force on Ethics and Law, 2003). The simplest way of reducing multiple gestation incidences is strict implementation of single embryo transfer (SET) strategy. However, this is related to significant declines of pregnancy rates. The development of advanced embryo culture media in the past two decades have allowed for extended, blastocyst cultivation of the embryos. Following the evolution of these media, many have advocated blastocyst transfer mainly due to better morphologic embryo assessment possibilities at blastocyst stage compared to cleavage stage embryos. Although the opinions on this subject are still not uniform, many recently performed studies have demonstrated significantly better outcome after blastocyst transfer (Papanikolau et al., 2008). Thus, a recent Cochrane review has shown a significant improvement in pregnancy and live birth rates for blastocyst transfer compared to transfer of cleavage stage embryos (Blake et al., 2007).

Currently, increasing number of legislation acts on MAR in developed countries impose mandatory single embryo transfer under certain circumstances (mostly in younger patients), in order to decrease the incidence of multiple gestations. Thus, the question remains; how to select the best embryos in order to achieve the highest success and at the same time lower the incidence of multiple gestations? With regards to these facts, additional studies should settle the issue in what scenario can the number of oocytes be a factor in decision for SET or multiple embryo transfer and whether embryos should be transferred at cleavage or blastocyst stage.

4. Influence of number of retrieved oocytes on embryo transfer success

A retrospective study of retrieved oocyte number on MAR outcome was performed at Department of Reproductive Medicine and Gynaecologic Endocrinology, University Medical Centre in Maribor. Totally, 6989 consecutive in vitro fertilisation (IVF) and intracytoplasmic sperm injection (ICSI) cycles resulting in follicle aspiration and oocyte pick-up were included. Ovarian stimulation protocols with combination of GnRH agonist/GnRH antagonist and recombinant FSH (Gonal-f®, Serono International SA, Geneva, Switzerland)/HMG (Menopur®, Ferring Pharmaceuticals Inc., Saint-Prex, Switzerland) were used and were previously described in detail (Vlaisavljević et al., 2000). Embryo quality was assessed by an experienced embryologist at day two and blastocysts were graded according to our established grading system at day five after oocyte pick-up (Kovačič et al., 2004). Embryo transfer was carried out three or five days after oocyte pick-up. Day five blastocyst transfer was performed if more than four fertilised oocytes were obtained and if more than three optimal embryos were available on day three according to our standard policies (Kovačič et al., 2002). After consultation with the patients, time of embryo transfer could be adjusted to day 3 or day 5 according to doctor-patient agreement. Clinical pregnancy was defined as the presence of fetal heartbeat on ultrasound examination at six weeks of gestation. Frozen-thawed embryo transfer cycles and cycles with preimplantation genetic diagnostics (PGD) or in vitro maturated (IVM) oocytes were excluded from the study.

Patients were stratified according to the number of oocytes collected at retrieval. Categorical variables were tested using Chi-Square test. Numerical values were tested bivariately using Student's *t*-test or Mann-Whitney *U* test. The analysis of variance test (ANOVA) with Tukey HSD or Games-Howell post-hoc test was used for analysing differences in continuous variables between groups stratified by the number of retrieved oocytes. To further explore the association between the number of oocytes and clinical pregnancy rate, a logistic regression model was constructed. The model was adjusted for confounding variables that affected pregnancy rate in univariate analysis (the history of previous MAR attempts, age and dose of gonadotrophins). Data were analysed using SPSS 17.0 (SPSS Inc., Chicago IL) statistical software package.

4.1 Distribution of retrieved oocytes per cycle

In 6989 studied cycles, 61793 oocytes were collected at retrieval. The median number of retrieved oocytes was 8 [interquartile range (IQR) 4-12] and the median number of embryos created was 4 [IQR 2-7]. Figure 1 represents the distribution of collected oocytes in cycles resulting in oocyte pick-up.

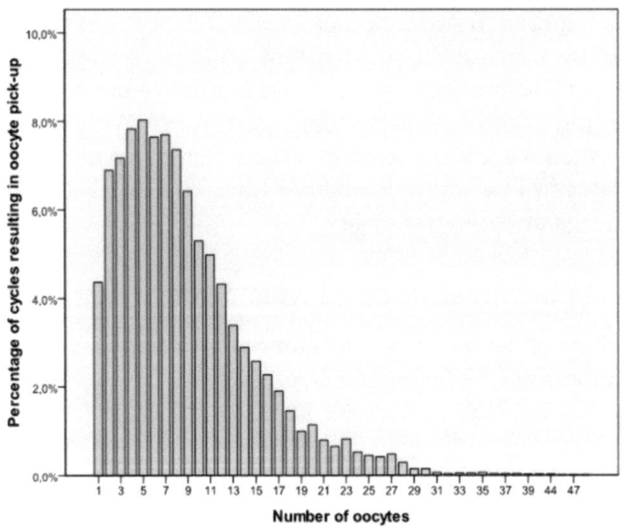

Fig. 1. Distribution of retrieved oocytes.

4.2 Outcome of MAR cycles

Cycles were stratified according to the number of retrieved oocytes. Overall clinical pregnancy rate per cycle was 37.1%, calculated pregnancy rate per embryo transfer was 41.0%. Delivery rates per cycle and per embryo transfer were calculated to be 29.8% and 32.9%, respectively. Clinical outcomes are summarized in Table 1.

No. of oocytes	1-5	6-10	11-15	16-20	>20	TOTAL
No. of cycles	2396	2405	1269	544	375	6989
Age (SD)	36.1 (4.6)[a]	33.8 (4.6)[b]	32.6 (4.2)[c]	32.2 (4.4)[c]	32.0 (4.2)[c]	34.2 (4.7)
No of previous MAR attempts (SD)	2.0 (2.4)[a]	1.6 (2.1)[b]	1.5 (1.9)[bc]	1.4 (1.9)[c]	1.3 (1.6)[c]	1.7 (2.2)
No. of oocytes collected	7765	18823	16061	9571	9573	61793
Fertilised oocytes (2PN)	4910	11552	9668	5686	5510	37326
Day 2 embryos	4837	11352	9454	5565	5381	36589
ET(s)	2027	2241	1213	513	332	6326
Percentage of day 5 ETs	14.0%[a]	69.4%[b]	86.7%[c]	92.6%[d]	94.3%[d]	58.2%
Cancelled ET	15.4%[a]	6.8%[b]	4.4%[c]	5.7%[bc]	11.5%[ab]	9.5%
Transferred embryos	3502	4040	2123	828	489	10982
Cryopreserved embryos	295	2212	2544	1982	2150	9183
Clinical Pregnancies	532	954	638	286	184	2594
Avg. Fertilisation rate	75.6%[a]	77.2%[ab]	77.6%[ab]	79.3%[ab]	83.8%[b]	77.3%
Pregnancy rate/cycle	22.2%[a]	39.7%[b]	50.3%[c]	52.6%[c]	49.1%[c]	37.1%
Pregnancy rate/ET	26.3%[a]	42.6%[b]	52.6%[c]	55.8%[c]	55.4%[c]	41.0%
Cycles with blastocyst cryopreservation	8.3%[a]	38.9%[b]	58.3%[c]	73.0%[d]	83.5%[e]	37.0%

[abcde] Within each category, numbers with different letter superscripts are significantly different from each other, numbers with the same letter superscript are not significantly different (p<0.05).

Table 1. Outcome of MAR treatment according to the number of retrieved oocytes

4.3 Clinical pregnancy & delivery rates in relation to the number of retrieved oocytes

Clinical pregnancy and delivery rates were calculated per each number of collected oocytes. Clinical pregnancy rate rises constantly to peak at 11-15 oocytes and from then on remains constant until it declines slightly at high responders with more than 20 oocytes (Table 1 & Figure 2). Nonetheless, there are no statistically significant changes in pregnancy rates in groups of patients with more then 11-15 harvested oocytes. However, the risks related to ovarian stimulation increase with rising oocyte count, which is partially reflected in higher cycle cancellation rates, especially in patients with more than 20 harvested oocytes (Table 1). Published data about the number of oocytes influencing embryo transfer outcome are not consistent. Whilst some scientists claim that oocyte number plays no role in achievement of pregnancy after embryo transfer (Letterie et al., 2005; Yoldemir et al., 2010), others report of increasing pregnancy rates with increasing number of oocytes. The optimal numbers reported in these studies are usually in the range of 5 to 15 oocytes (van Gast et al., 2006; Meniru & Craft, 1997; Timeva et al., 2006). Most of these studies are however single-centre analyses performed on a fairly low number of patients. Recently though, Sunkara et al performed a large scale review of UK national IVF data and concluded that 15 is the optimal number of oocytes to be collected at retrieval (Sunkara et al., 2011). Results of our study that included nearly 7000 cycles suggest that the optimal number of oocytes to aim for at ovarian stimulation in order to achieve clinical pregnancy should be between 11 and 15.

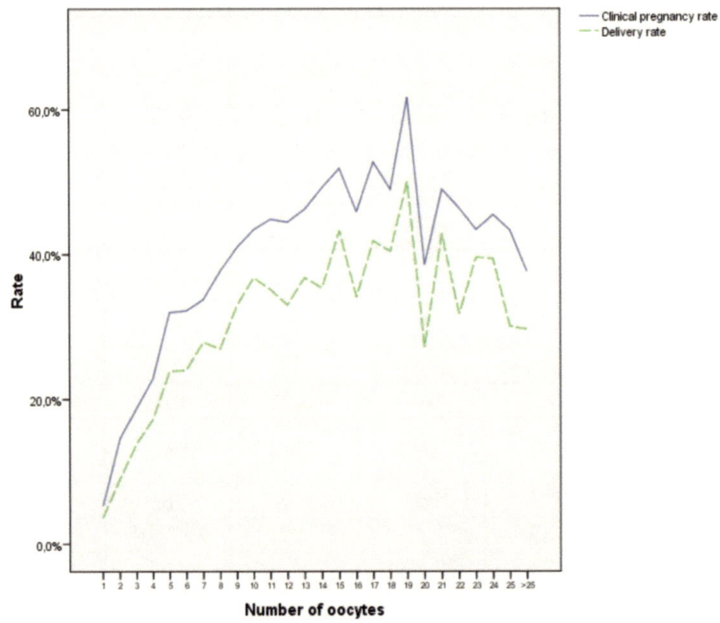

Fig. 2. Clinical pregnancy and delivery rates in relation to the number of retrieved oocytes

4.3.1 Low number of oocytes

As noted above, pregnancy and delivery rates are significantly lower in cycles where less than 5 oocytes are retrieved at pickup. Accordingly, these cycles were analysed more thoroughly. Significant changes can be observed in pregnancy rates among each of the groups (Table 2). These differences remain significant even after controlling for the age factor and history of previous MAR attempts in multivariate analysis.

It has been demonstrated that low oocyte numbers after ovarian stimulation are related to ovarian ageing and the depletion of primordial follicle pool (Tarlatzis et al., 2003). Ovarian stimulation for women with low ovarian reserve has remained one of the most frustrating aspects of IVF (Revelli et al., 2011). However, direct correlation with pregnancy rate has not been thoroughly investigated.

Low oocyte number coupled with high gonadotrophin dose in conventional stimulation methods can imply lower oocyte quality. Furthermore, endometrial quality can also be hampered in high-dose stimulating protocols (Gougeon, 1996; Pal et al., 2008). On the other hand, higher number of oocytes simply allows for better selection of quality embryos from a larger cohort of available embryos (Devreker, 1999; Pal et al., 2008).

On the opposite, it has been theorised that milder forms of ovarian stimulation allow for higher quality oocytes and embryos with lower incidence of chromosome aneuploidies that can result in comparable pregnancy rates in spite of the lower number of harvested oocytes (Verberg et al., 2009). However, studies on this subject are relatively sparse and a recently performed meta-analysis included only three studies featuring low number of participants (Verberg et al., 2009). All of the studies included report of relatively low pregnancy rates, 15-21%. What is more, the studies did not account for possible added benefits of embryo cryopreservation, which could shift the scale to the side of classic ovarian stimulation even further if adding freeze-thaw cycles to the analysis. In theory, mild stimulation seems a feasible choice that could be especially indicated in poor responding patients. Because of lower gonadotrophin dose, higher quality of oocytes and endometrium could be expected. But since there is very limited data available, current reports do not provide enough supporting evidence and in the end, additional studies are needed in order to define the role of mild stimulation protocols in routine MAR treatment.

Number of oocytes	1	2-3	4-5	TOTAL	
No. of cycles	305	983	1108	2396	
Age (SD)	37.9 (4.2)[a]	36.7 (4.4)[b]	35.2 (4.6)[c]	36.1 (4.6)	$p<0.001$
No of previous MAR attempts (SD)	2.0 (2.4)[a]	2.1 (2.7)[a]	1.9 (2.2)[a]	2.0 (2.4)	$p>0.05$
Gonadotrophin used (IE)	2979[a]	2789[b]	2518[c]	2692	$p<0.001$
No of oocytes collected	305	2467	4993	7765	
Fertilised oocytes (2PN)	212	1574	3124	4910	
Day 2 embryos	205	1532	3100	4837	
ET(s)	185	828	1014	2027	
Percentage of day 5 ETs	0.5%	3.0%	25.4%	14.0%	
Cancelled ET	39.34%[a]	15.77%[b]	8.48%[c]	15.40%	$p<0.001$
Transferred embryos	186	1368	1948	3502	
Cryopreserved embryos	0	41	254	295	
Clinical Pregnancies	16	184	332	532	
Avg. Fertilisation rate	78.2%[a]	75.0%[a]	75.8%[a]	75.6%	$p>0.05$
Pregnancy rate/cycle	5.30%[a]	18.70%[b]	30.00%[c]	22.20%	$p<0.001$
Pregnancy rate/ET	8.70%[a]	22.20%[b]	32.70%[c]	26.30%	$p<0.001$
Cycles with blastocyst cryopreservation	0%[a]	3.30%[b]	15.10%[c]	8.30%	$p<0.001$

[abc] Within each category, numbers with different letter superscripts are significantly different from each other, numbers with the same letter superscript are not significantly different.

Table 2. Cycle characteristics in "poor" and "low" responders (<5 oocytes collected)

4.4 Effect of age

Besides the number of oocytes, age was found to be one of the most important factors in predicting the success of the started cycle in our data. In further analysis, cycles were stratified according to the age of female patients. Advancing age significantly adversely affects the outcome of MAR cycles independently of oocyte count. Average clinical pregnancy rate was the highest in the youngest group of patients (20-34 years) at 45.6% and decreased to 16.8% in women over 40 years of age. On the other hand, mean oocyte count was also significantly lower in older women (20-34 years; 10.4 oocytes, 35-37 years; 8.5 oocytes, 38-39 years; 6.9 oocytes, 40-44 years; 5.7 oocytes, $p<0.001$). The results are illustrated in Figure 3.

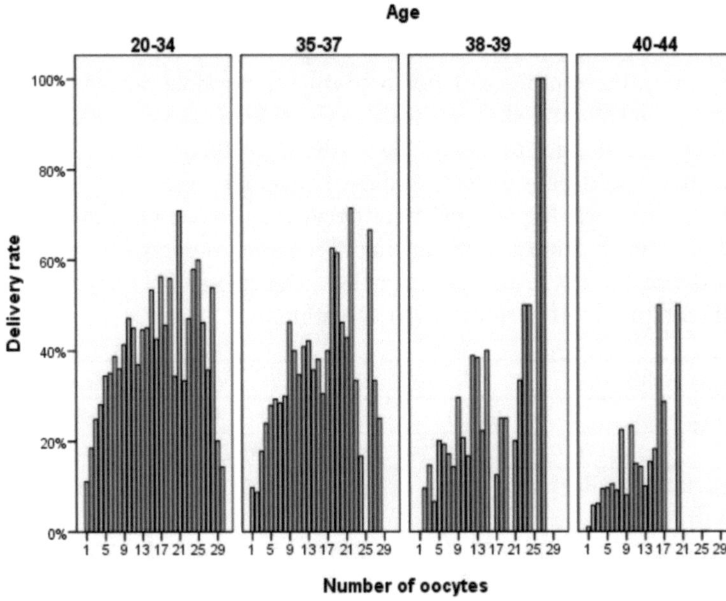

Fig. 3. Association between oocyte number and delivery rate stratified by the female patient age.

With ovarian ageing, the depletion of ovarian reserve usually involves adjusting stimulation protocols with higher doses of gonadotrophins that result in negative effects as discussed in previous topic. Although our study did not consider antral follicle count (AFC) and anti-Müllerian hormone (AMH) as a measure of ovarian reserve, it can be clearly seen from our results that age is independent predictor of lower oocyte count at retrieval. But even in the case of normal response to gonadotrophin treatment in older women, pregnancy rates are lower compared to younger patients. This could be related to the high proportion of embryo aneuploidies in these patients. This problem grows quickly after 40 years of age and after the age of 45 the birth of a healthy baby after MAR is very rare in spite of normal ovarian reserve tests (Forman et al., 2011).

4.5 Embryo cryopreservation

Although the birth of a live baby preceded by the successful achievement of clinical pregnancy is the single most important outcome of MAR treatment, several other surrogate indicators were evaluated in order to assess the quality of MAR cycles.

Embryo transfer was performed in 91.5% of cycles after oocyte pick-up. In approximately 9.5% cycles transfer had to be cancelled. The rate of transfer cancellation is the highest in "poor" responding patients and approximately 40% of transfers were cancelled when only 1 oocyte was retrieved (Table 1 & Table 2). This can be contributed to the fact that there are fewer embryos available for transfer and also to the lower quality of oocytes available for treatment (Tarlatzis et al., 2003). On the other hand, cycle cancellation again increases significantly in high responding patients, with more than 20 oocytes collected at retrieval. Together with the higher rate of cycle cancellation, a drop in pregnancy and delivery rates is also observed beyond 20 harvested oocytes (Table 1 & Figure 2). In concordance with these results, recently performed studies argue that the simple aim to harvest as many oocytes as possible is simply not justified (van der Gast et al., 2006; Sunkara et al., 2011). Our analysis has some limitations due to the fact that incidence of OHSS could not be analysed and cycles with cryopreservation of the whole embryo cohort due to high OHSS risk could not be excluded from the analysis. It could be reasoned that lower pregnancy rates and high embryo transfer cancellation can be attributed to ovarian hyperstimulation syndrome risk. But considering data in the literature, approximately 15% incidence of OHSS can be predicted at 20 collected oocytes and the risk increases with rising oocyte count (Reljič et al., 1999; Verwoerd et al., 2008). In addition, there is also evidence that high estradiol levels may negatively impact developmental potential of the embryos (Ertzeid & Storeng, 2001) and interfere with endometrial receptivity in the early luteal phase (Devroey et al., 2004; Horcajadas et al., 2008). Thus, pregnancy rates can be hampered in high responders even in the absence of ovarian hyperstimulation syndrome risk.

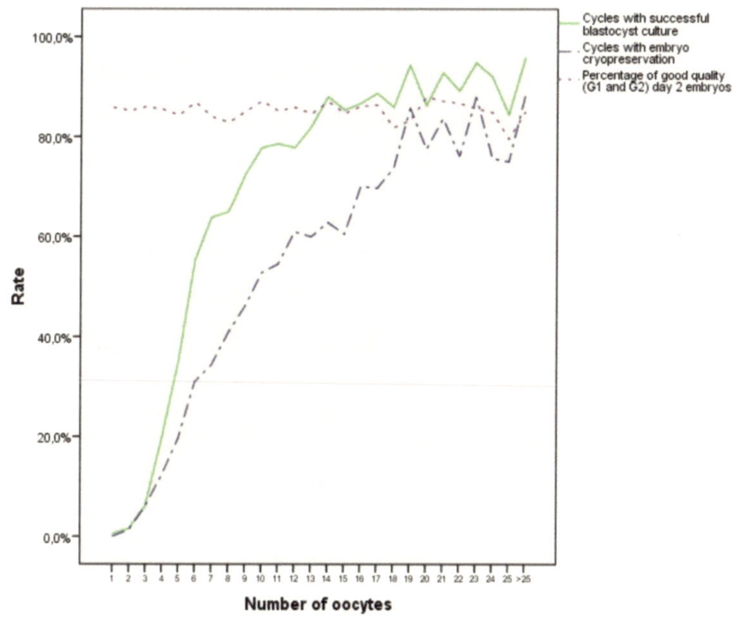

Fig. 4. Association of the number of retrieved oocytes to embryo cryopreservation, successful blastocyst culture and proportion of good quality embryos on day two.

Nonetheless, an increase in proportion of cycles with embryos available for freezing can be observed up until ~20 oocytes (Table 1 & Figure 4). The relationship was evident also in multivariate analysis after controlling for possible confounding variables (age, history of previous MAR attempts and dosage of gonadotrophins). Somewhat lower pregnancy rates in these patients could theoretically be recovered in subsequent cryo-thawed cycles. It should be noted though, that this group of patients included also couples with cancelled embryo transfer and cryopreservation of the whole embryo cohort due to high OHSS risk. Due to our study design, linkage between fresh and cryo-thawed cycles was not possible and the analysis of cumulative pregnancy rates could not be performed. Our results are comparable with findings of the research by Hamoda et al in which there was no increment in cycles with available oocytes for freezing beyond 18 harvested oocytes (Figure 4).

Furthermore, the storage of high numbers of cryopreserved embryos can also lead to logistic, administrative and ethical problems. Even so, in a unit with a successful cryopreservation programme, especially with the advances of embryo vitrification, cumulative pregnancy rates can be substantially improved (Kolibianakis et al., 2009).

Additionally, blastocyst transfer was performed significantly more frequently with rising number of harvested oocytes. Because day 5 blastocyst transfer allows for enhanced embryo selection and can optimize the chance of embryo transfer success (Blake et al., 2007; Kovačič et al, 2002; Papanikolaou et al., 2008), further analysis was aimed toward the comparison of different embryo cultivation and transfer policies.

4.6 Embryo cultivation protocol

Couples were stratified according to the stage at which embryos were replaced in the uterus. At blastocyst stage, single embryo or two embryos were transferred, at cleavage stage one to three embryos were transferred depending on the age, history of the patients and embryo quality. Results of embryo transfer after different protocols are illustrated in Table 3.

In the beginnings of MAR, cleavage stage embryo transfer was traditionally performed. Physiology and energy metabolism of early embryos were not well understood and thus media could not be used to culture embryos beyond the four-cell stage. However, with scientific advances, new improved, sequential blastocyst media have enabled longer in vitro cultivation of embryos (Menezo et al., 1998). There are two central reasons why this should theoretically improve embryo transfer results. First of all, it is considered that blastocyst transfer mimics natural conception physiology as the embryo travels through Fallopian tubes and reaches the uterine cavity no sooner than the fourth day after conception. The uterus provides different nutritional conditions for the embryo and this may cause homeostatic stress and reduce embryo implantation rates after cleavage stage transfer (Blake et al., 2007). The second reason lies in the before mentioned chance of better morphologic selection of the embryos at blastocyst stage. However, in our previous studies, it was demonstrated that in the case of low number of embryos this advantages did not help to improve success rates of embryo transfer. Extended blastocyst culture did not prove to be of any value in improving pregnancy rates in the scenario when fewer than three embryos were available at day two after oocyte pickup. On the other hand, although transfer cancellation was significantly higher when waiting until day five for transfer, pregnancy and delivery rates per started cycle were comparable (Kovačič et al., 2002; Vlaisavljević et al., 2001). According to the present study, clinical and ongoing pregnancy rates were significantly higher in the case of blastocyst transfer compared to day three cleavage stage embryo transfer (52.7% vs. 25.3% and 43.1% vs. 18.6% respectively). Even in the multivariable logistic regression model, adjusting for the age of the patients and the number of harvested oocytes, these differences remained statistically significant. These results should however be interpreted in the light of the fact that these groups were composed of patients with uneven characteristics. Generally, patients with less than five harvested oocytes and fewer than three embryos on day two that have effectively worse prognosis underwent cleavage stage transfer on day three. The number of harvested oocytes was significantly lower in day 3 group transfer as compared to day 5. In spite of this, considering data in the literature (Blake et al., 2007; Papanikolaou et al., 2008), our data confirm that blastocyst transfer provides a higher chance of embryo implantation and subsequent clinical pregnancy.

Additionally, it can clearly be seen that double blastocyst transfer does not improve pregnancy rates compared to transfer of a single blastocyst. This can be observed even when analysing only cycles with at least one optimal blastocyst transferred. On the other hand, the incidence of twin deliveries rises dramatically with double embryo, especially double blastocyst transfer (38.1%).

	Day 5	SBT	DBT	Day 3	SET	DET	TET	TOTAL
No. of cycles	**3572**	1452	2120	**2647**	798	1377	472	**6219**
Age (SD)	**32.8 (4.3)**	31.8 (4.2)[a]	33.4 (4.3)[b]	**35.8 (4.6)**	35.7 (4.7)[c]	35.3 (4.5)[c]	37.5 (4.3)[d]	
Avg. no of oocytes (SD)	**11.8 (5.6)**	12.5 (6.5)[a]	11.3 (5.1)[b]	**5.2 (3.7)**	3.5 (2.8)[c]	5.6 (3.6)[d]	6.9 (4.0)[e]	**8.8 (6.1)**
% transfers with optimal quality blastocyst	**53.2%**	60.6%	48.2%		.	.	.	.
Clinical pregnancy/ET	**52.7%**	52.2%[a]	53.1%[a]	**25.3%**	15.2%[b]	30.5%[c]	27.3%[c]	**41.1%**
Implantation rate	**43.9%**	53.1%[a]	37.6%[b]	**16.6%**	15.1%[cd]	19.2%[c]	11.3%[d]	**31.2%**
Ongoing pregnancy/ET	**43.1%**	(625) 43.1%[a]	(912) 43.2%[a]	**18.6%**	(92) 11.6%[b]	(313) 22.8%[c]	(84) 17.9%[c]	**(1663) 32.9%**
Twins	**24.5%**	(8) 1.7%	(303) 38.1%	**17.6%**	(1) 1.4%	(49) 20.1%	(19) 25.3%	**(380) 22.8%**
Triplets	**0.4%**	0	(5) 0.8%	**0.3%**	0	(1) 0.4%	0	**(6) 0.4%**

[abcde] Within each row, numbers with different letter superscripts are significantly different from each other, numbers with the same letter superscript are not significantly different ($p<0.05$)

Legend: »SBT«: single blastocyst transfer
»DBT«: double blastocyst transfer
»SET«: single cleavage stage embryo transfer
»DET«: double cleavage stage embryo transfer
»TET«: triple cleavage stage embryo transfer

Table 3. Embryo cultivation strategies and clinical outcome

The detailed investigation of the incidence of multiple gestations reveals that the incidence of higher order multiple pregnancies was low, as only 6 triplet pregnancies were observed during the ten-year study period. Conversely, birth of twins was recorded in 22.8% of deliveries and as mentioned before, this was especially high in the transfer of two blastocysts. In our publications, it was demonstrated that the age of the female patient and additional spare blastocysts available for cryopreservation are an important risk factor for multiple gestation after blastocyst transfer (Vlaisavljević et al., 2004). Our current data has shown, that even in the group of patients older than 40 years, after double blastocyst transfer, there were 27.7% twin gestations. This exemplifies the fact that the only option to minimize the risk of multiple gestations is strict implementation of single embryo transfer, even in the case of dealing with older patients.

5. Conclusion

Introduction of exogenous gonadotrophins to ovarian stimulation represents one of the most important events in MAR that substantially improved the results of infertility treatment. The first successful pregnancies achieved with MAR were the result of a natural cycle IVF. Since then, ovarian stimulation protocols using GnRH agonists or antagonists in the combination with recombinant or highly purified gonadotrophins have become an everyday routine in MAR practice. Our results show that current protocols of ovarian stimulation should be used in a way to avoid excessive follicular development and to achieve moderate stimulation of the ovaries. This approach provides superior results compared to either aggressive or mild stimulation protocols. According to our study, oocyte pick-up resulting in eleven to fifteen harvested oocytes presents the optimal outcome of ovarian stimulation. Day five blastocyst transfer enables for higher pregnancy rates compared to transfer of cleavage stage embryos, especially when high number of developed embryos is available on day three after oocyte pick-up. Extended blastocyst culture also allows for transfer of reduced number of embryos without decreasing the overall pregnancy rate. However, only strict implementation of single embryo transfer can lead to a decrease in the incidence of multiple gestations. These steps, coupled with successful laboratory embryo cryopreservation programme, present as an optimal choice for MAR.

6. References

Asch, RH. Li, HP. Balmaceda, JP. Weckstein LN & Stone, SC. (1991). Severe ovarian hyperstimulation syndrome in assisted reproductive technology: definition of high risk groups. *Human Reproduction*, Vol.6, No.10, pp. 1395–1399

Blake, D. Farquhar, C. Johnson, N. & Proctor, M. (2007). Cleavage stage versus blastocyst stage embryo transfer in assisted reproductive technology. *Cochrane Database Systemic Reviews*, No.4, Art. No.: CD002118. DOI: 10.1002/14651858.CD002118.pub3.

Brinsden, PR. Wada, I. Tan, SL. Balen, A & Jacobs, HS. (1995). Diagnosis, prevention and management of ovarian hyperstimulation syndrome. *British Journal of Obstetrics and Gynaecology*, Vol.102, No,10, pp.767-772

Devreker, F. Pogonici, E. De Maertelaer, V., Revelard, P., Van den Bergh, M. & Englert Y. (1999) Selection of good embryos for transfer depends on embryo cohort size: implications for the 'mild ovarian stimulation' debate. *Human Reproduction*, Vol.14, No.12, pp. 3002-8

Devroey, P. Bourgain, C. Macklon, NS. & Fauser, BC. (2004). Reproductive biology and IVF: ovarian stimulation and endometrial receptivity. *Trends Endocrinology and Metabolism*, Vol.15, pp. 84–90

Edwards, RG. Steptoe, PC. & Purdy, JM. (1980). Establishing full-term human pregnancies using cleaving embryo grown in vitro. *British Journal of Obstetrics and Gynaecology*, Vol.87, pp. 737–755

Edwards, RG. (2007). IVF, IVM, natural cycle IVF, minimal stimulation IVF - tome for a rethink. *Reproductive Biomedicine Online*, Vol.15, No.1, pp. 106-19

Ertzeid, G & Storeng, R. (2001). The impact of ovarian stimulation on implantation and fetal development in mice. *Human Reproduction*, Vol.16, pp. 221–225

Fauser, BC. & van Heusden, AM. (1997). Manipulation of human ovarian function: physiological concepts and clinical consequences. *Endocrine Reviews*, Vol.18, No.1, pp. 71–106

Fauser, BC. Devroey, P. Yen, SSC. Gosden, R. Crowley, WC. Baird, DT. & Bouchard P. (1999). Minimal ovarian stimulation for IVF: appraisal of potential benefits and drawbacks. *Human Reproduction*, Vol.14, No.11, pp. 681-686.

Forman, EJ. Treff, NR. Scott, RT. (2011). Fertility after age 45: From natural conception to Assisted Reproductive Technology and beyond. Review. *Maturitas*, Vol.70, pp. 216-221

Gougeon, A. (1996). Regulation of ovarian follicular development in primates: facts and hypotheses. *Endocrine Reviews*, Vol.17, No.2, pp. 121-155.

Hamoda, H. Sunkara, S. Khalaf, Y. Braude, P. & El-Toukhy, T. (2010). Outcome of fresh IVF/ICSI cycles in relation to the number of oocytes collected: a review of 4,701 treatment cycles. *Human Reproduction*, Vol.25, p. 417

Horcajadas, JA. Mínguez, P. Dopazo, J. Esteban, FJ. Domínguez, F. Giudice, LC. Pellicer, A. & Simón C. (2008). Controlled ovarian stimulation induces a functional genomic delay of the endometrium with potential clinical implications. *Journal of Clinical Endocrinology and Metabolism*, Vol.93, No.11, pp. 4500-4510

Humaidan, P. Kol, S. & Papanikolaou, E. (2011). Copenhagen GnRH Agonist Triggering Workshop Group. GnRH agonist for triggering of final oocyte maturation: time for a change of practice? *Human Reproduction Update*, Vol.17, No.4, pp. 510-524

Inge, GB. Brinsden, PR. & Elder, KT. (2005). Oocyte number per live birth in IVF: were Steptoe and Edwards less wasteful? *Human Reproduction*, Vol.20, No.3, pp. 588-592

Kolibianakis, EM. Venetis, CA. & Tarlatzis, BC. (2009). Cryopreservation of human embryos by vitrification or slow freezing: which one is better? *Current Opinion in Obstetrics & Gynecology*, Vol.21, No.3, pp. 270-274

Kovačič, B. Vlaisavljević, V. Reljič, M. & Gavrič-Lovrec V. (2002). Clinical outcome of day 2 versus day 5 transfer in cycles with one or two developed embryos. *Fertility Sterility*, Vol.77, No.3, pp. 529-536

Kovačič, B. Vlaisavljević V. Reljič M. & Čižek-Sajko M. (2004). Developmental capacity of different morphological types of day 5 human morulae et blastocysts. *Reproductive Biomedicine Online*, Vol.8, No.6, pp. 687-694.

Letterie, G. Marshall, L. & Angle, M. (2005). The relationship of clinical response, oocyte number, and success in oocyte donor cycles. *Journal of Assisted Reproduction and Gentics*, Vol.22, No.3, pp. 115-117

Macklon, NS. Stouffer, RL. Giudice, LC. & Fauser BC. (2006). The science behind 25 years of ovarian stimulation for in vitro fertilization. *Endocrine Reviews*, Vol.27, No.2, pp. 170–207

Menezo, YJR. Hamamah, S. Hazout, A. & Dale, B. (1998). Time to switch from co-culture tosequential defined media for transfer at the blastocyst stage. *Human Reproduction*, Vol.13, No.8, pp. 2043-2044.

Meniru, GI. & Craft, IL. (1997). Utilization of retrieved oocytes as an index of the efficiency of superovulation strategies for in-vitro fertilization treatment. *Human Reproduction*, Vol.12, No.10, pp. 2129-2132

Pal, L. Jindal, S. Witt, BR. & Santoro, N. (2008). Less is more: increased gonadotrophin use for ovarian stimulation adversely influences clinical pregnancy and live birth after in vitro fertilization. *Fertility Sterility*, Vol.89, No.6, pp. 1694-1701

Papanikolaou, EG. Kolibianakis, EM. Tournaye, H. Venetis, CA. Fatemi, H. Tarlatzis, B. & Devroey P. (2008). Live birth rates after transfer of equal number of blastocysts or cleavage-stage embryos in IVF. A systematic review and meta-analysis. *Human Reproduction*, Vol.23, No.1, pp. 91-99

Reljič, M. Vlaisavljević, V. Gavrić, V. & Kovačič, B. (1999). Number of oocytes retrieved and resulting pregnancy. Risk factors for ovarian hyperstimulation syndrome. *The Journal of Reproductive Medicine*, Vol.44, No.8, pp. 713-718

Revelli, A. Cassano, S. Salvagno, F. & Delle Piane L. (2011). Milder is better ? advantages and disadvantages of "mild" ovarian stimulation for human in vitro fertilization. *Reproductive Biology and Endocrinology*, Vol.9, No.25, pp. 1-9

Sharma, V. Allgar, V. & Rajkhowa, M. (2002). Factors influencing the cumulative conception rate and discontinuation of in vitro fertilization treatment for infertility. *Fertility Sterility*, Vol.78, No.1, pp. 40-46.

Sunkara, SK. Rittenberg, V. Raine-Fenning, N. Bhattacharya, S. Zamora, J. & Coomarasamy, A. (2011). Association between the number of eggs and live birth in IVF treatment: an analysis of 400 135 treatment cycles. *Human Reproduction*, Advance Access; Vol.0, No.0, pp. 1-7

Tarlatzis, BC. Zepiridis, L. Grimbizis, G. & Bontis J. (2003). Clinical management of low ovarian response to stimulation for IVF: a systematic review. *Human Reproduction Update*, Vol.9, No.1, pp. 61-76

The ESHRE Task Force on Ethics and Law. (2003). 6. Ethical issues related to multiple pregnancies in medically assisted procreation. *Human Reproduction*, Vol.18, No.9, pp. 1976-1979

Timeva ,T. Milachich, T. Antonova, I. Arabaji, T. Shterev, A. & Omar, HA. (2006). Correlation between number of retrieved oocytes and pregnancy rate after in vitro fertilization/intracytoplasmic sperm injection. *The Scientific World Journal*, Vol.6, pp. 686-690

van der Gaast, MH. Eijkemans, MJC. van der Net, JB. de Boer, EJ. Burger, CW. van Leeuwen, FE. Fauser, BCJM. & Macklon, NS. (2006). Optimum number of oocytes for a successful first IVF treatment cycle. *Reproductive Biomedicine Online*, Vol.13, No.4, pp. 476-480

Verberg, MFG. Eijkemans, MJC. Macklon, NS. Heijnen, EMEW. Baart, EB. Hohmann, FP. Fauser, BCJM. & Broekmans, FJ. (2009). The clinical significance of the retrieval of a low number of oocytes following mild ovarian stimulation for IVF: a meta-analysis. *Human Reproduction Update*, Vol.15, No.1, pp. 5-12

Verwoerd, GR. Mathews, T. & Brinsden, PR. (2008). Optimal follicle and oocyte numbers for cryopreservation of all embryos in IVF cycles at risk of OHSS. *Reproductive Biomedicine Online*, Vol.17, No.3, pp. 312-317

Vlaisavljević, V. Kovačič, B. Gavrić-Lovrec, V & Reljič, M. (2000). Simplification of the clinical phase of IVF and ICSI treatment in programmed cycles. *International Journal of Gynaecology and Obstetrics*. Vol.69, pp. 135-142

Vlaisavljević, V. Kovačič, B. Reljič, M. Gavrić-Lovrec, V. & Čižek Sajko M. (2001). Is there any benefit from the culture of a single oocyte to a blastocyst-stage embryo in unstimulated cycles? *Human Reproduction*, Vol.16, No.11, pp. 2379-2383

Vlaisavljević ,V. Čižek Sajko, M. Reljič, M. Gavrić-Lovrec, V. Kovač, V. & Kovačič B. (2004). Analysis of prognostic factors influencing multiple pregnancy. *Human Reproduction* Vol.19, Suppl.1, p. 196

Yoldemir, T. & Fraser, IS. (2010). The effect of retrieved oocyte count on pregnancy outcomes in assisted reproduction program. *Archives of Gynecology and Obstetrics*, Vol.281, No.3, pp. 551-556

4

Prevention and Treatment of Ovarian Hyperstimulation Syndrome

Ivan Grbavac, Dejan Ljiljak and Krunoslav Kuna
University Hospital Center "Sisters of Mercy", Zagreb
Croatia

1. Introduction

Ovarian hyperstimulation syndrome (OHSS) is a clinical symptom complex associated with ovarian enlargement resulting from exogenous gonadotropin therapy. In severe cases, a critical condition develops with massive ascites, marked ovarian enlargement, pleural effusion, electrolyte imbalance, hypovolemia with hypotension, oliguria, hemoconcentration, and thromboembolism (Madill JJ et al., 2008). Moderate to severe ovarian hyperstimulation syndrome (OHSS) has been calculated to occur in 0.2% to 2% of all ovarian stimulation cycles (Binder H et al., 2007).

Severe OHSS can be a life-threatening complication. The prognosis is usually worse in patients who get pregnant and have this syndrome.

2. Pathophysiology

The cause of OHSS is unknown, but it may be mediated by vasoactive cytokines secreted in excess by hyperstimulated ovaries (Goldsman MP et al., 1995). Human chorionic gonadotropin (hCG), either exogenous or endogenous (derived from a resulting pregnancy), is believed to be an early contributing factor. Increased vascular permeability is believed to result from vasoactive substances produced by the corpus luteum in response to hCG stimulation (Chen SU et al., 2010).

The pathophysiology of OHSS is characterized by increased vascular permeability with loss of fluid, protein, and electrolytes into the peritoneal cavity (Tollan A et al., 1990).

Gastrointestinal system findings include ascites (third-spacing of fluid), paralytic ileus, and enlarged ovaries. Pulmonary system findings include pleural effusions, restrictive lung disease from ascites or paralytic ileus, and ARDS. Cardiovascular system findings include decreased intravascular volume, decreased blood pressure, decreased central venous perfusion, and compensatory increased heart rate and cardiac output with arterial vasodilation. Coagulation abnormalities include hemoconcentration, increased estrogen level leading to hypercoagulability, and thrombosis. Renal system findings include decreased renal perfusion with subsequent oliguria or renal failure. Hepatic system findings may include hepatic edema.

Hematologic findings include increased hematocrit (secondary to increased capillary permeability and fluid loss) and elevated white blood cell count, a multifactorial finding associated with elevated estrogen level, prostaglandins, and dilution.

Gynecologic findings include enlarged ovaries which may torse or rupture. Finally, electrolyte findings classically include hyponatremia (secondary to increased antidiuretic hormone due to decreased intravascular volume) and hyperkalemia (secondary to the renal sodium/potassium pump alterations).

3. Hemodynamic changes

The clinical manifestations originate from the combination of decreased intravascular space and the accumulation of protein-rich fluid into body cavities and interstitial space. Loss of intravascular volume leads to hemodynamic changes manifested as hypotension, severe tachycardia, and decreased renal perfusion as well as hemoconcentration.

Because hypotension leads to decreased venous pressure and reduced venous return, a decreased cardiac output (CO) might be expected; however, it was found the CO was increased in OHSS. These findings led to the determination that there is accompanying arterial vasodilation in OHSS (Manau D et al., 1998).

Decreased renal perfusion leads to a decreased glomerular filtration rate (GFR), and can result in oliguria. Changes in perfusion can affect liver function, including synthesis of proteins, of which anticlotting factors are among the first to become depleted (Fabreuges F et al., 1999).

Hemoconcentration with increase in blood coagulability is responsible for arterial and venous thrombotic phenomena in patients with OHSS (Chan WS et al., 2009).

Loss of intravascular volume combined with decreased renal perfusion results in electrolyte abnormalities (hyperkalemia, hyponatremia), increase in hematocrit and white cell count, and decrease in creatinine clearance.

Abdominal discomfort is the most common symptom of OHSS because of the development of ascites. Accumulation of protein-rich fluid in the peritoneal cavity leads to abdominal distention and increased intra-abdominal pressure (IAP). Increased IAP may compromise respiratory, cardiovascular, renal, gastrointestinal and hepatic system homeostasis (Selgas R et al., 2010).

More reccently, vascular endothelial growth factor (VEGF), has emerged as one of the factors most likely to be involved in the patophysiology of OHSS. VEGF is a vasoactive glycoprotein (cytokine) which stimulates endothelial cell proliferation, cell permeability, and angiogenesis.

Recent studies indicate that hCG is the main factor that triggers OHSS and seems to be the main stimulus of the syndrome because elimination of hCG will prevent the full-blown picture of the syndrome (Soares SR et al., 2008). It has been clearly demonstrated that hCG increases VEGF and its VEGF-2 receptors (VEGFR-2) in human granulosa-lutein cells and raises serum VEGF concentration.

VEGF causes an increase in vascular permeability by rearranging endothelial junction proteins, including cadherin and claudin 5. When evaluating human endothelial cells from umbilical veins (used as an in vitro model of OHSS), hCG and VEGF caused changes in the actin fibers that are indicative of increased capillary permeability, and cadherin concentration was elevated when hCG and VEGF were added, but not with the addition of estradiol (Villasante A et al., 2007). Cadherin is a soluble cell adhesion molecule that may play a key role in the pathophysiology and progression of vascular hyperpermeability (Villasante A et al., 2007).

4. Classification of OHSS

Conventional OHSS staging has relied on clinical symptoms and laboratory findings to categorize severity of disease. The most popular classification system for staging OHSS is that of Golan et al., 1989. This system incorporated the use of transvaginal sonography for both estimating of ovarian enlargement and detection of ascites. The detection of ascites establishes the diagnosis of moderate OHSS which may deteriorate to a severe form and is therefore of major importance. Subsequent modifications defined a group of critical OHSS and added to the severe category of the syndrome (Jenkins JM et al., 2006).

Grade	Symptoms
Mild OHSS	Abdominal bloating Mild abdominal pain Ovarian size usually <8cm*
Moderate OHSS	Moderate abdominal pain Nausea +/- vomiting Ultrasound evidence of ascites Ovarian size usually 8-12 cm*
Severe OHSS	Clinical ascites (occasionally hydrothorax) Oliguria Haemoconcentracion hematocrit >45% Hypoproteinaemia Ovarian size usually >12 cm*
Critical OHSS	Tense ascites or large hydrothorax Haematocrit >55% Whitw cell count >25 000/ml Oligo/anuria Tromboembolism Acute respiratory distress syndrome (ARDS)

*Ovarian size may not correlate with severity of OHSS in cases of assisted reproduction because of the effect of follicular aspiration

Table 1. Classification of severity of OHSS

Depending on the time of onset, a division of OHSS into 'early' and 'late' may be useful in determining the prognosis. OHSS presenting within 9 days after the ovulatory dose of hCG is likely to reflect excessive ovarian response and the precipitating effect of exogenous hCG administered for final follicular maturation. OHSS presenting after this period reflects endogenous hCG stimulation from an early pregnancy. Late OHSS is more likely to be severe and to last longer than early OHSS (Mathur RS et al., 2000).

5. Risk factors

The following factors increase the risk independently for the development of OHSS (Enskog A. et al., 1999):

- young age
- low body mass index (BMI)
- polycystic ovarian syndrome (PCOS)
- allergic history
- high antral follicle count
- high doses of gonadotropins
- high or rapidly rising estradiol levels
- large numbers of large and medium-sized follicles
- large numbers of oocytes retrieved
- high or repeated doses of hCG
- pregnancy
- prior OHSS

High or rapidly rising estradiol levels are particularly unreliable and over-rated predictors of OHSS (Papanikolau EG et al., 2006).

An estradiol cut-off of 3,000 pg/mL will miss 2/3 of patients with severe OHSS. Counting the number of 12mm follicles is actually a better predictor of OHSS than serum estradiol levels, and the combination of an estradiol level of 5,000 pg/mL and eighteen 12mm follicles was found to be the best predictor of OHSS in this study, yielding a sensitivity of 83% and specificity of 84 %(Papanikolau EG et al., 2006).

6. Prevention

The keys to preventing OHSS are experience with ovulation induction therapy and recognition of risk factors for OHSS.

Caution is indicated when any of the following indicators for increased risk of OHSS are present (Practice Committee of American Society for Reproductive Medicine, 2008) :

- rapidly rising serum E_2 levels
- E_2 concentration in excess of 2500 pg/ml
- the emergence of a large number of intermediate sized follicles (10-14mm)
- OHSS prevention has historically included the following strategies:

6.1 Cycle cancellation

IVF cycle cancellation with withholding of hCG trigger is the most effective preventative technique, but is emotionally and financially stressful for all involved. Cycle cancellation is generally reserved for patients with a history of severe OHSS in a prior cycle and in cases of total loss of control of the cycle.

6.2 Coasting

Coasting involves temporarily stopping gonadotropin administration and postponing the hCG trigger until the estradiol (E_2) level is lower. The proposed mechanism of coasting is as follows: lower gonadotropin stimulation leads to decreased LH receptors, leading to decreased luteinization, and subsequent decreased VEGF levels. Lower gonadotropin stimulation may also increase the rate of granulose cell apoptosis, especially of smaller follicles. Coasting lowers the level of follicular fluid VEGF, thereby potentially preventing the development of OHSS (Tozer AJ et al., 2004).

It is a good alternative that can be used to avoid cycle cancellation in extremely high responders to ovulation induction, who have high risk of developing severe OHSS. Even if OHSS develops after coasting, both incidence and severity will be diminished. However, prolonged coasting has a drawback of a reduced pregnancy rate (Garcia-Velasco JA et al., 2006).

6.3 Decreasing the dose of hCG trigger

Although theoretically it makes sense to reduce the dose of hCG, there is little data to support this practice and studies are either limited by small sample size or not powered to detect a difference.

6.4 Agonist trigger

Using an agonist medication to trigger ovulation has been proposed as another strategy to prevent OHSS. Agonist trigger can only be used in the setting of an antagonist protocol.

Comparing pregnancy rate per patient randomized to GnRH agonist vs. hCG trigger identified no difference in number of oocytes retrieved, fertilization rate, or embryo score.

No patients randomized to either GnRH agonist or hCG trigger developed OHSS; but there was the suggestion of a lower pregnancy rate in patients who had GnRH agonist trigger, possibly due to a luteal support problem (Griesinger G et al, 2006).

6.5 Cryopreservation of all embrios

Certainly the concept of cryopreservation of all embryos seems logical as a strategy to prevent OHSS given that OHSS is more common and more severe with pregnancy due to hCG-induced intrinsic ovarian stimulation.

Sills et al. in 2008 analyzed outcomes in patients undergoing elective embryo cryopreservation to prophylax against the development of OHSS (Sills ES et al., 2008).

Elective transfer of a single zona-free day 5 embryo and freezing of the supernumerary embryos or cryopreservation of all embryos for postponement of transfer can prevent the occurrence of late OHSS from pregnancy. However, it does not prevent early OHSS development due to exogenous hCG administration. The management based on elective 2 pronucleate embryo cryopreservation with subsequent thaw and grow-out to blastocyst stage for trasnsfer did not appear to compromise embryo viability or overall reproductive outcome.

The mean number of days from embryo cryopreservation to date of thaw embryo transfer was 115 (range 30–377), and embryo blastulation rate was 88%. Finally, the live birth rate per embryo transfer was an excellent 43.6% in these patients.

However, the Cochrane review found insufficient evidence in the literature to support the routine practice of embryo cryopreservation to prevent OHSS (D' Angelo A et al., 2002). As with all methods, it may reduce but not eliminate OHSS.

6.6 Intravenous albumin at the time of oocyte retrieval

Albumin is a low molecular weight plasma compound with a major impact on oncotic pressure. Human albumin has been used on the day of hCG administration in high-risk women to prevent OHSS. However, in a recent prospective randomized study, it was found that human albumin did not seem either to prevent or to reduce the incidence of severe OHSS. Without a concomitant reduction in vascular permeability, however, the effect of albumin on intravascular volume and hematocrit may be of short duration due to its diffusion into extravascular space, exacerbating both ascites and pleural effusions (Isikoglu M et al., 2007).

6.7 Non-steroidal anti-inflammatory administration

Low-dose aspirin therapy (100 mg daily, beginning on the first day of ovarian stimulation) was shown to be effective in preventing OHSS among high risk women in a recent study (Varnagy A et al., 2010). This study evaluated 2,425 cycles in which gonadotropin-releasing hormone agonist was used. Among 1,192 women at a high risk for developing OHSS, 780 randomly received aspirin, and the incidence of OHSS was 0.25% compared with 8.4% among the 412 women who did not receive aspirin. The pregnancy rates were similar.

6.8 Dopamine agonist

The most recently suggested strategy to prevent the development of OHSS is the use of dopamine agonists such as Cabergoline. The proposed mechanism is inhibition of phosphorylation of the VEGF receptor by Cabergoline, thereby preventing increased capillary permeability, the main action of VEGF.

In study by Alvarez et al. (2007), patients were assigned to receive either Cabergoline 0.5mg/day for 8 days starting on the day of hCG (35 patients) or placebo (32 patients). All patients underwent evaluation for OHSS, including serum hematocrit, ultrasound to evaluate for ascites, and magnetic resonance imaging (MRI) for ovarian venous permeability. They found that in the women who received Cabergoline, the ascites volume was statistically significantly lower than in those who received placebo. They also found that the percentage of women who developed moderate OHSS was statistically significantly lower in those patients who received Cabergoline. There was no difference in the percentage of patients in each group who developed severe OHSS.

In spite of these beneficial effects of the dopamine agonist cabergoline on vascular permeability without compromising implantation and pregnancy rates, this treatment would complement the ongoing progress with ither procedures such as in vitro maturation and oocyte vitrification and enable physicians to predict and prevent OHSS (Garcia-Velasco Ja et al., 2009).

6.9 *In vitro* maturation of oocytes (IVM)

The safest way to prevent OHSS would be by not stimulating the ovaries. During an IVM cycle, immature oocytes are retrieved from barely stimulated or completely unstimulated ovaries. The oocytes are matured in defined culture media for 24–48 h and then fertilized by in vitro fertilization or intracytoplasmatic sperm injection. The embryo transfer is performed as usual; normally two embryos are transferred in two or three days after fertilization. The lack of ovarian stimulation during IVM cycles brings many benefits, including the following: reduction in medication cost, no risk for OHSS, and a reduction in the total number of patient visits for clinical and laboratory evaluations (Lazendorf SE et al., 2006).

Clinical trials evaluating IVM performed in women with PCOS demonstrated good pregnancy ratio per embryo transferred (20–54%) and good implantation rates (5.5–34.5%) (Suikkari aM et al., 2008). When evaluating IVM performed in ovulatory women, the results were a little worse, with pregnancy per embryo transfer rates between 15 and 33.3% and implantation rates between 8.8 and 22.6%.

Although good results have been reported by some clinics, IVM has not yet become a mainstream fertility treatment. The most important reasons are: technical difficulties for retrieving immature oocytes from unstimulated ovaries and to cultivate them, lower chance of a live birth per treatment compared with conventional in vitro fertilization, the report of higher rates of meiotic spindle and chromosome abnormalities from immature human oocytes (Lazendorf SE et al., 2006).

7. Management

7.1 Outpatient management

Patients with mild manifestation of OHSS do not require any specific treatment. Outpatient surveillance is, nevertheless, mandatory to detect cases that may progress to moderate or severe OHSS. Most patients with moderate OHSS still can be managed on an outpatient basis, but they require more careful evaluation including daily weight and abdominal girth measurement, physical and ultrasound examination to detect increasing ascites, and to measure ovarian size. Oral fluid intake should be maintained at no less than 1 L per day. Women should be encouraged to drink to thirst, rather than to excess. Strenuous exercise and sexual intercourse should be avoided. Strict bed rest is unwarranted and may increase risk of thromboembolism. Progesterone supplementation is continued in the luteal phase, but supplementation is never done with hCG.

Discomfort may be relieved with acetaminophen or opiate medications if severe. Nonsteroidal anti-inflammatory agents are not recommended because they may compromise renal function in patients with OHSS.

Laboratory investigations that are helpful in assessing the severity of OHSS are haemoglobin,haematocrit, serum creatinine and electrolytes and liver function tests. Baseline values may help track the progress of the condition.

Review every 2-3 days is likely to be adequate. However, urgent clinical review is necessary if the woman develops increasing severity of pain, increasing abdominal distension, shortness of breath and a subjective impression of reduced urine output (Jenkins JM et al., 2006).

7.2 Hospital management

Women with serious illness or severe OHSS require hospitalization for more careful monitoring and aggressive treatment. Careful and frequent reevaluation of the hospitalized patient with severe OHSS is essential. Clinical examination includes an assessment of hydration and cardiorespiratory system. Abdominal circumference and weight should be recorded at admission and daily until resolution. Fluid intake and output should be recorded and monitored on at least a daily basis. Urine output of less than 1,000 mL/day is a matter of concern.

Biochemical monitoring should include serum electrolytes, renal and liver function tests, a coagulation profile, and blood count. Sonographic examination provides assessment of ovarian size and the presence of ascites as well as pleural, or pericardial effusions. A chest X-ray and pulse oximetry are mandatory for any patient with respiratory symptoms and signs suggestive of hydrothorax, pulmonary infection, or pulmonary embolism. Assay of b-hCG will help to diagnose pregnancy as early as possible. Pain and ascites can easily mask adnexal torsion, ovarian rupture, and acute intra-abdominal hemorrhage. Serial clinical and laboratory evaluations provide the means to monitor progression of illness and to recognize evidence of resolution (Jenkins et al., 2006).

Antiemetic drugs used should be those appropriate for the possibility of early pregnancy, such as prochlorperazine, metoclopramide and cyclizine.

The management of OHSS is essentially supportive until the condition resolves spontaneously.

Symptomatic relief is important, particularly regarding pain and nausea. Discomfort may be relieved with paracetamol or opiate medications if severe. If opiates are used, particularly in women with reduced mobility, care should be taken to avoid constipation. Nausea is usually related to the accumulation of ascites and so measures described to reduce abdominal distension should provide relief. Counselling support for both the woman and her partner provides reassurance and information to allay anxiety.

Regarding fluid management, it is critical to correct hemoconcentration. It is recommended to start with an initial IV fluid bolus of 500–1,000cc normal saline (NS) over the first hour of admission, followed by rehydration at a decreased rate of 30cc/hour using D5NS titrated to urine output. Oral fluid intake should be reduced to thirst and patient comfort. Albumin (25%) may be needed for intravascular volume repletion, in which case 50 -100gm of IV albumin is infused over 4 hours and repeated at 4–12 hour intervals as needed.

Hyperkalemia is treated in the standard manner with Kayexelate, insulin/glucose, sodium bicarbonate, or albuterol as needed. Rarely, diuretics can be given, but extreme caution is used in the administration of diuretics to patients with OHSS given their known intravascular volume depletion. Other inpatient management strategies include paracentesis if needed. Thromboembolism prevention is critical given the hypercoagulatory state of OHSS. It is generally recommended both venous support stockings and anticoagulants such as heparin 5,000 U subcutaneously twice daily. Occasionally, patients may need intensive care unit admission for thromboembolic complications, renal failure, or if invasive hemodynamic monitoring is indicated (central venous pressure, pulmonary capillary wedge pressure) (Alper MM et al., 2009).

8. References

Alper MM, Smith LP, Sills ES. Ovarian hyperstimulation syndrome: current views on pathophysiology, risk factors, prevention, and management. J Exp Clin Assist Reprod. 2009 Jun 10;6:3.

Alvarez C, Marti-Bonmati L, Novella-Maestre E, Sanz R, Gomez R, Fernandez-Sanchez M, Simon C, Pellicer A. Dopamine Agonist Cabergoline Reduces Hemoconcentration and Ascites in Hyperstimulated Women Undergoing Assisted Reproduction. J Clin Endocrinol Metab 2007;92(8):2931–2937.

Binder H, Dittrich R, Einhaus F, Krieg J, Muller A, Strauss R, et al. Update on ovarian hyperstimulation syndrome: Part 1—incidence and pathogenesis. Int J Fertil Womens Med 2007;52:11–26.

Chan WS. The 'ART' of thrombosis: a review of arterial and venous thrombosis in assisted reproductive technology. Curr Opin Obstet Gynecol 2009;21:207-18.

Chen SU, Chen RJ, Shieh JY, Chou CH, Lin CW, Lu HF, et al. Human chorionic gonadotropin up-regulates expression of myeloid cell leukemia-1 protein in human granulosa-lutein cells: implication of corpus luteum rescue and ovarian hyperstimulation syndrome. J Clin Endocrinol Metab 2010;95:3982-92.

D'Angelo A, Amso N. Embryo Freezing for Preventing Ovarian Hyperstimulation Syndrome. *Cochrane Database Syst Rev* 2002;2:CD002806.

Enskog A, Henriksson M, Unander M, Nilsson L, Brannstrom M. Prospective study of the clinical and laboratory parameters of patients in whom ovarian hyperstimulation syndrome developed during controlled ovarian hyperstimulation for in vitro fertilization. Fertil Steril 1999;71(5):808–814.

Fabregues F, Balasch J, Gines P, Manau D, Jimenez W, Arroyo V, et al. Ascites and liver test abnormalities during severe ovarian hyperstimulation syndrome. Am J Gastroenterol 1999;94:994–9.

García-Velasco JA, Isaza V, Quea G, Pellicer A. Coasting for the prevention of ovarian hyperstimulation syndrome: much ado about nothing? Fertil Steril. 2006 Mar;85(3):547-54.

Gracia-Velasco JA. Reprod Biomed Online. 2009;18 Suppl 2:71-5.

Golan A, Ron-El R, Herman A, Soffer Y, Weinraub Z, Caspi E. Ovarian hyperstimulation syndrome: an update review. Obstet Gynecol Surv 1989;44:430-40.

Goldsman MP, Pedram A, Dominguez CE, Ciuffardi I, Levin E, Asch RH. Increased capillary permeability induced by human follicular fluid: a hypothesis for an ovarian origin of the hyperstimulation syndrome. Fertil Steril 1995;63:268-72.

Griesinger G, Diedrich K, Devroey P, Kolibianakis EM. Gnrh Agonist for Triggering Final Oocyte Maturation in the GnRH Antagonist Ovarian Hyperstimulation Protocol: a Systematic Review and Meta-Analysis. Hum Reprod Update 2006;12(2):159–168.

Isikoglu M, Berkkanoglu M, Senturk Z, Ozgur K. Human albumin does not prevent ovarian hyperstimulation syndrome in assisted reproductive technology program: a prospective randomized placebo-controlled double blind study. Fertil Steril. 2007;88:982–5.

Jenkins JM, Drakeley AJ, Mathur RS. The management of ovarian hyperstimulation syndrome. Green-top Guideline 2006 September;(5):1–11.

Lanzendorf SE. Developmental potential of in vitro- and in vivomatured human oocytes collected from stimulated and unstimulated ovaries. Fertil Steril. 2006;85:836–7.

Madill JJ, Mullen NB, Harrison BP. Ovarian hyperstimulation syndrome: a potentially fatal complication of early pregnancy. J Emerg Med 2008;35(3):283-6.

Manau D, Balasch J, Arroyo V, Jimenez W, Fabregues F, Casamitjana R, Creus M, et al. Circulatory dysfunction in asymptomatic in vitro fertilization patients. Relationship with hyperestrogenemia and activity of endogenous vasodilators. J Clin Endocrinol Metab 1998;83:1489–93.

Mathur RS, Akande AV, Keay SD, Hunt LP, Jenkins JM.Distinction between early and late ovarian hyperstimulation syndrome. Fertil Steril 2000;73:901–7.

Papanikolaou EG, Pozzobon C, Kolibianakis EM, Camus M, Tournaye H, Fatemi HM, et al. Incidence and prediction of ovarian hyperstimulation syndrome in women undergoing gonadotropin-releasing hormone antagonist in vitro fertilization cycles. Fertil Steril 2006;85:112–120.

Practice Committee of American Society for Reproductive Medicine. Ovarian hyperstimulation syndrome. Fertil Steril 2008;90:188-93.

Selgas R, Del Peso G, Bajo MA. Intra-abdominal hypertension favors ascites. Perit Dial Int 2010;30:156-7

Sills ES, McLoughlin LJ, Genton MG, Walsh DJ, Coull GD, Walsh AP. Ovarian Hyperstimulation Syndrome and Prophylactic Human Embryo Cryopreservation: Analysis of Reproductive Outcome Following Thawed Embryo Transfer. *J Ovarian Res* 2008;1(1):7.

Soares SR, Gomez R, Simon C, Garcia-Velasco JA, Pellicer A. Targeting the vascular endothelial growth factor system to prevent ovarian hyperstimulation syndrome. Hum Reprod Update 2008;14:321-333.

Suikkari AM. In-vitro maturation: its role in fertility treatment. Curr Opin Obstet Gynecol. 2008;20:242–8

Tollan A. Holst N, Forsdahl F, Fadnes HO, Oian P, Maltau JM. Transcapillary fluid dynamics during ovarian stimulation for in vitro fertilization. Am J Obstet Gynecol 1990;162:554-8.

Tozer AJ, Iles RK, Iammarrone E, Gillott CM, Al-Shawaf T, Grudzinskas JG. The Effects of "Coasting" on Follicular Fluid Concentrations of Vascular Endothelial Growth Factor in Women at Risk of Developing Ovarian Hyperstimulation Syndrome. Hum Reprod 2004;19(3):522–528.

Varnagy A, Bodis J, Manfai Z, Wilhelm F, Busznyak C, Koppan M: Low-dose aspirin therapy to prevent ovarian hyperstimulation syndrome. Fertil Steril. 2010;93(7):2281-4.

Villasante A, Pacheco A, Ruiz A, Pellicer A, Garcia-Velasco JA. Vascular endothelial cadherin regulates vascular permeability: Implications for ovarian hyperstimulation syndrome. J Clin Endocrinol Metab. 2007;92:314–21.

Part 3

Advances in Insemination Technology

5

Sperm Cell in ART

Dejan Ljiljak[1], Tamara Tramišak Milaković[2], Neda Smiljan Severinski[2], Krunoslav Kuna[1] and Anđelka Radojčić Badovinac[2]
[1]University Hospital Center "Sisters of Mercy", Zagreb
[2]University Hospital Center Rijeka, Rijeka
Croatia

1. Introduction

Infertility today represents a global problem. Male factor contributes in approximately 50% of infertile couples. In the last decade we are witnesses of the decreased quality of semen and the increased frequency of testicular cancer and cryptorchidism. Currently, the assessment of semen quality is based on the routine semen analysis including sperm count, morphology and motility. Although variation and combination among these three main factors articulate few diagnosis, nowadays developed assisted reproduction techniques (ART), especially intracytoplasmatic sperm injection (ICSI) may be used to treat most of the male infertility problems. In general we can say that traditional semen parameters provide a limited degree of diagnostic information, thus we are aware that these indexes of diagnosis should be revisited, which includes more specific test of sperm assessments, such as DNA tests and sperm proteome.

Spermatogenesis is a process that includes physiological, morphological and biochemical changes. After a complex process from the round diploid spermatogonia to haploid spermatozoa, a mature sperm just has an ability to fertilize a mature oocyte. If any errors occur during spermatogenesis process, appropriate sperm will not be produced. Thus, in our ART practice, it is important to understand normal physiology of spermatogenesis and find the reason of abnormal situation. In this chapter we will review today knowledge about:

- - Spermatogenesis
- - Sperm chromatin structure (sperm nucleus proteins),
- - DNA damage through spermatogenesis,
- - Apoptosis,
- - Oxidative stress (testicular and postesticulars factors),
- - Y chromosome microdeletions,
- - Centrosome (epigenetic factors)
- - New techniques of sperm selection in ART

2. Spermatogenesis

The sperm cell is composed of a sperm head, a sperm neck and a sperm tail. Whole sperm is covered by the sperm plasma membrane called plasmalemma (Picture 1.). The sperm head

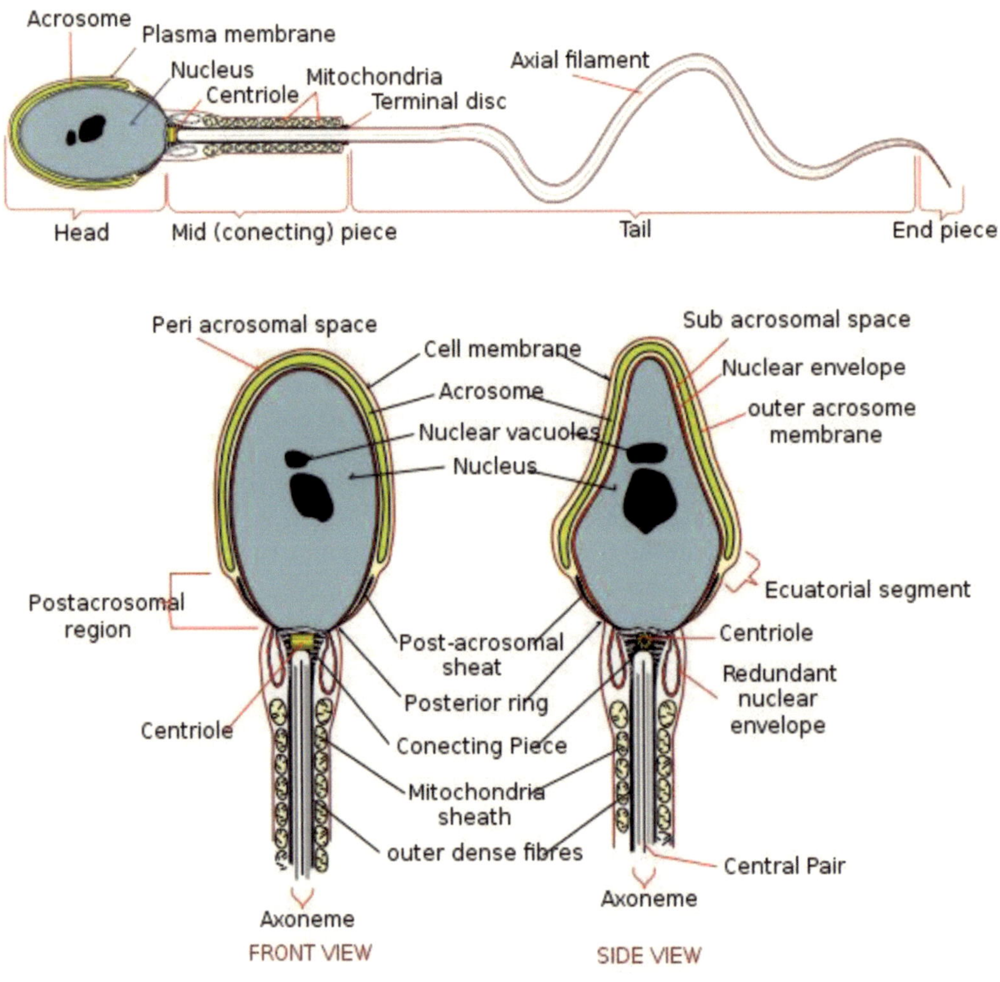

Picture 1. Diagram of human spermatozoon

is composed of a nucleus and an acrosome. The nucleus contains sperm DNA (half number of chromosomes) and the acrosome has important enzymes for fertilization. The sperm neck or midpiece has 100 sperm mitochondria which generate energy for the sperm tail. The sperm tail is based on 9 + 2 microtubules. The microtubule doublets are connected doublet-to-doublet by dynein arms.

A spermatogenesis basically includes the mitotic expansion of stem cells, the meiotic recombination of genetic information and the haploid spermatid production (Picture 2.). The aim of the process is to produce a highly specialized mature sperm cell which can bind to the oocyte. The paternal inherited centrosome is essential for normal fertilization, chromatin packaging and early embryogenesis. The complete matured spermatozoon must undergo acrosome development, nuclear elongation and condensation, the formation of middle piece and tail, and the reduction of cytoplasm.

The primordial germ cells in fetal testis are enclosed in tubules which form very proliferative active cells called the gonocytes. The meiotic prophase is inhibited. Spermatogonia are positioned on seminiferous tubules and have a connection with the Sertoli cells. The basement membrane and Sertoli cells form the blood-testis barrier. After birth, gonocytes rise to a population of spermatogonia which constitute the stem cell pool. The spermatogonia are characterized by mitotic division and they are inactive until the puberty. The diploid spermatogonia differentiate into primary spermatocytes. The primary spermatocytes undergo first meiotic division and create secondary spermatocytes. After the second meiotic division four haploid spermatids are created. After the morphological differentiation a mature sperm is formed. The Leydig cells are responsible for the production of testosterone which is necessary for spermatogenesis. Some other hormones are also responsible for spermatogenesis. The Luteinising hormone and the follicle stimulating hormone have important influence on right spermatogenesis as well. The first one (FSH) stimulates the Leydig cells to make testosterone and maintain mitotic division. The second one (FSH) is obligated for the influence on Sertoli cells. Sertoli cells produce inhibin B. Spermatogenesis process takes about 3 weeks.

Cell	Ploidy / number of chromosomes	Process
Spermatogonium	Diploid / 46	Spermatocytogenesis
Primary spermatocyte	Diploid / 46	Spermatidogenesis (Meiosis I)
Secondary spermatocyte	Haploid / 23	Spermatidogenesis (Meiosis II)
Spermatid	Haploid / 23	Spermiogenesis
Mature sperm cell	Haploid / 23	Spermiogenesis

Table 1.

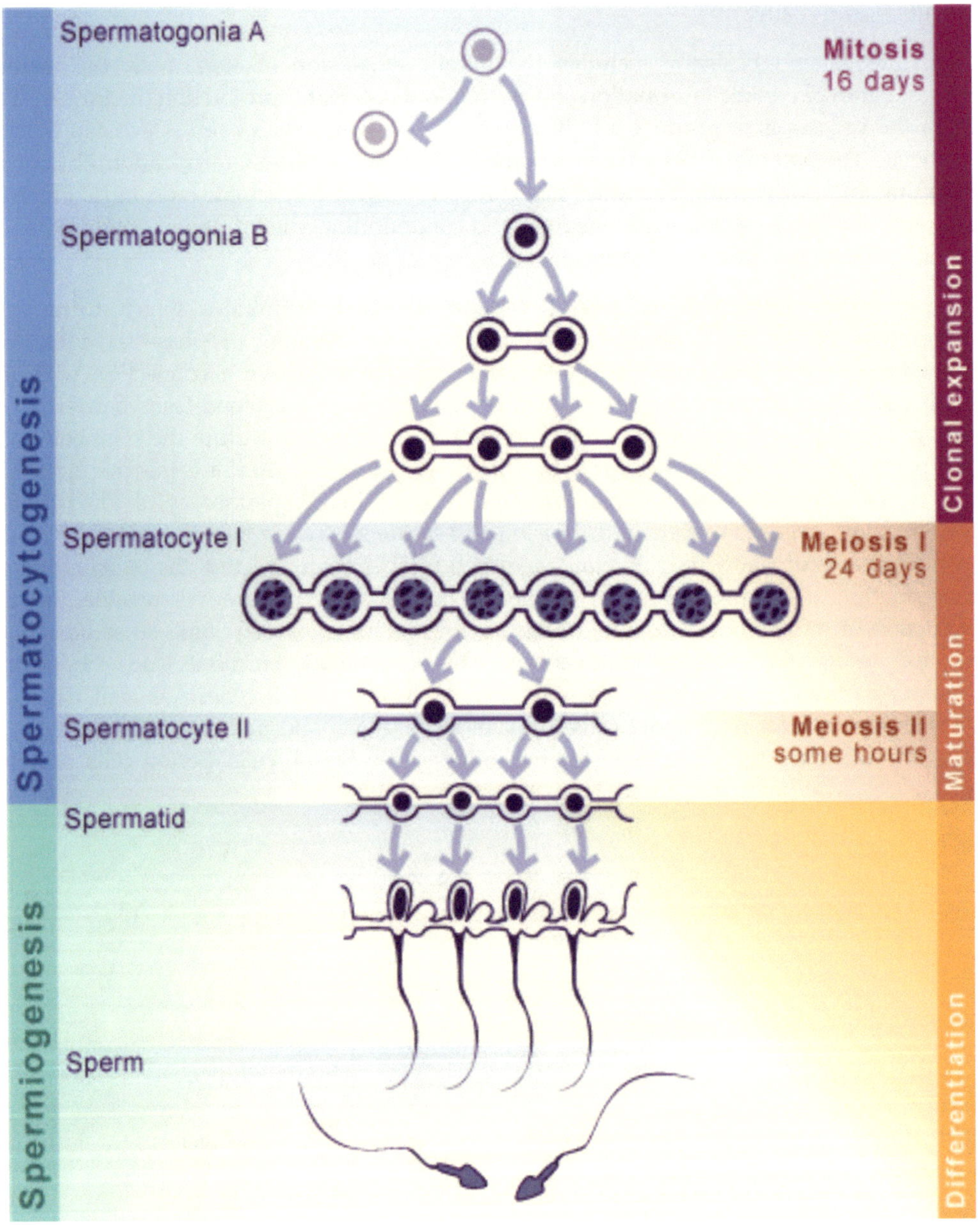

Picture 2. Spermatogenesis

3. Sperm chromatin structure

The sperm chromatin is very tightly compacted and the result is a paternal genome inactivation. Nuclear proteins and DNA are connected in a unique way. Nuclear remodelling and condensation in the spermatid combine with histone modification and displacement with transition proteins and then by protamines. However, around 15% of sperm DNA remains packaged by histones. The reason lays in the specific manner of oocyte activation after sperm entry. Disulfide cross-links between the cysteine-rich protamines are responsible for the compaction of chromatin and the stabilization of paternal genome. The genome is protected from oxidation or temperature elevation in the female reproductive tract. Human testis express two protamines: protamine 1 (P1) and protamine 2 (P2). Equal amounts of P1 and P2 are considered normal for human spermatozoa. Any unbalance of P1 and P2 ratio is associated with male infertility. Mouse knockout models demonstrate that the sperm protamine haploinsufficiency directly impairs spermatogenesis and embryo development. Through evolution protamines have increased the number of positively charged residues. These positively charged residues create highly condensed complex with DNA.

The protamine 1 is synthesized as a mature protein and protamine 2 as a precursor and protamine 1 and 2 differ from each other only by the N-terminal extension of 1-4 residues.

Protamine 2 is zinc-finger protein with one Cys2-His motif and they are expressed only in some mammals. Both, P1 and P2 undergo post-transcriptional modifications before binding to the DNA. After binding, protamines and DNA make highly compact nucleoprotamine complex. Khara et al., (1997) showed first comparison P1/P2 ratio related to IVF and found a P1/P2 ratio between 0.55 and 0.29 in the group with fertilization index (FI) ≥50% and three of the infertile patients who had a F1 below 50% had a ratio outside this range (Khara et al., 1997). Carrel and Liu (2001) describe the undetectable protamine 2 in infertile males.

4. DNA damage during spermatogenesis

The sperm DNA damage is clearly associated with male infertility. Small part of spermatozoa from fertile men also has detectable levels of DNA damage. Factors that cause the DNA damage include protamine deficiency, apoptosis, chemotherapy, ROS, cigarette smoking and varicoceles. The DNA fragmentation is characterized by single and double strand breaks. Oxidative stress is a result of the production of reactive oxidative species (ROS). Spermatozoa are vulnerable to ROS because they have a small amount of cytoplasm which does not contain antioxidant molecules and repair system. The DNA fragmentation is associated with diminished motility, morphology and sperm count. Also the DNA fragmentation has predictive value for unsuccessful IVF cycle. The most interesting group of patients which go to IVF is idiopathic infertility. Significant paternal contribution to sex chromosome trisomy has been described. Spermatozoa with numerical chromosome abnormalities are able to fertilize oocyte. The increase of sperm aneuploidy rate is associated with lower implantation and pregnancy rate. The sperm mitochondria represent the biggest source of reactive oxygen species. Oxidative stress induces activation of free radicals by the mitochondria which later induce oxidative DNA damage and DNA fragmentation. The majority of DNA damage is caused by oxidative stress.

5. Apoptosis

The apoptosis represents normal physiological process in spermatogenesis. About 75% potential spermatozoa are destructed by the programmed cell death. The apoptosis acts like selective factor of the early germ cells and prevents overproliferation of germ cells. Also the abnormal sperm formation is excluded from spermatogenesis. Sertoli cells can support a specified number of germ cells. Some spermatozoa with DNA damage or fragmentation escaped apoptosis and exist in the semen. Men with abnormal sperm parameters have higher levels of apoptotic protein Fas. Apoptotic protein Fas is strongly correlated with poor sperm concentration and abnormal sperm morphology. Also some other apoptotic markers can be found in human sperm such Bcl-x, p53, caspase and anexin V.

6. Oxidative stress

Reactive oxygen species (ROS) are the product of the normal metabolism in a cell. Free radicals are highly chemically reactive because of the unpaired electrons. Also ROS are produced by leukocytes in phagocytic process. ROS can effect on sperm DNA integrity. High levels of reactive oxygen species are detected in the semen of infertile men. Reactive oxygen species cause hypercondensation of DNA as a result of the oxidation of sperm protein sulfhydryl groups. The post-testicular genital infection results in the leukocytospermia and the increased levels of DNA damage. ROS can damage the DNA by causing deletions and mutations. Antioxidant therapy has shown a decreasing sperm DNA fragmentation.

7. Y chromosome microdeletions

Microdeletions in the Y chromosome genes are associated with impaired or absent spermatogenesis. Three regions of the Y chromosome azoospermic factor AZFa, AZFb and AZFc are crucial for an adequate process of spermatogenesis. Deletions in AZFa region are associated with Sertoli cells only, deletions in AZFb region with spermatogenic arrest and deletions in AZFc region are associated with the spermatogenic arrest at the spermatid stage. The frequency of Y chromosome microdeletions affects approximately 5-15% infertile men. Previous studies have shown that boys born from oligozoospermic men treated using ICSI have an increased risk of carrying Y chromosome deletions.

8. Centrosome

The centrosome consists of two centrioles in a perpendicular arrangement and pericentriolar material. After the fusion of sperm and oocyte, sperm tail is incorporated into ooplasm and centriolar region forms the sperm aster which acts to guide the female pronucleus towards the male pronucleus. The maternal centrosome is fully degradeted, thus the centrosome of zygote is mainly inherited from the sperm. After fertilization normally formed centriole is an essential proper cell division. The centrosome disfunction may lead to the numerical chromosomal abnormalities. The human sperm centrosome is responsible for normal syngamy and an early embryonic development.

9. New techniques of sperm selection in ART

The routine sperm preparation techniques are density gradient centrifugation and swim-up. They depend on the sedimentation or migration ways to separate spermatozoa. The sperm characteristics such as apoptosis, DNA integrity and membrane maturation are not directly targeted by routine sperm preparation techniques. At this moment magnet activated cell sorting (MACS) becomes novel technique for sperm separation based on presence of anexin V as apoptotic marker. Also modified ICSI called PICSI is commonly used for single sperm selection on the level of membrane maturity for sperm binding on hyaluron acid binding sites. Generally, sperm selection can be based on the sperm surface charge (electrophoresis-based technology), non-apoptotic sperm selection, selection based on the sperm membrane maturity and selection based on the sperm ultramorphology. Electrophoresis-based technology separates spermatozoa based on the size and electronegative charge. The externalization of phosphatidylserine (apoptotic marker) allows binding with Annexin-V-conjugated paramagnetic microbeads which separates apoptotic spermatozoa using a magnetic-activated cell sorting system (MACS, Miltenyi Biotec GmbH, Germany).

10. References

[1] Oliva R, Dixon GH. Vertebrate protamine genes and the histone-to-protamine replacement reaction. Prog Nucleic Acid Res Mol Biol 1991;40:25-94.

[2] Lewis JD, Song Y, de Jong ME, Bagha SM, Ausio J. A walk though vertebrate and invertebrate protamines. Chromosoma 2003;111:473-482.

[3] Vilfan ID, Conwell CC, Hud NV. Formation of native-like mammalian sperm cell chromatin with folded bull protamine. J Biol Chem 2004;279:20088-20095.

[4] Oliva R. Protamines and male infertility. Hum Reprod Update 2006;4:417-435.

[5] Corzett M, Mazrimas J, Balhorn R. Protamine 1: protamine 2 stoichiometry in the sperm of eutherian mammals. Mol Reprod Dev 2002;61:519-527.

[6] Aoki VW, Moskovtsev SI, Willis J, Liu L, Mullen JBM, Carrell DT. DNA integrity is compromised in protamine-deficient human sperm. J Androl 2005;26:741-748.

[7] Cho C, Jung-Ha H, Willis WD i sur. Protamine 2 deficiency leads to sperm DNA damage and embryo death in mice. Biol Reprod 2003;69:211-217.

[8] Balhorn R. The protamine family of sperm nuclear proteins. Genome Biology 2007;8:227-234.

[9] Fernandez JL, Muriel L, Rivero MT, Goyanes V, Vazquez R, Alvarez JG. The sperm chromatin dispersion test: a simple method for the determination of sperm DNA fragmentation. J Androl 2003;1:59-66.

[10] Larson KL, DeJonge C, Barnes A, Jost L, Evenson DP. Relationship between assisted reproductive techniques (ART) outcome and status of chromatin integrity as measured by the sperm chromatin structure assay (SCSA). Hum Reprod 2000;15:1717-1722.

[11] Zini A, Sigman M. Are tests of sperm DNA damage clinically useful. J Androl 2009;3:219-229.

[12] Kutchino Y i sur. Misreading of DNA templates containing 8-hydroxydeoxyguanosine at the modified base and at adjacent residues. Nature 1987;327:77-79.

[13] Aoki VW, Carrell DT. Human protamines and the developing spermatid: their structure, function, expression and relationship with male infertility. Asian J Androl 2003;5:315-324.

[14] Sakkas D, Alvarez JG. Sperm DNA fragmentation: mechanisms of origin, impact on reproductive outome, and analysis. Fertil Steril 2010;4:1027-1036.

[15] Burrello N i sur. Morphologically normal spermatozoa of patients with secretory oligo-asthenoteratozoospermia have an increased aneuploidy rate. Hum Reprod 2004; 19:2298–302.
[16] Glander HJ, Schaller J. Localization of enzymes in live spermatozoa by cellprobe reagents. Andrologia 1999;31:37-42.
[17] Oosterhius GJ, Mulder AB, Kalsbeek-Batenburg E, Lambalk CB, Schoemaker J, Vermes I. Measuring apoptosis in human spermatozoa: a biological assay for semen quality. Fertil Steril 2000;74:245-250.
[18] Picture Number 1 was taken from: http://en.wikipedia.org/wiki/File:Complete_diagram_of_a_human_spermatozoa_en.svg
[19] Picture Number 2 was taken form: http://www.embryology.ch/anglais/cgametogen/spermato03.html
[20] Tamer MS, Land JA. Effects of advanced selection methods on sperm quality and ART outcome: a systematic review. Hum Rep Update 2011; 719-733.

Meiotic Chromosome Abnormalities and Spermatic FISH in Infertile Patients with Normal Karyotype

Simón Marina, Susana Egozcue, David Marina, Ruth Alcolea and Fernando Marina
Instituto de Reproducción CEFER. ANACER member, Barcelona Spain

1. Introduction

It is generally accepted that infertility affects 15% of couples at reproductive ages. The causes of infertility are 38% female, 20% male, 27% mixed and 15% unknown (Ferlin et al., 2007). The male factor is the sole responsible party or a copartner in infertility in 50% of couples. About 7-8% of men have infertility problems or are the cause of miscarriages. Chromosomal causes rank high among the causes of infertility. 50% of first-trimester abortive eggs have aneuploidy (Hassold et al., 1980). In second and third-trimester miscarriages, the aneuploidy rate drops to 15% and 5%, respectively (Simpson, 2007). Among living newborns, 0.5% to 1% shows aneuploidy (Gardner and Sutherland, 2004). Among the infertile population, 15% of infertility is due to chromosomal or genetic reasons (Griffin and Finch, 2005).

The prevalence of chromosomal alterations that are only meiotic, with a normal mitotic karyotype, is unknown. Checking for sperm chromosomal alterations requires testicular biopsy, which is an invasive procedure because meiotic cells, spermatocytes I and II present in ejaculate does not tend to be valid, due to their scarcity and poor condition. Unlike mitosis, which can affect other organs and functions, chromosomal alterations of solely meiosis may have an impact on reproductive capacity. Meiotic chromosomal anomalies can cause alterations to one or more of the basic seminal parameters including sperm count, motility and morphology, even lead to the formation of aneuploid gametes. At a clinical level, men with meiotic anomalies will have primary or secondary infertility or produce gestations with miscarriages. Secondary infertility or difficulty in having another child can be explained by the coexistence of altered cell lines and other normal cell lines (mosaicism).

The meiotic chromosomal anomalies may be studied by directly observing meiotic cells obtained from testicular biopsies. Understanding impact on fertility requires: 1) ascertaining the patient's reproductive history with his current and past partners, if there were any; 2) semen analysis, which can be normal with regard to its three basic parameters, have somewhat severe alterations in some or all sperm parameters, or even azoospermia; 3) studying the testicular histopathology that, at an optical level, can swing between complete blockage at the level of spermatocyte I or II, through apparently normal spermatogenesis and 4) studying aneuploidy present in sperm.

Genetic–not chromosomal– alterations that have an impact on fertility such as Kallmann Syndrome, cystic fibrosis, globozoospermia, 9+0 Syndrome, Y-chromosome microdeletions, etc. will not be the focus of this chapter. Nonetheless, the limits between genetic and chromosomal alterations are more academic than real, as genetic alteration of meiosis tends to be the grounds for chromosomal meiotic alteration.

This chapter will set forth the results of FISH on sperm and of the study on meiotic chromosomes in testicular biopsy for infertile patients. Among the patients on whom both studies were conducted -testicular biopsy and sperm-FISH- we present the findings for 60 with more precise clinical data on semenology for FISH and testicular meiosis.

The aims of this paper are two: a) to know the incidence and types of spermatic aneuploidies and testicular meiotic anomalies in general infertile men, and b) to correlate the results of both studies: spermatic aneuploidies with meiotic chromosomes.

2. Spermatogenesis

The spermatogenesis process lasts some 64 days (Heller and Clermont, 1964) and takes place inside the seminiferous tubules in adult testes. There are three different stages:

2.1 Spermatogonial stage

In this phase, the spermatogonia divide by mitosis. Some remain as cell reserves to divide again later and others enter meiosis. The spermatogonia are located in the basal compartment of the seminiferous tubule between the tubular wall, the Sertoli cells and the inter-Sertolian tight junctions. The Sertoli cells and the tight junctions form the hemato-testicular barrier and create an avascular space (the luminal compartment) in the centre of the seminiferous tubule. The spermatogonia that go into meiosis move from the basal to luminal compartment through the spaces between the Sertoli cells, thanks to the dissolution and reformation of the tight junctions (Byers et al., 1993).

2.2 Spermatocytal or meiotic stage

During this phase, meiosis has two cell divisions that take place in spermatocytes I and II. In the first meiotic division, the spermatocyte I gives rise to two spermatocytes II. The division of the spermocyte II, the second meiotic division or equational divisions, gives rise to two spermatids. This process usually lasts about two weeks (Heller and Clermont, 1964). Finally, each spermatid spawns one spermatozoon.

2.3 Spermiogenesis stage

There is no cell division in this stage, but cell differentiation of spermatid into spermatozoon.

2.4 Spermiation

The sperm detach from the Sertoli cells and are released into seminiferous tubule lumen.The meiotic and spermiogenic stages take place in the luminal compartment of the seminiferous tubule. There, specific hormonal conditions are created, among which the high concentration of testosterone must be pointed out. This chapter will only deal with the meiotic stage.

3. Meiosis

During the meiotic process, two essential and specific events occur: genetic recombination and reductional cell division. Genetic recombination is produced by the exchange of genes between homologous chromosomes that form a pair, with one inherited from the father and the other from the mother. This interchange of genes gives rise to an astronomical genetic variability of spermatozoa (and also the oocytes), on the order of 2^{23} per gamete and $2^{23} \times 2^{23}$ per embryo. Thus, the process facilitates the appearance of gene combinations that are different than the ones the man and woman have. Some of these new gene combinations can be advantageous for the individual and for the species. Others can be more or less pathological. Meiosis is the physical foundation of Mendelian genetic inheritance. The second crucial event that occurs during meiosis is reductional cell division. Meiosis means reduction in Greek. All of the body's nucleated cells contain 46 chromosomes (23 pairs). Only the cells from meiosis I: spermatocytes II, spermatids and spermatozoa, have 23 chromosomes instead of 23 pairs. Spermatocyte II chromosomes contain two chromatids and spermatids and spermatozoa chromosomes contain a single chromatid. The opposite of meiosis is fertilization. In this process, the chromosomes of the haploid spermatozoon (n=23) join with those from the oocyte, also haploid (n=23) and through syngamy form a zygote, which is diploid, with 23 pairs of chromosomes (n=46).

Sexual reproduction is based on meiosis and fertilization. Meiosis assures that the number of chromosomes remains constant from one generation to the next, from parents to children, and that they have different gene combinations than their progenitors. Each chromosome, except for the sexual XY pair, has its homologous chromosome: one of paternal and the other of maternal origin. The X chromosome is always maternal and the Y is always of paternal origin. A chromosome is determined by a centromere and can have one or two chromatids -called sisters- depending on the phase of the cell cycle. There is no genetic recombination between them, as one is a copy of the other. Genetic recombination takes place between homologous chromatids, not sisters.

3.1 First meiotic division

Premeiotic or preleptotene phase: During premeiotic synthesis (phase S), two chromatids are produced in each chromosome via DNA replication with identical genetic content, called sister chromatids, which remain joined, bound, through the G2 phase of the cellular cycle. Premeiotic synthesis is particularly long, lasting some 24 hours. When the S phase ends, the DNA content of each homologous chromosome pair is a tetrad, namely, each pair has four chromatids. The two chromatids from the same chromosome are called sisters. They are termed homologous with respect to the chromatids in the homologous chromosome. The union of the sister chromatids is maintained by a ring-shaped structure that mediates cohesion between them (Gruber et al., 2003) and is formed of proteins from the cohesin complex. At a centromeric level, it is formed by the cohesins shugoshin and sororin. Shugoshin has been located in the pericentromeric region (Lee et al., 2008).

3.1.1 Prophase I

Attachment of chromosomes to the internal nuclear membrane

Dispersed throughout the nucleus, when meiosis begins the chromosomes start to move towards the nuclear membrane, attaching by their telomeres (Fig. 1A). The karyotheca is denser at the sites where the telomeres attach. The telomeres move along the internal face of the karyotheca and congregate around the centrosome, shaping a bouquet (Fig. 1B) (Zickler and Kleckner, 1998; Scherthan, 2001; Bass, 2003). The formation of the bouquet requires actin (Trelles-Sticken et al., 2005). Each chromosome approaches its homologue, which it recognizes.

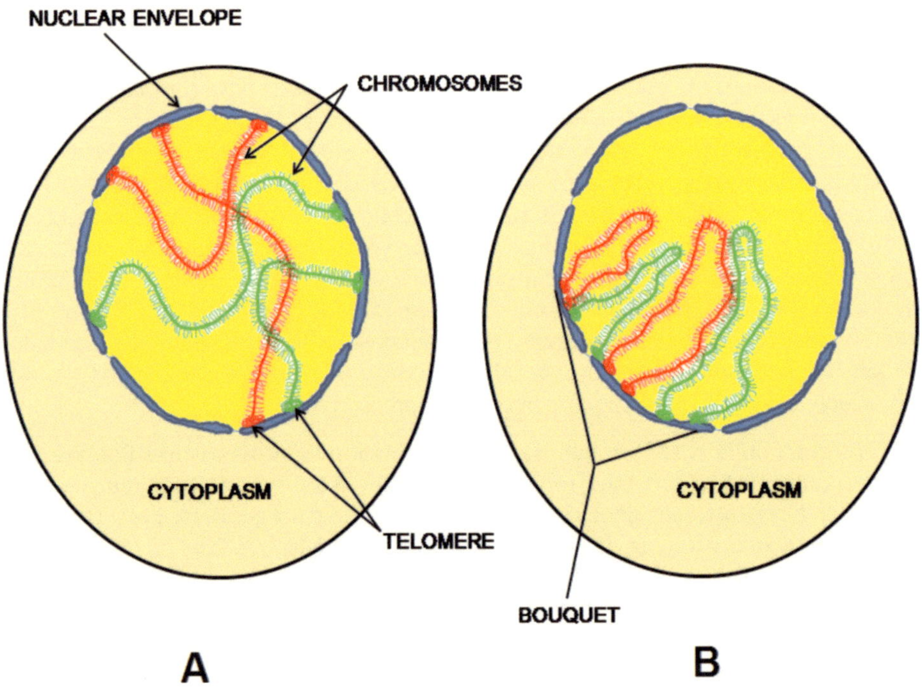

Fig. 1. Fixing the telomere to the nuclear envelope (A). Formation of the bouquet (B)

If the telomeres do not attach to the karyotheca and/or do not form a bouquet, pairing and genetic recombination are altered (Trelles-Sticken et al., 2000). The bouquet shape is seen at the end of the leptotene stage and during the zygotene stage and disappears in the pachytene phase. The chromosomes, already paired and after genetic recombination has taken place between homologous chromatids, disperse over the entire surface of the karyotheca, but are still attached to it. The telomeres detach from the nuclear envelope and the cells proceed to diakinesis (review: Alsheimer, 2009).

Leptotene: The alignment of homologous chromosomes

Almost in parallel to the grouping of the telomeres, the homologous chromosomes align, which is conditioned by the formation of long thin strands along the chromosomes during the first stage of prophase I, or leptotene. These are the lateral elements (LE). Each LE is associated with a pair of sister chromatids. The LEs expand when attaching to the internal nuclear membrane.

Zygotene: The pairing of homologous chromosomes, or synapsis

The leptotene stage is followed by the zygotene, during which the chromosomes thicken and each one pairs up with its homologue. The XY sex pair forms the sex body.

Pairing, or synapsis, requires the formation of the synaptonemal complex (SC) described by Fawcett with the electronic transmission microscope (Fawcett, 1956). The SC (Fig. 2) is a protein structure with three longitudinal elements, two lateral elements (LE), already seen in the previous leptotene stage, and a central element (CE), which provides stability to the SC (Hamer et al., 2006; Bolcun-Filas et al., 2007). The LEs are parallel and equidistant from the CE. The LEs stick to the nuclear envelope. The SC's structure is completed by fine transverse filaments (TFs), which connect the LEs and are perpendicular to the LEs and CE. Each LE is associated with a pair of sister chromatids. The homologous chromosomes are intimately associated at a distance of 100 nm (Zickler, 2006).

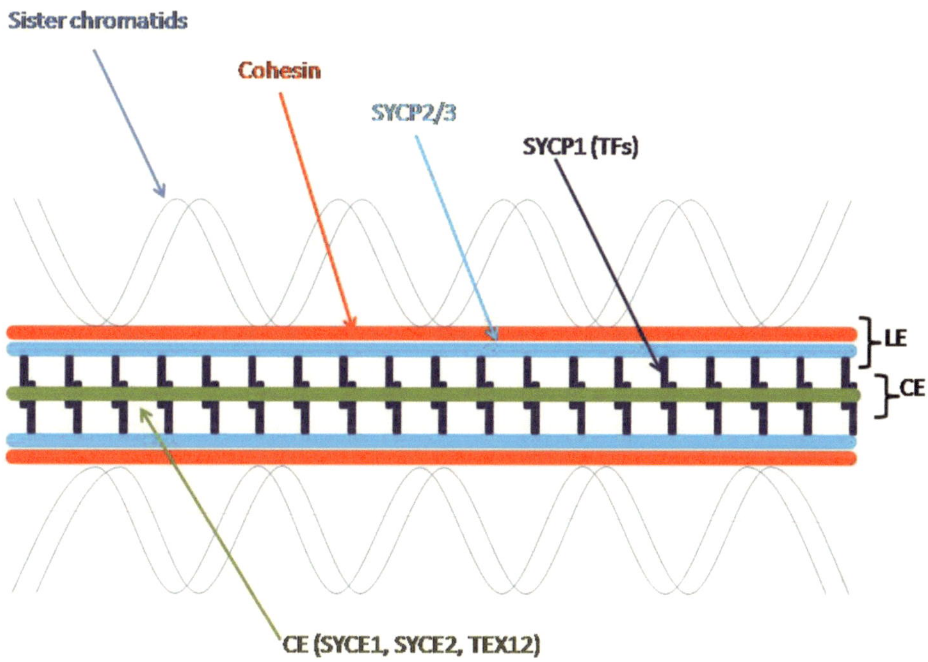

Fig. 2. Diagram of the synaptonemal complex (SC)

LEs are made up of the proteins SYCP2 and SYCP3 and cohesin complexes, which include SMC1 beta, REC8 and STAG3, specific to meiosis (Revenkova and Jessberger, 2006). The specific proteins SYCE1, SYCE2 and TEX12 have been identified in the CE (Costa et al., 2005; Hamer et al., 2006). The protein SYCP1 has been identified in the TFs (Meuwissen et al., 1997). The chromatin is attached to the LEs, forming a series of loops.

Pachytene: Genetic exchange or recombination

Genetic exchange or recombination starts in the DNA double-strand break (DSB) that initiates in the preleptotene and leptotene phases, generated by the enzyme topoisomerase II (Lichten, 2001; Keeney and Neale, 2006). Genetic recombination takes place between homologous chromatids, not sisters. This process is independent in each spermatocyte, which explains the differences between siblings. It takes place predominantly in genomic loci, termed hotspots, close to the telomeres (Lynn et al., 2004). The DSB is an indicator of high genetic exchange activity in the hotspots and is not distributed either randomly or uniformly (Petes, 2001; Nishant and Rao, 2006; Buard and de Massy, 2007).

There is proof of epigenetic control in genetic recombination, as hotspot activity is not determined by the local DNA sequence (Neumann and Jeffreys, 2006). The factors and mechanisms that determine the location of hotspots in the genome are unknown. The hotspot is believed to be the minimum functional unit of recombination. To detect hotspots, a resolution power between 100-200 kb is needed. Crossovers are more frequent close to the telomeres (Lynn et al., 2004). They are the basis of chiasmata (crossings) observed with the optical microscope (Nishant and Rao, 2006). Only two homologous chromatids intersect in each chiasma. The other two do not participate. The number of chiasmata observed in the pachytene and diplotene is similar. This number oscillates from 50 to 53, with an inter- and intra-individual variation of 3-10% (Codina-Pascual et al., 2006). During the pachytene stage, homologous chromosomes are attached only by the crossovers or chiasmata. A single chiasma is observed in the XY pair in the pseudoautosomal region. This pair of sexual chromosomes has a condensed chromatin and forms a corpuscle, termed the sex body, glued to the internal face of the spermatocyte's karyotheca (Solari, 1974). The breaking of the DNA chain needed for genetic exchange must be repaired. The broken DNA chain that ends in 3′ remains free. It associates with recombinases and starts searching for complementary base sequences in another DNA molecule corresponding to the homologous chromatid.

Diplotene: Desynapsis

The SC is dismantled in the following diplotene stage. The homologous chromosomes desynapse, separate, but remain connected by chiasmata and the sister chromatids continue to be attached.

3.1.2 Metaphase I

The nuclear membrane disappears in this phase and the homologous chromosome pairs (bivalent) align along the equator of the meiotic spindle. A bivalent chromosome has two centromeres and four chromatids. Each homologous chromosome has at least one chiasma required for correct segregation.

3.1.3 Anaphase I

During anaphase I, the arms of the homologous chromosomes lose cohesion, with the chiasmata disappearing and segregating. The centromeres attach to the spindle's microtubules, which pull each homologue towards an opposite pole. Half of the chromosomes are attracted towards each opposite pole by the spindle fibres. Homologous chromosomes separate completely, without separation of the sister chromatids. Each chromosome has two chromatids. Centromeres do not duplicate or divide. The segregation of homologous chromosomes in anaphase I requires the release of the REC8 cohesin by the separase enzyme (Kudo et al., 2009). Cohesion between the arms of the sister chromatids is lost, although cohesion is maintained at a centromeric level.

3.1.4 Telophase I

Each spermatocyte II has a haploid number of chromosomes (n=23), but each chromosome is formed of two chromatids. All the homologous chromosomes are pulled towards opposite poles and the nuclear membrane is formed.

3.1.5 Interphase or interkinesis

Interkinesis, or interphase, between the first meiotic cell division and the second is very short. The second meiotic division is not preceded by DNA synthesis. It is a quick phase, similar to mitotic cell division. The division of the cytoplasm is incomplete and the two cells remain in communication via intercellular bridges.

3.2 Second meiotic division

During anaphase II, the shugoshin cohesin becomes inactive and the centromeres' cohesion is lost (Marston and Amon, 2004). The two kinetochores, elliptical disks on each side of the centromere, separate. The kinetochores have an anphitelic orientation (biorientation, namely, each one is pulled towards an opposite pole). They attach to the spindle microtubules and the chromatids segregate by action of the separase enzyme, like during anaphase I (Kudo et al., 2009; review: Barbero, 2011).

The resulting cells -spermatids- only contain one set of haploid chromosomes (n=23), where each chromosome has one chromatid. Through cell differentiation, spermatids give rise to spermatozoa.

Of the approximate two weeks that meiosis lasts, prophase I takes some 12 days, and the other phases of meiosis happen in one to two days.

During the two weeks of meiosis, two cell divisions have taken place and four haploid cells have been generated from a cell with tetrad DNA, each one with a different genetic content. Both genetic recombination and haploidization have occurred.

4. Causes of meiotic chromosome abnormalities

Meiotic alterations can be due to different causes and different mechanisms. To summarise, we can group them into the sections below.

4.1 Mitotic alterations of spermatogonia that have an impact on meiosis

In Klinefelter Syndrome with a 47, XXY karyotype, XY pairing is altered. At least part of the spermatogonia in patients with euploid spermatozoa seems to be euploid (Bergère et al., 2002). Robertsonian and reciprocal translocations produce trivalents and tetravalents at a meiotic level, respectively.

4.2 Alterations of genes involved in meiosis

More than 200 genes are expressed in meiosis. If there is gene expression in other organs and tissues as well, man will exhibit other pathologies. These may be revealed in alterations of the cohesins (cohesinopathies) that intervene in meiosis, in DNA repair (Watrin and Peters, 2006), and in gene expression (Dorsett, 2007). Roberts' Syndrome is due to a cohesinopathy (Gerkes et al., 2010). The alteration of SC proteins can lead to infertility. Patients with heterozygosis mutation in the SYCP3 protein gene exhibit azoospermia (Miyamoto et al., 2003). The absence of the REC8 cohesin also causes infertility by altering synapsis (Bannister et al., 2004; Xu et al., 2005). Shugoshin and sororin are proteins from the cohesin group needed to maintain the cohesion of the centromere. The inactivation of shugoshin in meiosis II allows the separation of the sister chromatids. If there is no inactivation, then there is no disjunction of these chromatids and aneuploid gametes are produced. Infertility in mice has been described owing to the lack of the cohesin SMC1 beta that causes blockage during pachytene (Revenkova et al., 2004). The lack of the SYCP1 protein on TFs lets the chromosomes align, but they do not create pairs (de Vries et al., 2005).

4.3 Epigenetics

Epigenetic entails temporary inheritable changes in gene expression without changes to the DNA base sequence. Gene expression is influenced by the degree of DNA methylation. Methylation can be affected by cadmium chloride, arsenic and nickel compounds. There are claims that incorrect DNA methylation can induce aneuploidy (review: Pacchierotti and Eichenlaub-Ritter, 2011).

4.4 Organophosphate pesticides

Organophosphate pesticides pass through the hemato-testicular barrier, interfere with chromosome segregation and affect fertility (Perry, 2008). This effect depends on exposure time and pesticide concentration (Härkonen, 2005).

4.5 Folate deficiency

This acid provides methyl groups for DNA methylation. Deficiency causes an alteration to chromosome segregation (Pacchierotti and Eichenlaub-Ritter, 2011).

5. Diagnosis of meiotic chromosome alterations

Diagnosing meiotic alterations with normal mitotic karyotype requires a direct study of the testicle or spermatic aneuploidy as a consequence of meiotic anomalies, but testicular biopsy is invasive and has some limitations. The fragment of testicular parenchyma may not contain meiotic cells, may have a reduced number of them, reveal only cells in prophase I but not in metaphase I or particularly, in metaphase II, given the brevity of the second meiotic division (Hultén et al., 1992). (Fig. 3). The most frequent result is to observe cells in prophase I, which is the meiotic stage that lasts longest. Another limitation of the meiotic study is that the specific chromosomes are not identified.

The study of meiotic chromosomes only reveals if the affected chromosomes are large, medium or small sized. It is not uncommon to see two cell lines, one with normal meiosis and another with altered meiosis, and then assess the percentage from each of them.

The study of spermatic aneuploidy using FISH is not possible in cases of azoospermia. The value drops in patients with cryptozoospermia, as a minimum of 500 to 1000 spermatozoa must be studied in order for the results to have statistical value.

FISH with the used probes only provides information on the studied chromosomes, normally five: 13, 18, 21, X and Y. If aneuploidy affects any of the 19 remaining chromosomes, it is not detected. It is possible to study all chromosomes with FISH or array CGH (comparative genomic hibrization) but the cost is very expensive. Despite these limitations, this test is the one most often employed to diagnose meiotic alterations, as it is non-invasive. If the FISH is altered, a testicular biopsy does not need to be done. Reproductive history can let meiotic anomalies be ruled out. For example, if the patient has had healthy children that he wanted with a past partner.

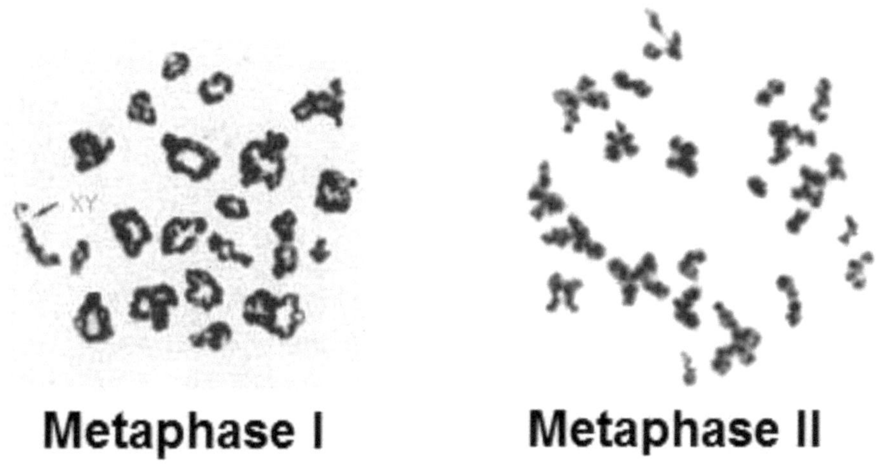

Fig. 3. Normal spermatocytes I and II

Physical examination does not provide representative data on meiotic alterations. Standard semen analysis does not reveal specific alterations of meiotic anomalies, although their frequency is higher with low total spermatic counts (TSC) and in patients with severe teratozoospermia.

6. Repercussions of chromosome alterations limited to meisois

The complex meiotic process requires the precise function and coordination of a large number of genes and their proteins. Some genes are expressed only in the testicles and are specific to meiosis and these gene alterations could impact reproductive ability. Another some genes are expressed not only in testis, but also in other tissues and organs, which is the case of the genes in the cohesin complex. These gene alterations may affect reproduction and also exhibit other pathologies. All men, including fertile ones, have meiotic anomalies. Depending on the type of anomaly and the quantity of affected meiotic cells, the impact on reproductive capacity will range from insignificant to different degrees of severity. Meiotic chromosome alterations can have an impact on testicular histology, blocking meiosis in different phases of the process and preventing it from finishing. Using an optical microscope, maturation blocks can be identified at a spermatocyte I and spermatocyte II level, albeit much less frequently. In parallel, the blocking of meiotic maturation can be complete or incomplete (Fig. 4). In this case, meiosis progresses but is quantitatively reduced.

There may be meiotic alterations without meiotic blockage. In these cases, the testicular histology at an optical level is normal. At a semen level, the repercussions of meiotic alterations may be: 1) azoospermia if meiotic blocking is complete, 2) greater or lesser reduction of total spermatic count (TSC) related to the severity of the maturation block, 3) normal or even high TSC (polyzoospermia) or 4) more or less severe teratozoospermia.

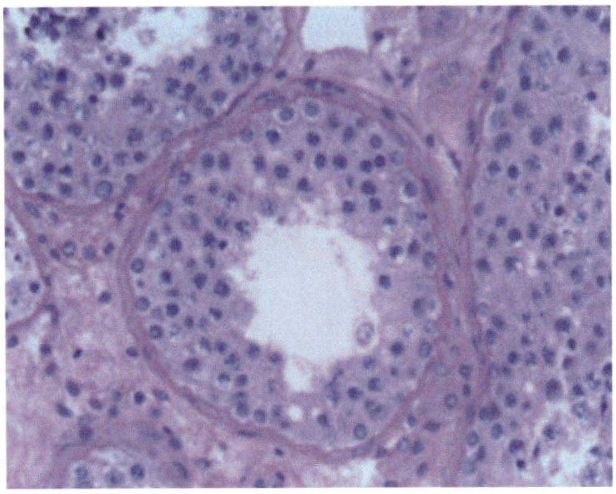
Fig. 4. Seminiferous tubule H&E stain (X200).

- 32-year-old patient seeking treatment for infertility.
- Anamnesis without pathological data of note.
- Physical examination: Testicles - 25 ml. Rest of the andrological examination normal.
- Ejaculate: 4.6ml. Azoospermia.
- Normal mitotic karyotype.
- Normal micro-deletion of Y.
- FSH: normal (5.2mUI/ml).
- TESE: No sperm were observed in the right or left testicle.
- Biopsy of the testicle. Pathological anatomy: Complete blockage at spermatocyte I. General desynapsis

In meiotic chromosome studies during testicular biopsies, the alterations observed are primarily in prophase I (pairing anomalies); in metaphase I (desynapsis) (Fig. 5). In metaphase II (diploidy, hyperploidy), they are less frequent. The absence of cells in metaphase II is not considered a meiotic alteration. The meiotic chromosomal anomalies can produce gametes with aneuploidies, chromosomal translocation, deletion, inversion, etc.... We will focus on aneupliodies.

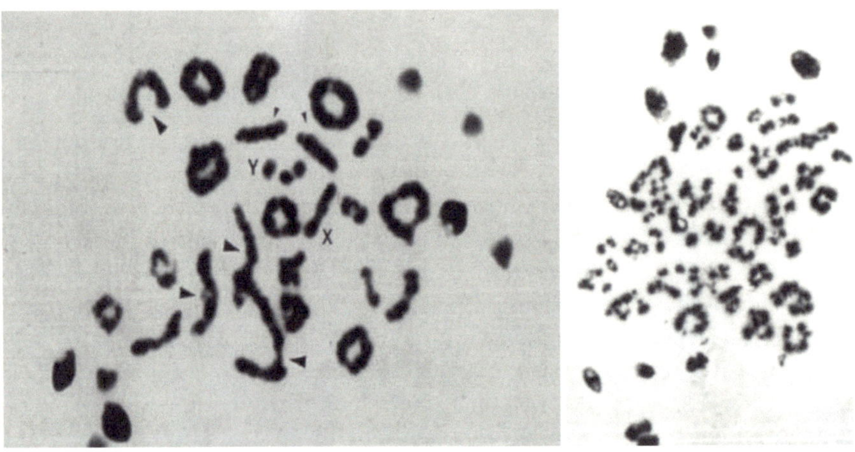

Fig. 5. Desynapsis of bivalent (left) and general desynapsis (right)

At a clinical level, men with complete meiotic blockage and azoospermia are sterile. Patients with incomplete meiotic blocks and reduced TSCs will have reduced reproductive capacity depending on the TSC and the number of aneuploid gametes. They can lead to a lack of gestation; gestation and subsequent miscarriage; or having a healthy child and difficulty having another (including having a sick child).

The quantification of these situations is complex, given the multitude of factors that intervene in attaining gestation, as well as female fertility.

IVF-ICSI treatments are useful in patients with low TSC if they have euploid spermatozoa. IVF-ICSIs do not resolve the problem if gametes are aneuploid. This is why it is crucial to know if the patients' spermatozoa that we treat are aneuploid or not, and what percentage of them.

7. Our experience

The data given here correspond to studies carried out on patients treated in the Barcelona CEFER Reproduction Institute. The sperm FISH study and/or biopsy of testicles with meiotic chromosome were not indicated for all patients. Not all the patients in whom the FISH technique and/or biopsy was indicated actually went through with it.

The sperm FISH and/or testicular biopsy indication criteria were not the same for the entire trial. At the beginning, the FISH study was not indicated if the patient had a healthy son or if the seminogram was normal. It was indicated more frequently in patients with oligoasthenoteratozoospermia (OAT). The patients were divided into three groups.

7.1 Groups of patients

Group 1. Patients with FISH (n= 1813; 100%)

All infertile patients had a normal mitotic karyotype and sufficient sperm in the semen for FISH analysis.

Group 2. Patients with testicular biopsy (n= 216; 100%)

This group included all patients with the meiotic biopsy study in the last three years. All of these sought consultation due to infertility or miscarriage and had normal mitotic karyotype. The seminogram varied from azoospermia to normal semen.

Group 3. Patients with FISH and testicular biopsy (n=60; 100%)

This group includes sterile patients or patients prone to miscarriage with the sperm FISH and meiotic study on the testicular biopsy.

However, the following patients were excluded: i) patients with healthy children from their current partner or a previous one; ii) patients whose karyotype showed morphological variations not considered to be of pathological significance, such as pericentric inversion of chromosome 9. All the patients included in our study had normal mitotic karyotypes; iii) patients with a total sperm count below 0.10 x 10^6; these patients were not included because of the difficulty of evaluating the FISH results, given the reduced number of sperm available; and iv) patients whose semen contained many non-gamete cells; these patients were rejected due to the difficulty of interpreting the FISH results.

7.2 Semen analysis

Semen analysis was carried out following WHO recommendations (WHO, 1999). In some cases, analysis was done using the sample provided closest to the date of the sample used for FISH; in the majority of patients, semen analysis and FISH were performed on the same semen sample.

7.3 The FISH technique

The semen samples were fixed in a methanol/acetic acid solution (3:1). Sperm nuclei were decondensed by incubating the slides in dithiothreitol (DTT) (5 mM) and Triton X-100 (1%). The details of semen fixation, nuclear decondensation and FISH have been described (Vidal et al.,1993). Three-colour FISH was performed using centromeric probes for all patients (Vysis Inc., Downers Grove, IL, USA) for chromosomes 18 (spectrum aqua), X (spectrum green) and Y (spectrum orange), and two-colour FISH was performed with locus-specific probes for chromosomes 13 (spectrum green) and 21 (spectrum orange). The incubation and detection protocol suggested by the manufacturer (Vysis) was followed. Evaluation was carried out using an Olympus BX51 microscope fitted with specific FITC, TRITC, Aqua and DAPI/FITC/PI filters. Only nuclei identified as decondensed sperm nuclei (either by their oval shape and/or the presence of a tail) were evaluated. The following criteria were used to avoid subjective observation: 1) overlapping sperm or those without a well-defined contour were not evaluated; 2) in the case of disomy and diploidy, the signals had to have the same intensity and be separated by a distance equivalent to the diameter of one of them (Blanco et al., 1996). The hybridization efficiency had to be greater than or equal to 98% and was calculated as a percentage of the haploid sperm plus twice the percentage of disomic sperm plus the percentage of diploid sperm (Blanco et al., 1996).

A minimum of 1000 sperm were analysed per patient (500 sperm for each of the two kinds of probes studied: centromeric and locus-specific probes) The chi-square test was used for statistical analysis. Results were considered to be statistically significant when $P<0.05$. The frequency of chromosomal abnormalities was expressed as a percentage with a 95% confidence interval. The control group has been published (Blanco et al., 1997).

7.4 Study of meiotic cells in testicular biopsies

Open testicular biopsies, only on one testicle, were carried out under local anaesthesia on an outpatient basis. The testicular tissue was placed in a hypotonic solution of potassium chloride (0.075 M). Fixation was carried out in accordance with the described technique (Egozcue et al., 1983).Treating meiotic cells with hypotonic solution produces swelling, breaks down the cells' nuclear membrane in prophase, causes the spindle to disappear, and the normal topography of bivalent chromosomes is lost. At diplotene, it is possible to see the cross-over sites, called chiasmata, where genetic exchange takes place. Differentiating between the chromosome figures at diakinesis (the last phase of prophase I) and metaphase I is not easy. We shall use the term metaphase I for both phases. The technique used does not allow for the identification of individual chromosomes, except for the pair of sex chromosomes and chromosome 9, due to its secondary constriction.

7.5 Results

7.5.1 Group 1. patients with FISH (n=1813)

From the 1813 (100%) patients that underwent sperm FISH, 1576 (86.9%) showed normal results; these results were altered in 237 patients (13%). Figures 6, 7 and 8 are box plots which showed a correlation between the FISH results and the semen parameters, count, motility and morphology.

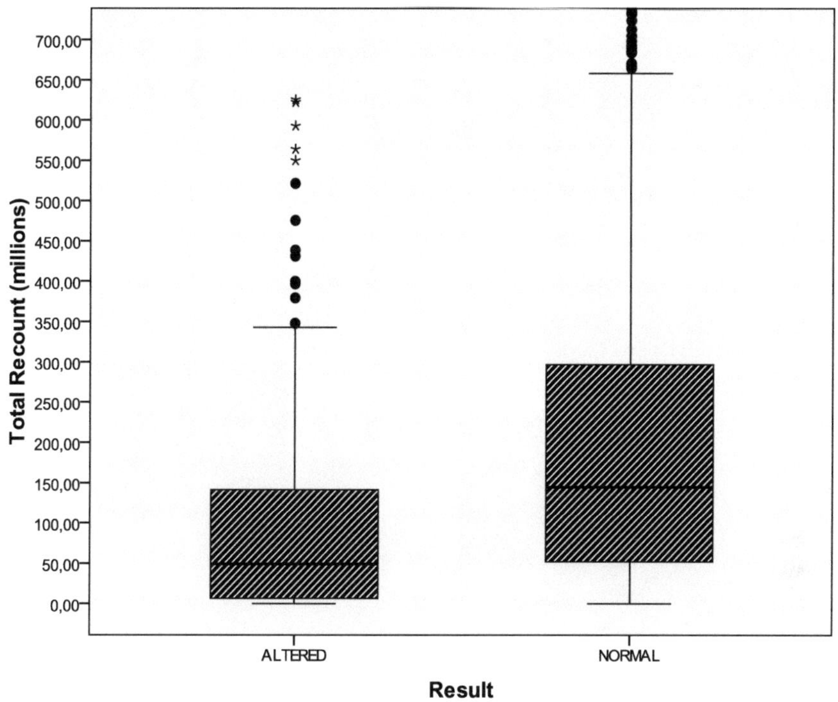

Fig. 6. Relationship between the FISH results and the overall spermatic count.

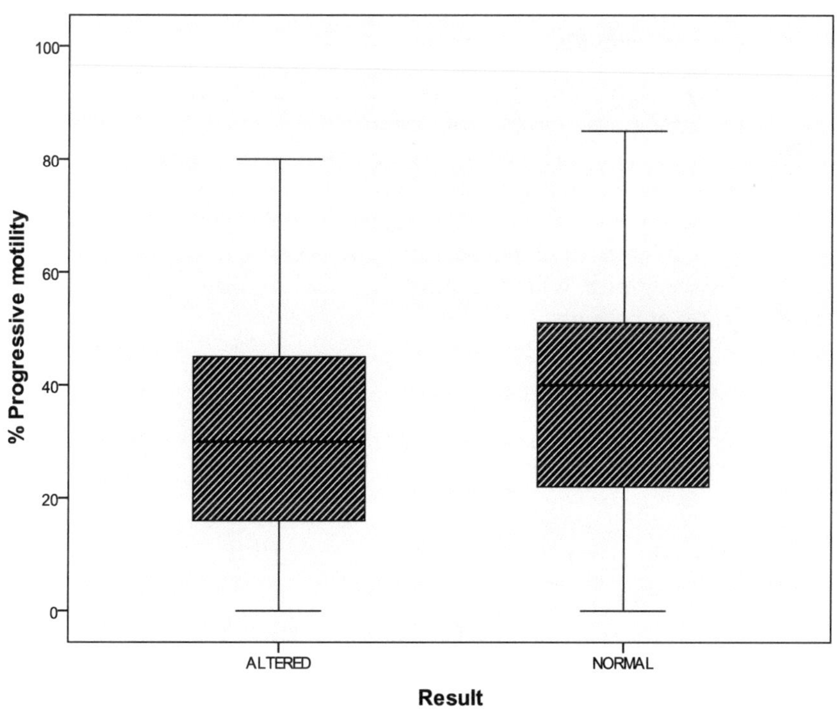

Fig. 7. Relationship between the FISH results and spermatic motility.

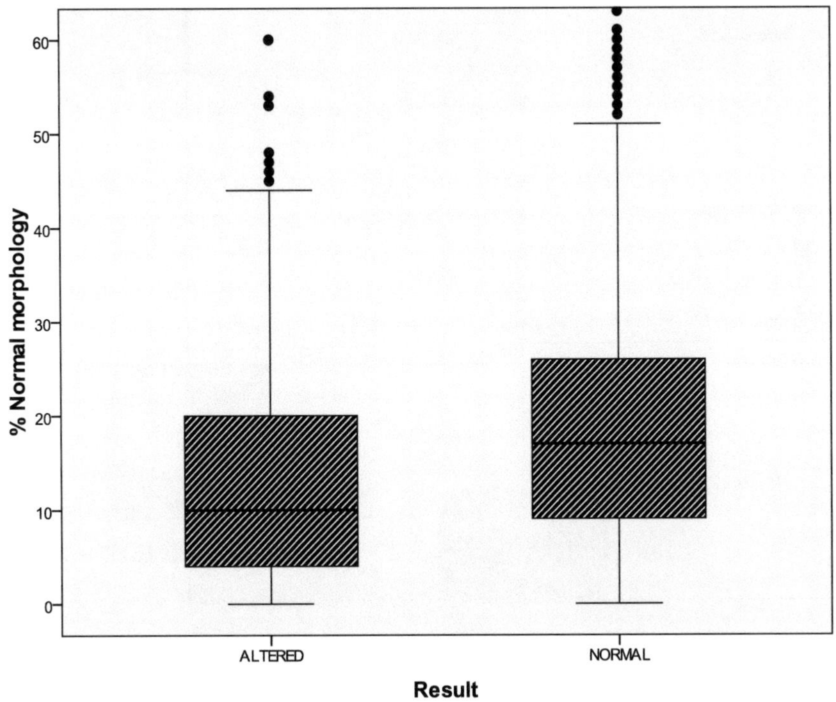

Fig. 8. Relationship between the FISH results and spermatic morphology.

7.5.2 Group 2. patients with testicular biopsy (n=216)

All patients sought consultation due to infertility or miscarriage and had normal mitotic karyotype. The seminogram varied from azoospermia to normal semen in the basic sperm count, motility and morphology parameters. All cases of spermatocytes in prophase I and metaphase I without alterations were considered normal. The absence of spermatocytes II was not considered pathological. The coexistence of normal and altered spermatocytes were diagnosed as mosaicism. Any cases with a variety of abnormalities were included in the group with the most frequent abnormalities. Table I gives the results for this group of patients.

DIAGNOSIS	No.	%
Normal meiosis	67	31
Only Sertoli cells	16	7.4
Only cells in prophase I	31	14.3
Altered meiosis	42	19.4
Mosaicism	60	27.7
Total	216	100

Table I. Results of the meiotic study on the testicular biopsy.

The types of meiotic abnormality observed in 42 patients (100%) are given in table II.

ABNORMALITIES	No	%
Abnormal mating in PI	6	14.2
Desynapsis of the bivalents	14[a]	33.3
Reduction in the number of chiasmata	3	7.1
Presence of univalents in MI	11[b]	26.2
XY separation	2	4.7
MI hyperploids	5	11.9
MII diploids	1	2.3
Total	42	100

a)we observed spermatocyte II diploids in 4 cases and 2 cases with general desynapsis, b) there were also 2 cases with separation of the XY pair.

Table II. Meiotic abnormalities. PI, MI and MII: Cells in prophase I, metaphase I and II.

7.5.3 Group 3. patients with FISH and testicular biopsy (n=60; 100%)

The study of FISH and meiosis in the testicular biopsies did not reveal any abnormalities in 18 of the 60 cases studied (30%) (table III). The partners of 13 patients in this group had experienced miscarriages (21.6%): six of 18 in the group with normal meiosis (33.3%); and seven of 42 in the two groups with altered meiosis (16.6%)(tables IV and V). These figures were low, but significant differences in the miscarriage rate were observed in both groups, with normal meiosis and with altered meiosis. An absence of figures in metaphase II in the fragment of testicular tissue studied was observed in 13 of the 18 cases with normal meiosis (72.2%). Of those 13 cases, nine had a normal total sperm count, which would seem to be incompatible with the total absence of figures in metaphase II. The shortness of this phase explains the frequent absence of figures observed in metaphase II in testicular-biopsy samples (Hultén et al., 1992).

The sperm FISH in 25 patients was normal and the testicular meiosis showed alterations. The seminological data and testicular meiosis are presented in table IV.

The data collected from the 17 patients with sperm FISH and testicular meiosis altered are contained in table V.

The abnormalities found in the FISH for this group of patients are given in table VI.

Of the 17 patients with altered FISH results and altered meiosis, the partner of only one had a history of miscarriages. Total sperm count was normal in nine cases (52.9%) Sperm motility was normal or moderately low (≥30%) in nine cases (52.9%); and sperm morphology was normal or moderately low (≥20%) in 11 patients (64.7%). Individual data with meiotic results are shown in table V.

The meiotic abnormalities observed (n=42; 70%) and the individual data for each case are summarized in tables IV and V. All these patients (n=42; 100%) had meiotic figures at prophase I and all of them had sex body. Pairing of homologous chromosomes at pachytene was normal in 24 cases (57.1%). At metaphase I the most common abnormality was incomplete desynapsis observed as bivalents with some but not all of their chiasmata, small univalents or an association of both abnormalities. It affected some metaphase figures in 29 out of 38 cases in which figures at metaphase I were observed (76.3%). Complete desynapsis was observed in four cases (10,5%).

	MISCARRIAGES	SEMEN ANALYSIS			STUDY OF MEIOSIS		
Case	n	TSC ($x10^6$)	Motility (%)	Morphology (%)	Prophase I	Metaphase I	Metaphase II
1	No	738	20	8	Normal	Normal	Normal
2	No	205	10	3	Normal	Normal	Normal
3	No	203	25	6	Normal	Normal	Normal
4	No	157	50	17	Normal	Normal	Normal
5[a]	No	121	15	3	Normal	Normal	No
6	No	116	30	40	Normal	Normal	No
7[b]	No	104	5	18	Normal	Normal	No
8	No	85	55	17	Normal	Normal	No
9	No	57	25	18	Normal	Normal	No
10	No	1.1	40	38	Normal	Normal	No
11[c]	No	0.7	0	4	Normal	Normal	No
12	No	0.13	0	8	Normal	Normal	No
13	6	564	60	47	Normal	Normal	No
14	2	495	50	16	Normal	Normal	Normal
15	4[d]	161	50	18	Normal	Normal	No
16	2[e]	154	40	23	Normal	Normal	No
17	2	90	30	16	Normal	Normal	No
18	3[f]	0.5	30	9	Normal	Normal	No

[a]left varicocele; [b]unilateral microorchidism; [c]unilateral cryptorchidism,[d]one with trisomy 13 and one with 46, XX; [e]one with trisomy 16; [f]one with 46, XX

TSC = total sperm count

Table III. Patients with normal FISH results and normal meiosis (18 out of 60; 30%):miscarriages, semen analysis and study of meiosis

	MISCARRIAGES	SEMEN ANALYSIS			STUDY OF MEIOSIS		
Case	Nº	TSC (x10[6])	Motility (%)	Morphology (%)	Prophase I	Metaphase I	Metaphase II
1	No	1721	45	19	PA (some)	2-3 desynaptic bivalents[bc]	No
2	No	670	45	17	Normal	2-4 univalents[a]	No
3	No	363	40	4	PA (some)	2-3 desynaptic bivalents[b]	No
4	No	330	40	9	Normal	2-4 desynaptic bivalents[b]	No
5	No	287	11	33	Normal	2-6 univalents[a] and 2-3 desynaptic bivalents[b]	No
6	No	265	3	3	Normal (70%); PA (30%)	Normal (70%), and complete desynapsis (30%)[d]	No
7	No	192	35	27	Normal	2 desynaptic bivalents[b]	No
8	No	159	40	7	Normal	23 bivalents[d]	No
9	No	88	15	5	PA (some)	1 desynaptic bivalent[be]	No
10	No	77	50	21	Normal	Normal (75%), and complete desynapsis (25%)[d]	No
11	No	42	30	5	Normal	1 extra bivalent: hyperploidy	No
12	No	28	35	4	PA	2 desynaptic bivalents[ace]	No
13	No	17	15	11	PA	No	No
14	No	10	25	34	Normal	No	No
15	No	9.6	60	15	Normal	2-3 desynaptic bivalents[bcd]	No
16	No	9	65	23	PA (some)	2-4 univalents [a]	No
17	No	4	16	2	Normal	2-3 desynaptic bivalents[ce]	No
18	No	0.2	8	10	Normal	23 bivalents[d]	No
19	No	0.18	50	8	PA and tetraploids[f]	Complete desynapsis	Diploids
20	3	1716	40	54	Normal	2-3 desynaptic bivalents[b]	No
21	5	489	40	25	Normal	2-4 univalents[a]	No
22	3	218	30	11	Normal	23 bivalents[d] and 23 normal bivalents	No
23	4	208	50	35	Tetraploids (12%)	Tetraploids (some)	1 diploid
24	5	198	15	19	PA (some)	2-4 univalents[a] and 2 desynaptic bivalents[abe]	No
25	4	73	55	20	PA (some)	2-3 desynaptic bivalents[c]	No

[a]small; [b]medium-sized; [c]big; [d]degenerative in appearance; [e]early separation of XY pair; [f]some tetraploid figures with two sex vesicles

TSC = total sperm count; PA = pairing anomalies

Table IV. Patients with normal FISH results and altered meiosis (25 out of 60; 41.6%): miscarriages, semen analysis and study of meiosis

	MISCARRIAGES	SEMEN ANALYSIS			FISH RESULTS	STUDY OF MEIOSIS		
Case	Nº	TSC (x10⁶)	Motility (%)	Morphology (%)	Alteration	Prophase I	Metaphase I	Metaphase II
1	No	260	45	23	Gonosomal disomies	Normal	2 univalents[ad]	No
2	No	250	15	39	Diploidies and disomies 21	Normal	2-6 univalents; 1 desynaptic bivalent[b]	No
3	No	202	35	22	Diploidies	Some tetraploids	2 univalents; 1-2 bivalents[abc]	Some diploids or hypoploids
4	No	176	45	45	Diploidies	Normal	Normal (25%); 2 desynaptic bivalents (75%)[c]; 2-4 univalents[a] (some)	No
5	No	80	3	9	Disomies 13	Normal	2 univalents[a]; 2-3 desynaptic bivalents[bcd]	No
6	No	74	30	20	Gonosomal disomies	PA	2-3 desynaptic bivalents[bc]	No
7	No	66	15	4	Diploidies and disomies 13	Normal	2-4 univalents[a]; desynaptic bivalent[b]	No
8	No	64	45	54	Diploidies	Normal	4 desynaptic bivalents[bc]	No
9	No	38	55	20	Diploidies	PA in 3 bivalents [bc]	No	No
10	No	15	35	33	Diploidies	Normal	4-6 univalents[a]; 2-3 desynaptic bivalents[bc]	No
11	No	9	20	46	Diploidies and disomies 13	Normal	2-3 desynaptic bivalents [b]	No
12	No	7	30	8	Diploidies and gonosomal disomies	Normal	2-4 univalents[a]; 1 desynaptic bivalent[b]	No
13	No	3	10	15	Diploidies and gonosomal disomies	Normal	univalents[a]; desynaptic bivalents[d]	No
14	No	1.2	16	10	Diploidies and gonosomal disomies	PA	Complete desynapsis	No
15	No	0.9	5	1	Diploidies	PA	No	No
16	No	0.46	15	22	Disomies 13	PA	2-4 univalents[a]; 1-2 desynaptic bivalents[bd]	Some hyperploids
17	2[e]	396	55	53	Diploidies	PA	10 univalents[a]; 4 desynaptic bivalents[bd]	Some diploids

TSC: total sperm count; PA: pairing anomalies; [a]small; [b]medium-sized; [c]large; [d]early separation of XY pair; [e]one with 92,XX,YY

Table V. Patients with altered FISH results and altered meiosis (17 out of 60; 28.3%):

FISH ABNORMALITIES	No.	(%)
Diploidies	7	41,1
Diploidies and gonosomic disomies	3	17,6
Diploidies and autosomic disomies [a]	3	17,6
Gonosomic disomies	2	11,7
Autosomic disomies [b]	2	11,7
TOTAL	17	100,0

[a] Chromosome 13 and 21 were affected
[b] Chromosome 13 was affected in both cases

Table VI. The anomalies observed with the FISH technique (n=17; 100%)

Incomplete desynapsis and/or the presence of small univalents was observed in patients with polyzoospermia and those with normal, low or very low total sperm counts: normal, low or very low sperm motility; and normal, low or very low sperm morphology (tables IV and V). No relationship was observed between incomplete desynapsis and more or less severe alterations of basic semen parameters. No relationship was detected between the type of meiotic abnormalities observed in the testes and the kind of gamete aneuploidy (diploidies, disomies). The synaptic process is controlled individually for each chromosome and not at cell level (Templado et al., 1981). The cases of complete desynapsis of all bivalents and in all cells had very low total sperm counts: 0.18 and 1.2 x 10^6 (Case 19 in table IV and Case 14 in table V). Cases six and ten in table IV, which had complete desynapsis but not in all cells (only in 30% and 25%, respectively) presented with normal total sperm counts: 265 and 77 million, respectively. No figures at metaphase II were observed in 37 of 42 cases (88%).

The meiotic report from the testicular biopsy cannot simply be extrapolated to the entire testicular parenchyma.

8. Remarks

When the first successful birth was achieved using the IVF-ICSI technique (Palermo et al., 1992) and one year later when this technique was used successfully on sperm extracted from the testicle (TESE) (Schoysman et al., 1993), andrology entered a new era. It simply became a matter of obtaining a dozen or so sperm from the semen or the testicle in order to have a child. These 20 years of experience in IVF-ICSI have come to show that the reality is not quite as straightforward as this. The few sperm used have to be euploids. IVF-ICSI cannot resolve the problem of infertility if the sperm introduced into the ooplasm is an aneuploid.

If the sperm selected for microinjection into the mature ovocyte is aneuploid, the oocyte may not be fertilized (Lee et al., 2002) or an aneuploid embryo may be produced but stops developing in the first few days after fertilization. Such embryos have higher levels of chromosomal abnormalities (Almeida and Bolton, 1998); another possibility is that the embryo does not implant; they can produce abortions (Giorlandino et al., 1998) or the child is born with a pathology.

In fertile men, around 0.1% of disomies were detected per chromosome; lower in chromosome 8 (0.03%) and higher in the gonosomes (0.27%) (Templado et al.,2011), including a very high level (0.43%) of disomies XY (de Massy, 2003). The total disomies detected via the FISH technique in fertile men is around 4.5% (Templado et al., 2011). It is worth noting then that all fertile men present meiotic abnormalities. It is simply a question of percentages. In infertile patients with normal mitotic karyotype, the level of spermatic aneuploidies is significantly higher in comparison to fertile men: 13% according to the data obtained and 14% according to Sarrate et al., (2010). The high number of patients included in both studies, in excess of 2000, gives added solidity to the data. The incidence of spermatic aneuploidies in infertile men is sufficiently high to recommend investigation in all patients with fertility problems.

Infertility is a symptom that can be brought on by a variety of causes, including causes that are not directly attributed to the man (female issues). The symptom of infertility (or a history of miscarriage) does not enable us to confirm or disregard the possibility that meiotic alterations form part of its etiology.

An increase in spermatic aneuploidies has been observed in patients with oligoasthenoteratozoospermia (OAT) (Devillard et al., 2002; Lee et al., 2002). Also in semen with isolated alterations of each of the basic semen parameters: low spermatic count (Templado et al., 2011); or altered morphology (Calogero et al., 2002). Not all the authors found a correlation between altered spermatic motility (Calogero et al., 2001) or morphology (Sbracia et al., 2002) and an increase in the level of aneuploidies.

The variability of the semen parameter results from one laboratory to another, one patient to another and one day to another only enables us to identify trends as opposed to establishing concrete percentages.

Expressing the spermatic count in concentration levels (per ml) instead of the total spermatic count is another variable that causes difficulties in comparing the results published.

The normality of the basic semen, count, motility and morphology parameters including polyzoospermia, does not enable us to rule out the presence of spermatic aneuploidies or testicular meiotic alterations (tables IV and V). The semen parameter that best correlates with gametic aneuploidies is TSC (Fig. 6); followed by spermatic morphology (Figure 8). The data obtained from group 3 refer to a small highly selective group of patients and cannot be applied to the general infertile population or people prone to miscarriage. There is high percentages of abnormalities detected with FISH (17 out of 60; 28.3%) in group 3 (table V) in comparison to the 13% in the more numerous group 2 (237 out of 1813; 13%). This is explained by the rigorous selection process for the cases.

Depending on the reproductive history (infertility, miscarriage, low fertilisation rate in IVF-ICSI cycles, including donated oocytes, embryonic blockages and embryonic implant failure) and the quality of the semen parameters, the incidence of spermatic aneuploidies and meiotic abnormalities will be different. The percentage published by Sarrate et al.,(2010) is very similar (26.5%) to ours (28.3%).

The FISH study of five chromosomes enabled us to detect a higher percentage of aneuploidies, specifically 11.7% of chromosome 13 in the data provided (table VI), than if only three probes were used, typically chromosomes 18, X and Y in this case.

Patients with altered FISH (100%) in this study presented meiotic abnormalities in the testicular biopsy. Sarrate et al., (2010) encountered the situation in 91.7% of patients. If the sperm FISH is altered, it is not necessary to carry out a meiotic study on the testicular biopsy as any gametic aneuploidy is considered to be caused by meiotic alteration. In a small percentage of patients, between 5 and 8%, according to both our not-published data and that published by Sarrate et al., (2010), the FISH is altered and testicular meiosis is normal. We did not observe any cells in metaphase II in the biopsy in our patients. Meiotic alteration causing gametic and aneuploidy could occur in the second meiotic division. Another possible explanation is the presence of mosaicism.

In patients with normal FISH, the meiosis is altered in 41.6% of cases (25 out of 60) in this study and reaches 73.6% in the Sarrate et al., (2010) publication. The data indicate that a normal FISH does not rule out the existence of meiotic abnormalities. This situation may be explained by the existence of altered meiotic cells that do not produce spermatozoa, along with normal meiotic cells that produce euploid gametes. Another possible explanation is that the spermatozoa are aneuploids but for other chromosomes than those studied with the probes used. If the FISH is normal then it will be necessary to consider whether to indicate the meiotic study or not on the testicular biopsy depending on the reproductive history and the semen parameters.

We did not find a correlation between the meiotic anomalies observed in the testicle and the type of FISH alteration: diploidies or disomies of one or other chromosome. We also did not observe an increase in gonosomic disomies in comparison to autosomic disomies. The number of cases presented is small (n=25) and not conclusive.

The detection of meiotic chromosomal abnormalities both with the FISH and by means of testicular biopsy, together with the reproductive history of the patients, has led the andrologist to indicate a study of the chromosomes in the embryos in order to avoid transferring aneuploids. Another option is to propose the use of a sperm bank. Repeating and re-repeating IVF cycles without studying possible meiotic alteration is not the most reliable option.

The meiotic study on the testicle biopsy was normal in 31% of cases and was not informative in 7.4%. The blockage in prophase I (14.3% of cases) may be due to genetic alterations with no translation of mating abnormalities at an optic level. Out of the alterations observed, the most frequent is desynapsis 33,3% (table II).

It is worth noting that 27.7% (60 out of 216) of patients presented mosaicism. This is the group that may benefit from IVF-ICSI. The use of the IMSI technique (Intracytoplasmic Morphologically Selected Spermatozoon Injection) will enable a better selection of spermatozoon for micro-injection. The selection of spermatozoon for introduction into the oocyte can be 16000x instead of 400x the standard ICSI. It has been correlated the presence of vacuoles in the spermatic nucleus with aneuploid spermatozoon. (Garolla et al., 2008)

The PGD technique, particularly the array comparative genomic hibridization (aCGH) technique that studies all chromosomes enables us to select euploid embryos that are suitable for transferring to the uterus.

9. Conclusions

We can draw the following conclusions from the data presented and quoted in the bibliography.

1. The incidence of spermatic aneuploidies is three times greater in the infertile population (13% - 14%) than the fertile population (4.5%).
2. None of the clinical or seminological data enable us to confirm or rule out the possibility that an infertile patient with normal mitotic karyotype may or may not produce aneuploid gametes. We have observed an inverted relationship in particular between the sperm count and the aneuploidy level.
3. The concordance of the results of the altered FISH and testicular meiosis is almost 100% and in this case there is no need to carry out a testicular biopsy.
4. In case of normal FSIH may be necessary to do testicular biopsy because in more than 40% of this patients we observed testicular meiotic abnormalities. It depends on reproductive history.
5. The FISH study must be carried out together with the seminogram for all infertile patients. The information is significant and cannot be obtained in a more straightforward fashion.

10. References

Almeida PA & Bolton VN. (1998). *Cytogenetic analysis of human preimplantation embryos following developmental arrest in vitro.* Reprod Fertil Dev 10:505-513.

Alsheimer M. (2009). *The Dance Floor of Meiosis: Evolutionary Conservation of Nuclear Envelope Attachment and Dynamics of Meiotic Telomeres.* In: Meiosis, Benavente R, Volff JN (Eds.), pp.81-93, S. Karger, Basel, Switzerland.

Bannister LA, Reinholdt LG, Munroe RJ & Schimenti JC. (2004). *Positional cloning and characterization of mouse mei8, a disrupted allele of the meiotic cohesin Rec8.* Genesis 40:184-194.

Barbero JL. (2011). *Sister Chromatid Cohesion Control and Aneuploidy.* In: Aneuploidy, Delhanty J D A, Pellestor F (Eds.), pp. 223-233, S. Karger, Basel, Switzerland.

Bass HW. (2003). *Telomere dynamics unique to meiotic prophase: formation and significance of the bouquet.* Cell Mol Life Sci 60:2319-2324.

Bergère M, Wainer R, Nataf V, Bailly M, Gombault M, Ville Y & Selva J. (2002). *Biopsied testis cells of four 47,XXY patients: fluorescence in-situ hybridization and ICSI results.* Hum Reprod 17:32-37.

Blanco J, Egozcue J & Vidal F. (1996). *Incidence of chromosome 21 disomy in human spermatozoa as determined by fluorescent in-situ hybridization.* Hum Reprod 11: 722-726.

Blanco J, Rubio C. Simón C, Egozcue J & Vidal F. (1997). *Increased incidence of disomic sperm nuclei in a 47, XYY male assessed by fluorescent in situ hybridization (FISH).* Hum Genet 99: 413-416.

Bolcun-Filas E, Costa Y, Speed R, Taggart M, Benavente R, De Rooij DG & Cooke HJ. (2007). *SYCE2 is required for synaptonemal complex assembly, double strand break repair, and homologous recombination.* J Cell Biol 176:741-747.

Buard J & de Massy B. (2007). *Playing hide and seek with mammalian meiotic crossover hotspots.* Trends Genet 23:301-309.

Byers S, Pelletier R-M. & Suárez-Quian C. (1993). *Sertoli cell junctions and the Seminiferous Epithelium Barrier.* In: The Sertoli Cell; L.D. Russell and M.D. Griswold (Eds.), pp. 431-446; Cache River Press. Clearwater F.L. U.S.A.

Calogero AE, De Palma A, Grazioso C, Barone N, Romeo R, Rappazzo G & D'Agata R. (2001). *Aneuploidy rate in spermatozoa of selected men with abnormal semen parameters.* Hum Reprod 16:1172-1179.

Calogero AE, Vicari E, De Palma A, Burrello N, Barone N, Grazioso C, Zahi M & D'Agata R. (2002). *Elevated sperm aneuploidy rate in patients with absolute polymorphic teratozoospermia.* Hum Reprod 17 (Abstract book 1), pp. 95–96.

Codina-Pascual M, Campillo M, Kraus J, Speicher M, Egozcue J, Navarro J & Benet .J (2006). *Crossover frequency and synaptonemal complex length: their variability and effects on human male meiosis.* Mol Hum Reprod 12:123-133.

Costa Y, Speed R, Ollinger R, Alsheimer M, Semple CA, et al. (2005). *Two novel proteins recruited by synaptonemal complex protein 1 (SYCP1) are at the centre of meiosis.* J Cell Sci 118:2755-2762.

de Massy B. (2003). *Distribution of meiotic recombination sites.* Trends Genet 19:514-521.

de Vries FA, de Boer E, van den Bosch M, Baarends WM, Ooms M, et al. (2005). *Mouse Sycp1 functions in synaptonemal complex assembly, meiotic recombination, and XY body formation.* Genes Dev 19:1376-1389.

Devillard F, Metzler-Guillemain C, Pelletier R, DeRobertis C, Bergues U, Hennebicq S, Guichaoua M, Sele B & Rousseaux S. (2002). *Polyploidy in large-headed sperm: FISH study of three cases.* Hum Reprod 17:1292-1298.

Dorsett D. (2007). *Roles of the sister chromatid cohesion apparatus in gene expression, development, and human syndromes.* Chromosoma 116:1-13.

Egozcue J, Templado C, Vidal F, Navarro J, Morer-Fargas F& Marina S. (1983). *Meiotic studies in a series of 1100 infertile and sterile males.* Hum Genet 65:185-188.

Fawcett DW. (1956). *The fine structure of chromosomes in the meiotic prophase of vertebrate spermatocytes.* J Biophys Biochem Cytol 2:403-406.

Ferlin A, Raicu F, Gatta V, Zuccarello D, Palka G & Foresta C. (2007). *Male infertility: role of genetic background.* Reprod Biomed Online 14:734-745.

Gardner RJ & Sutherland GR. (2004). *Chromosome Abnormalities and Genetic Counseling, 3rd ed.* (Oxford University Press, New York).

Garolla A, Fortini D, Menegazzo M et al. (2008). *High-power microscopy for selecting spermatozoa for ICSI by physiological status.* Reproductive BioMedicine Online 17:610-616.

Gerkes EH, van der Kevie-Kersemaekers AM, Yakin M, Smeets DF & van Ravensswaaij-Arts CM. (2010). *The importance of chromosome studies in Roberts syndrome/SC phocomelia and other cohesinopathies.* Eur J Med Genet 53:40-44.

Giorlandino C, Calugi G, Iaconianni L, Santoro ML & Lippa A. (1998). *Spermatozoa with chromosomal abnormalities may result in a higher rate of recurrent abortion.* Fertil Steril 70:576-577.

Griffin DK & Finch KA. (2005). *The genetic and cytogenetic basis of male infertility*. Hum Fertil (Camb) 8:19-26.

Gruber S, Haering CH & Nasmyth K. (2003). *Chromosomal cohesin forms a ring*. Cell 112:765-777.

Hamer G, Gell K, Kouznetsova A, Novak I, Benavente R & Höög C. (2006). *Characterization of a novel meiosis-specific protein within the central element of the synaptonemal complex*. J Cell Sci 119:4025-4032.

Härkönen K. (2005). *Pesticides and the induction of aneuploidy in human sperm*. Cytogenet Genome Res 111:378-383.

Hassold T, Chen N, Funkhouser J, Jooss T, Manuel B, et al. (1980). *Scytogenetic study of 1000 spontaneous abortions*. Ann Hum Genet 44:151-178.

Heller CG & Clermont Y. (1964). *Kinetics of the germinal epithelium in man*. Rec Progr Hormone Res 20:545-575.

Hultén MA, Goldman ASH, Saadallah N, Wallace BMN & Creasy MR. (1992). *Meiotic studies in man*. In: De Rooney and BH Czepulkowski, Hum Cytogenet. A practical approach., pp 193-221, Oxford University Press, Oxford, UK.

Keeney S & Neale MJ. (2006). *Initiation of meiotic recombination by formation of DNA double-stranded breaks: mechanism and regulation*. Biochem Soc Trans 34:523-525.

Kudo NR, Anger M, Peters AH, Stemmann O, Theussl HC, et al. (2009). *Role of cleavage by separase of the Rec8 kleisin subunit of cohesion during mammalian meiosis I*. J Cell Sci 122:2686-2698.

Lee MS, Tsao HM, Wu HM, Huang CC, Chen CI and Lin David PC (2002). *Correlations between sperm apoptosis and aneuploidy*. Hum Reprod 17 (Abstract book 1), pp. 112 - 113.

Lee J, Kitajima TS, Tanno Y, Yoshida K, Morita T, et al. (2008). *Unified mode of centromeric protection by shugoshin in mammalian oocytes and somatic cells*. Nat Cell Biol 10:42-52.

Lichten M. (2001). *Meiotic recombination: Breaking the genome to save it*. Curr Biol 11:R253-R256.

Lynn A, Ashley T & Hassold T. (2004). *Variation in human meiotic recombination*. Annu Rev Genomics Hum Genet 5:317-349.

Marston AL & Amon A. (2004). *Meiosis: cell-cycle controls shuffle and deal*. Nat Rev Mol Cell Biol 5:983-997.

Meuwissen RL, Meerts I, Hoovers JM, Leschot N &, Heyting C. (1997). *Human synaptonemal complex protein1 (SCP1): isolation and characterization of the DNA and chromosomal localization of the gene*. Genomics 39:337-384.

Miyamoto T, Hasuike S, Yogev L, Maduro MR, Ishikawa M, Westphal H & Lamb DJ. (2003). *Azoospermia in patients heterozygous for a mutation in SYCP3*. Lancet 362:1714-1719.

Neumann R & Jeffreys AJ. (2006). *Polymorphism in the activity of human crossover hotspots independent of local DNA sequence variation*. Hum Mol Genet 15:1401-1411.

Nishant KT & Rao MR. (2006). *Molecular features of meiotic recombination hotspots*. Bioessays 28:45-56.

Pacchierotti & Eichenlaub-Ritter. (2011). *Envioronmental Hazard in the Aetiology of Somatic and Germ Cell Aneuploigy.* In: Aneuploidy, Delhanty JDA and Pellestor F (Eds.), pp. 254-268,S. Karger, Basel, Switzerland.

Palermo G, Joris H, Devroey P & Van Steirteghem AC. (1992). *Pregnancies after intracytoplasmic injection of single spermatozoon into an oocyte.* Lancet 340:17-18.

Perry MJ. (2008). *Effects of environmental and occupational pesticide exposure on human sperm: a systematic review.* Hum Reprod Update 14:233-242.

Petes TD. (2001). *Meiotic recombination hot spots and cold spots.* Nat Rev Genet 2:360-369.

Revenkova E, Eijpe M, Heyting C, Hodges CA, Hunt PA, et al. (2004). *Cohesin SCM1 beta is required for meiotic chromosome dynamics, sister chromatid cohesion and DNA recombination.* Nat Cell Biol 6:555-562.

Revenkova E & Jessberger R. (2006). *Shaping meiotic prophase chromosomes: Cohesins and synaptonemal complex proteins.* Chromosoma 115:235-240.

Sarrate Z, Vidal F & Blanco J. (2010). *Role of sperm fluorescent in situ hybridization studies in infertile patients: indications, study approach, and clinical relevance.* Fertil Steril 93:1892-1902.

Sbracia M, Baldi M, Cao D, Sandrelli A, Chiandetti A, Poverini R & Aragona C. (2002). *Preferential location of sex chromosomes, their aneuploidy in human sperm, and their role in determining sex chromosome aneuploidy in embryos after ICSI.* Hum Reprod 17:320-324.

Scherthan H. (2001). *A bouquet makes ends meet.* Nat Rev Mol Cell Biol 2:621-627.

Schoysman R, Vanderzwalmen P, Nijs M, Segal L, Segal-Bertin G, Geerts L, van Roosendaal E & Schoysman D. (1993). *Pregnancy after fertilisation with human testicular spermatozoa.* Lancet 342:1237-1238

Simpson JL. (2007). *Genetics of spontaneous abortions.* In: Recurrent Pregnancy Loss. Howard J.A. Carp (Ed), pp.23-34, Informa Healthcare. London, U.K.

Solari AJ. (1974). *The behaviour of the XY pair in mammals.* Int Rev Cytol 38:273-317.

Templado C, Vidal F, Marina S, Pomerol JM & Egozcue J. (1981.) *A new meiotic mutation: Desynapsis of individual bivalents.* Hum Genet 59:345-348.

Templado C, Vidal F & Estop A. (2011). *Aneuploidy in human Spermatozoa.* In: Aneuploidy, Delhanty J D A, Pellestor F, (Eds.),pp.91-99, S. Karger, Basel, Switzerland.

Trelles-Sticken E, Dresser ME & Scherthan H. (2000). *Meiotic telomere protein Ndj1p is required for meiosis specific telomere distribution, bouquet formation and efficient homologue pairing.* J Cell Biol 151:95-106.

Trelles-Sticken E, Adelfalk C, Loidl J & Scherthan H. (2005). *Meiotic telomere clustering requires actin for its formation and cohesion for its resolution.* J Cell Biol 170:213-223.

Vidal F, Moragas M, Català V, Torelló MJ, Santaló J, Calderon G, Gimenez C, Barri P N, Egozcue J & Veiga A. (1993). *Sephadex filtration and human serum albumin gradients do not select spermatozoa by sex chromosome: a fluorescent in-situ hybridization study.* Hum Reprod 8:1740-1743.

Watrin E & Peters JM. (2006). *Cohesin and DNA damage repair.* Exp Cell Res 312:2687-2693.

WHO. (1999). *Laboratory manual for the examination of human semen and sperm-cervical mucus interaction.* 4th ed. Cambridge University Press, Cambridge, UK.

Xu H, Beasley MD, Warren WD, van der Horst GT & McKay MJ. (2005). *Absence of mouse REC8 cohesin promotes synapsis of sister chromatids in meiosis.* Dev Cell 8:949-961.

Zickler D. (2006). *From early homologue recognition to synaptonemal complex formation. Chromosoma* 115:158-174.

Zickler D & Kleckner N. (1998). *The leptotene-zygotene transition of meiosis.* Annu Rev Genet 32:619-697.

7

New Advances in Intracytoplasmic Sperm Injection (ICSI)

Lodovico Parmegiani, Graciela Estela Cognigni and Marco Filicori
GynePro Medical Centers, Reproductive Medicine Unit, Bologna
Italy

1. Introduction

In these last twenty years, intracytoplasmic sperm injection (ICSI) has efficiently permitted the treatment of male factor infertility (Van Steirteghem et al., 1993); the direct injection of spermatozoa into ooplasm has allowed the embryologist to overcome low sperm motility, poor sperm-Zona Pellucida (ZP) binding, and defective acrosome reaction. Although ICSI has been successfully applied worldwide for several years, nevertheless we have no real knowledge regarding the hypothetical long term side effects on ICSI adults. In fact, some doubts about the safety of this technique can arise (Oehninger, 2011) due to the fact that with ICSI some check points of natural fertilization are bypassed and that some steps differ considerably from the physiological process; For instance, the introduction of the sperm tail into the ooplasm may cause sperm nuclear decondensation problems (Dozortsev et al., 1995; Markoulaki et al., 2007). It should be considered that ICSI may increase the risk of injecting spermatozoa with genetic or functional anomalies (Sakkas et al., 1997; Bonduelle et al., 2002; Marchesi & Feng, 2007; Schatten & Sun, 2009; Heytens et al., 2009; Navarro-Costa et al., 2010). For these reasons and to minimize any risk related to ICSI, any new advance in this procedure which can help the operator to restore some of the basic physiological checkpoints and to simulate the natural fertilization process should be welcome (Parmegiani et al., 2010a).

2. Hyaluronic acid (HA) and Zona Pellucida: Two important human fertilization checkpoints

In nature, human oocytes are surrounded by:

- the cumulus oophorus-corona radiata complex (COC), made up of cells and an extracellular matrix of polymerized hyaluronic acid (HA) and proteins
- the Zona Pellucida (ZP), a thick elastic coat of glycoproteins located immediately next to the oocyte (Yanagimachi, 1994)

These layers have to be penetrated by spermatozoa before they fuse with the oolemma.

In the human testis, during spermiogenesis, the elongated spermatids undergo cytoplasmic extrusion and plasma membrane remodelling which determines the formation of the HA and ZP receptors, essential for sperm penetration into oocyte.

At the end of spermiogenesis, different expression levels of two specific proteins seem to be related to sperm maturity, DNA integrity, chromosomal aneuploidy frequency and fertilizing potential. These two proteins are:

- the heat shock protein HspA2 chaperone, involved in meiosis
- creatine kinase (CK), abundant in the sperm cytoplasm (Cayli et al., 2003)

Mature spermatozoa have high HspA2 (Huszar et al., 2000) and low CK (Cayli et al., 2003). In contrast, spermatozoa with arrested maturity have low HspA2 expression, which may cause meiotic defects and probably chromosomal aneuploidies, in fact, mature spermatozoa show a reduction of more than five fold in aneupliody rate than immature ones (Jakab et al., 2005). Immature spermatozoa also have higher levels of CK (Huszar & Vigue, 1993); this high level of CK in immature spermatozoa is due to a sperm defect in terminal spermiogenesis when in normal development the surplus cytoplasm is extruded from the elongating spermatid as 'residual bodies' (Cayli et al., 2003). In contrast, arrested/ diminished maturity spermatozoa show a higher retention of cytoplasm with CK and other cytoplasmic enzymes, increased levels of lipid peroxidation and consequent DNA fragmentation, and abnormal sperm morphology. Due to the lack of their membrane remodelling, these immature spermatozoa have deficiency in the ZP and HA binding sites and for this reason they are not able to fertilize the oocyte naturally.

3. Physiologic HA ICSI

In nature hyaluronic acid (HA), is involved in the mechanism of sperm selection because only mature spermatozoa which have extruded their specific receptors to bind to HA are able to reach the oocyte and fertilize it. The role of HA as "physiological selector" is also well recognized in-vitro. It has been demonstrated that the spermatozoa able to bind to HA in-vitro are those which have completed their plasma membrane remodelling, cytoplasmic extrusion and nuclear maturation (Cayli et al., 2003; Huszar et al., 2003; 2007). Furthermore, HA-bound spermatozoa have a better morphology (Prinosilova et al, 2009; Parmegiani et al., 2010a) and they show a reduced risk of being aneuploid (Jakab et al., 2005) or having fragmented DNA (Parmegiani et al., 2010a). Because of this, selection of spermatozoa by HA prior to ICSI helps to optimize the outcome of the treatment (Parmegiani et al., 2010 a, b) and also has a number of other advantages:

- in practical terms, HA-bound spermatozoa can be easily recovered using an injecting pipette (Balaban et al., 2003)
- HA-containing culture medium have no negative effects on post-injection zygote development (Van den Bergh et al., 2010)
- Because of its natural origin HA can be metabolized by the oocyte (Balaban et al., 2003; Barak et al., 2001; Van den Bergh et al., 2010)

At very least, HA represents a more natural alternative for handling spermatozoa prior to ICSI than the synthetic plastic polyvinylpyrrolidone (PVP), which is routinely used to reduce sperm motility during ICSI procedure in the majority of AR centres and has been hypothesized to have toxic effects on oocytes (Jean et al., 1996; 2001).

A "home made" HA-sperm selection system can be simply produced in any IVF lab (Huszar et al., 2003, Nasr-Esfahani et al. 2008). However at the present time, two ready-to-use systems specially designed for sperm-HA binding selection are currently available:

- a plastic culture dish with microdots of HA hydrogel attached to the bottom of the dish (PICSI® Sperm Selection Device, MidAtlantic Diagnostic - Origio, Måløv, Denmark), Figure 1.
- a viscous medium containing HA (Sperm Slow™, MediCult - Origio)

This new approach to ICSI with HA-bound spermatozoa, when using HA-viscous medium or HA-culture dishes, has been defined as "Physiologic ICSI" (Parmegiani et al., 2010a).

Since both these sperm-HA binding selection systems are easily available, efficient and approved for IVF use (Parmegiani et al., 2010 a; 2010 b; Mènèzo & Nicollet, 2004; Worrilow et al., 2007; 2010) IVF centres can choose the one best suited to their needs. The viscous medium requires a specific procedure of droplet preparation to optimize the selection of HA-bound spermatozoa (Parmegiani et al., 2010b); conversely, it is more versatile than PICSI as it can be used also on a glass-bottom culture dish for high magnification sperm evaluation: "physiologic IMSI" (Parmegiani et al., 2010 a) -*see also paragraph 5, IMSI*. On the other hand, PICSI HA-bound spermatozoa can be easily recognized even by non-trained embryologists.

3.1 PICSI procedure

PICSI dishes are conventional plastic culture dishes pre-prepared with 3 microdots of powdered HA. The powdered HA is re-hydrated by adding a 5 μL droplets of fresh culture medium to each of the three microdots. A 2 μL droplet with suspension of treated spermatozoa is then connected with a pipette tip to these culture medium droplets. The PICSI dish is incubated under oil; within 5 minutes the bound spermatozoa are attached by their head to the surface of the HA-microdots and are spinning around their head (Figure 1).

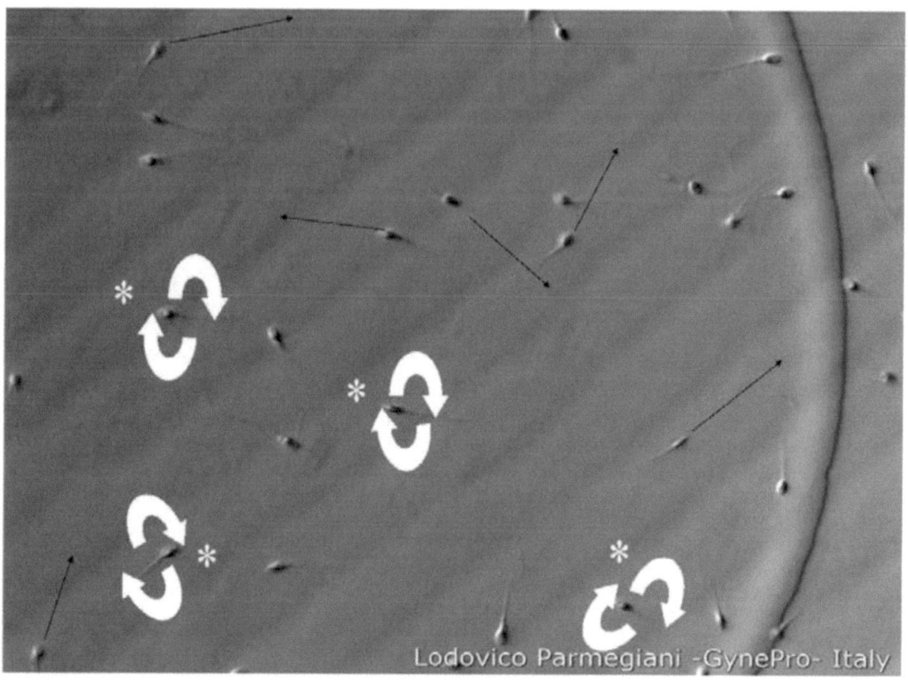

Fig. 1. Spermatozoa in PICSI dish (magnification 400 X)

An ICSI injecting pipette is used to pick the best motile HA-bound sperm up and inject them one by one into an oocyte. The ICSI injecting pipette can be previously loaded with viscous medium (PVP or Sperm Slow) to facilitate sperm micromanipulation.

In PICSI, HA-sperm (*) are bound by the head to the bottom of the dish and have vigorous motility with the tail spinning around their head. HA-unbound spermatozoa, in contrast, swim free all around the droplet of culture medium with varied motility.

3.2 Sperm slow procedure (*Parmegiani et al., 2010b*)

On a culture dish (plastic or glass bottomed), a 2 µL droplet with suspension of treated spermatozoa is connected with a pipette tip to a 5 µL droplet of fresh culture medium. Simultaneously, a 5 µL droplet of Sperm Slow is connected with a pipette tip to the 5 µL droplet of fresh culture medium (Figure 2). The spermatozoa on this culture dish are incubated for 5 min at 37°C under oil. Spermatozoa bound to HA are slowed (as if trapped in a net) in the junction zone of the 2 droplets, these spermatozoa are selected and detached by injecting pipette and subsequently injected into oocytes. In Sperm Slow, HA-bound sperm tail appears stretched, its motility is dramatically slowed and its beats have narrow amplitude. HA non-bound spermatozoa swim all around the medium droplet, they are less slowed by the viscosity of the medium and their tail-beats have wider amplitude.

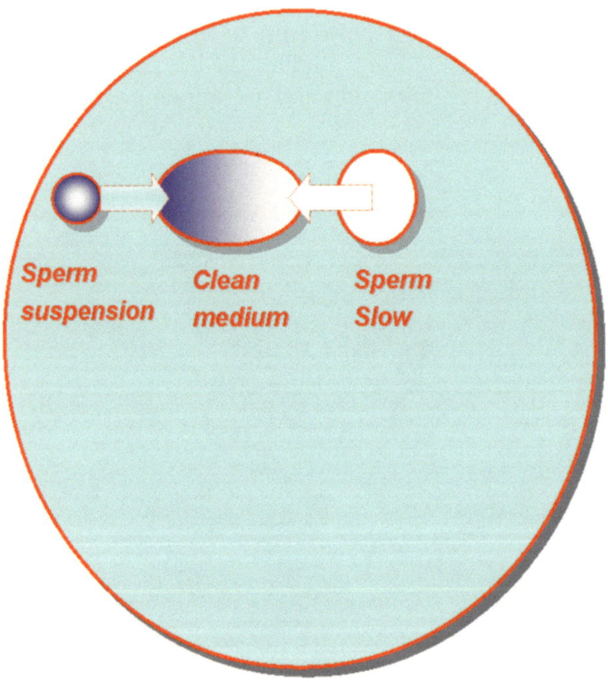

Fig. 2. Sperm Slow droplet preparation

A 2 µL droplet with suspension of treated spermatozoa is connected with a pipette tip to a 5 µL droplet of fresh culture medium. Simultaneously, a 5 µL droplet of Sperm Slow is connected with a pipette tip to the 5 µL droplet of fresh culture medium.

3.3 Clinical efficiency of "physiologic ICSI"

It has been demonstrated that the injection of HA-bound spermatozoa improves embryo quality and development by favouring selection of spermatozoa with normal nucleus and intact DNA: in fact, top-quality embryo rate is higher in HA-ICSI than in conventional PVP-ICSI and embryo development rate has also been found to be significantly increased (Parmegiani et al., 2010 a). Furthermore, HA-ICSI may speed up the time-consuming IMSI (Parmegiani et al., 2010 a). The largest study published to date as full article (428 patients) comparing physiologic HA-ICSI to conventional PVP-ICSI (Parmegiani et al., 2010 b) revealed that injection of HA-bound spermatozoa determines a statistically significant improvement in embryo quality and implantation.

A positive trend in fertilization and pregnancy rates - when injecting HA-bound spermatozoa – has been reported (Mènèzo & Nicollet, 2004). Nasr-Esfahani et al. (2008) have also published a study showing a higher fertilization rate when injecting oocytes with HA-selected spermatozoa.

A statistically significant improvement in fertilization rate and embryo quality and a reduction in the number of miscarriages were found by Worrilow et al. (2007) performing PICSI versus conventional ICSI. In a subsequent study, the same authors demonstrated that PICSI significantly improves embryo quality, significantly reducing embryo fragmentation rate on day 3 and favours good blastocyst formation and clinical pregnancy rate (Worrilow et al., 2010).

In contrast, one report found no differences in fertilization, pregnancy and implantation rates (Sanchez et al., 2005); this lack of significant clinical improvements after the injection of HA-bound spermatozoa may be due to the small number of patients studied (18). Recently, a historical comparison between 2014 HA-ICSI and 1920 PVP-ICSI showed no statistically significant increase in embryo quality and pregnancy rate for physiologic ICSI (Mènèzo et al., 2010).

Van den Berg et al., (2010) found no difference in zygote score when injecting, in a prospective randomized way, 407 sibling metaphase II oocytes, with either HA bound (HA+) or non-bound (HA-) spermatozoa. Our group (Parmegiani et al., 2010 c) questioned the ethical aspect of this study, which was based on the injection of HA non-bound spermatozoa, due to the risk of transmission of chromosomal anomalies.

In conclusion, most of the studies cited above showed an improved clinical outcome of physiologic ICSI using HA-viscous medium or HA-dish (Parmegiani et al., 2010 a; 2010b; Worrilow et al., 2007; 2010; Nasr-Esfahani et al., 2008). At the very least, in all the studies physiologic ICSI never caused a detrimental effect on ICSI outcome parameters (Table 1). If larger multi-centre prospective-randomized studies confirm the suggested beneficial effects on ICSI outcome, HA should be considered the first choice for "physiologic" sperm selection prior to ICSI because of its capacity to reduce genetic complications and for its total lack of toxicity (Parmegiani et al., 2010 c).

FR: fertilization rate; EQ: embryo quality; PR: pregnancy rate; IR: implantation rate; MR: miscarriage rate; ND: not described.

Authors	*HA-System*	*N° of treatments or patients*	*HA-ICSI determines :*
Menezo et Nicollet, 2004	Sperm Slow	92 HA-ICSI vs 110 PVP-ICSI	No differences
Sanchez et al, 2005	N.D.	18 HA-ICSI versus control group	No differences
Worrilow et al, 2007	PICSI	240 couples: PICSI vs PVP-ICSI	Improvement in FR, EQ, MR
Nasr-Esfahani et al, 2008	home-made	50 couples: sibling oocytes; HA-ICSI vs PVP-ICSI	Improvement FR
Van Den Berg et al, 2009	Sperm Slow	44 couples: sibling oocytes; HA+ vs HA- sperms	No differences
Parmegiani et al, 2010 a	Sperm Slow	125 HA-ICSI vs 107 PVP-ICSI	Improvement in EQ
Parmegiani et al, 2010 b	Sperm Slow	331 HA-ICSI vs 97 PVP-ICSI	Improvement in EQ, IR
Worrilow et al, 2010	PICSI	215 couples: PICSI vs PVP-ICSI	Improvement in EQ
Menezo et al, 2010	Sperm Slow	2014 HA-ICSI vs 1920 PVP-ICSI	No differences

Table 1. Studies on injection of HA-bound spermatozoa

4. Zona - Bound spermatozoa

Immature spermatozoa have a low density of ZP binding sites as well as HA receptors (Huszar et al., 2003). Human sperm bound to ZP exhibit attributes similar to those of HA-bound sperm, including minimal DNA fragmentation, normal shape, and low frequency of chromosomal aneuploidies (Yagcy et al., 2010). Furthermore, in some mammals, the same sperm membrane protein is involved firstly in hyaluronidase activity and subsequently in ZP binding (Hunnicutt et al., 1996). These findings suggest that the spermatozoa–ZP binding process plays an important role in the natural selection of spermatozoa as well as HA.

A spermatozoa-ZP binding test can be performed by culturing spermatozoa for a couple of hours with immature metaphase I oocytes; the spermatozoa bound to ZP can be recovered with an injecting pipette and used for ICSI: when using this system Paes de Almeida Ferreira Braga et al. (2009) found that the injection of ZP-bound spermatozoa increases embryo quality. Black et al. (2010) observed a trend in implantation and clinical pregnancy rates when injecting ZP-bound spermatozoa in a study on ZP-ICSI versus conventional ICSI. Liu et al. (2011) observed a significant improvement in top embryo quality rate comparing ZP-ICSI with conventional ICSI.

Even though at the present time there is little information regarding all the factors involved in sperm-ZP binding and its mechanism, these last studies suggest that the spermatozoa–ZP binding test may be an efficient method for identifying competent spermatozoa for ICSI. ZP selection could then be coupled to HA selection in order to replicate the natural path of the spermatozoa towards the oocyte.

5. Intracytoplasmic morphologically selected sperm injection (IMSI)

The conventional magnification for sperm evaluation at ICSI is a maximum 400 X. Some studies demonstrate that sperm morphology according to strict criteria (Kruger et al., 1986; 1988):

- has little prognostic value in ICSI cycle outcomes (Svalander et al., 1996; French et al., 2010)
- does not influence embryo development or morphology (French et al., 2010)

But, it seem logical that the goal of obtaining the most viable embryo and reducing diseases in newborns is dependent on the selection of ideal gametes, both oocytes and spermatozoa (Parmegiani et al., 2010 c). Unfortunately, when observed at 400-1000 magnification, sperm dimension and shape are no reliable attributes for predicting chromatin integrity or presence of numerical chromosomal aberrations (Celik-Ozenci et al., 2004). To improve "imaging" sperm selection, the group of Bartoov (1994, 2001, 2002) developed a method of unstained, real-time, high magnification evaluation of spermatozoa (MSOME: motile sperm organelle morphology examination). MSOME is performed using an inverted light microscope equipped with high-power Nomarski optic enhanced by digital imaging to achieve a magnification of up to 6300 X (Figure 3). Application of MSOME selection in patients undergoing ICSI demonstrated that morphological integrity of the human sperm nucleus is an important parameter associated with pregnancy rate (Bartoov et al., 2003, Berkovitz et al., 2005). The modified ICSI procedure based on MSOME criteria was defined as IMSI: intracytoplasmic morphologically selected sperm injection (Bartoov et al., 2003). A matched study (Bartoov et al., 2003) revealed that pregnancy rate was significantly increased in IMSI as compared with routine ICSI, and implantation rate was even the 3-fold higher. Berkovitz et al., 2005 found an increase in abortion rate from 10% (no spermatozoa with normal nuclei) to 57% if no normal sperm for ICSI was available. In fact, ICSI outcome is significantly improved by the exclusive microinjection into the oocyte of spermatozoa with a strictly defined, morphologically normal nucleus, in couples with previous ICSI failures (Bartoov et al., 2003; Berkovitz et al., 2005; Hazout et al., 2006; Antinori et al., 2008; Franco et al., 2008; Mauri et al., 2010; Souza Setti et al., 2010) or with severe male factor (Balaban et al., 2011, Souza Setti et al., 2011). IMSI positive effect is not evident on day 2 embryos (Mauri et al., 2010) but, conversely, the injection of spermatozoa with abnormal sperm head or with nuclear vacuoles negatively affects embryo development in day 5-6 (Vanderzwalmen et al., 2008) and ICSI outcome (Berkovitz et al., 2006a; 2006b; Cassuto et al., 2009; Nadalini et al., 2009). The positive effect on ICSI outcome given by the injection may be due to the significantly better mitochondrial function, chromatin status and reduced aneuploidy rate of spermatozoa without nuclear vacuoles when compared with vacuolized spermatozoa (Garolla et al., 2008; Boitrelle, et al., 2011). In addition, spermatozoa free of nuclear morphological malformations are related with lower incidence of aneuploidy in derived embryos (Figueira et al., 2011).

It should be mentioned that IMSI is a time-consuming procedure: selecting a "normal" MSOME spermatozoon requires 60-120 minutes (Antinori et al., 2008). Furthermore, the process of searching for spermatozoa at high magnification may itself damage sperm cytoplasm: sperm nucleus vacuolization significantly increases after 2 hours on the microscope's heated stage (Peer et al., 2007). IMSI procedure can be speeded up by merging of high magnification microscopy together with HA-sperm selection. In fact, a HA-medium may help to select a sub-population of spermatozoa with normal nucleus according to MSOME criteria: Parmegiani et al (2010a) found that nucleus normalcy rate was significantly higher in HA-bound spermatozoa than in spermatozoa in PVP.

It can be concluded that, despite the time consuming procedure and the cost of the instrument for high magnification microscopy, IMSI has proved itself a valid tool for safe, non-invasive sperm selection and it can be widely applied in the near future.

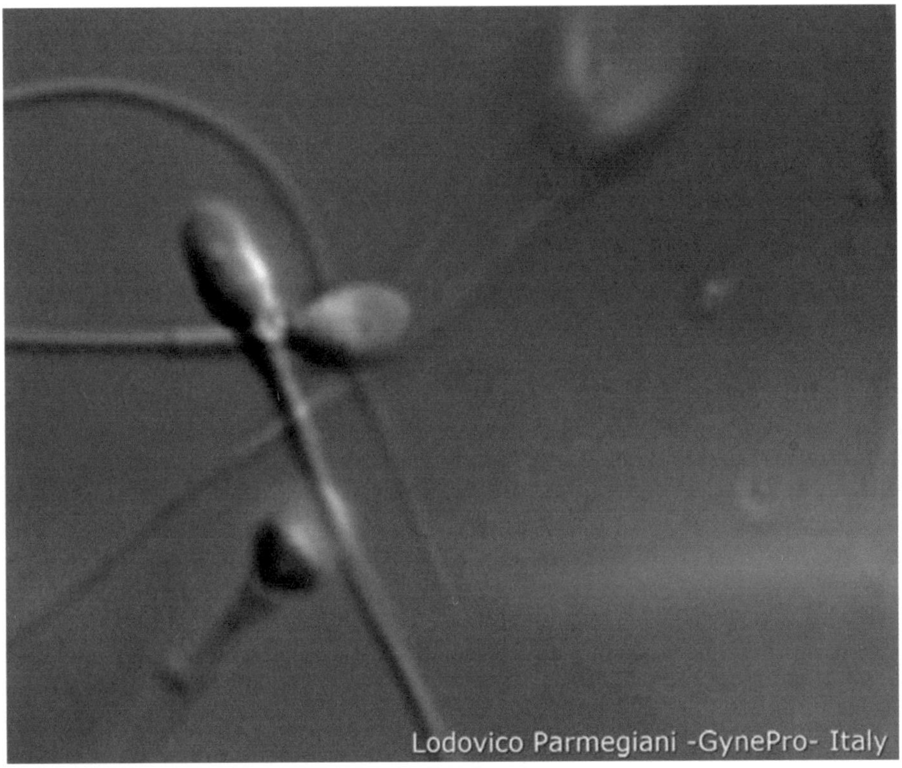

Fig. 3. Human Spermatozoa (magnification >6300 X)

5.1 IMSI procedure

Spermatozoa are generally first treated with a density gradient system. Then, the prepared sperm suspension is put into a PVP (or Sperm Slow in case of "Physiologic IMSI", *Parmegiani et al., 2010 a*) droplet, on a glass-bottom culture dish under oil. In order to choose the best spermatozoa to inject, sperm "nucleus normalcy" is evaluated. The nucleus normalcy is assessed in real time according to Motile Sperm Organelle Morphology Examination (MSOME) criteria. According to MSOME criteria, normally-shaped sperm nucleus is smooth, symmetric, and with oval configuration. Average lengths and widths (± Standard Deviation) must be 4.75±0.28 μm and 3.28 ±0.20 μm, respectively. Nuclear chromatin content is considered abnormal if sperm head contains one or more vacuoles (diameter of 0.78±0.18) that occupy more than 4% of the normal nuclear area. To be considered morphologically normal, a sperm nucleus has to have both normal shape and normal chromatin content. For rapid evaluation of nuclear normalcy, a fixed, transparent, celluloid form of a sperm nucleus fitting MSOME criteria for length and widths can be superimposed on the examined cell on the screen: the nuclear shape is considered abnormal if it differs in length or width by 2 standard deviations from the normal mean axes values; vacuoles can be examined using a similar celluloid form (Figure 4). Alternatively, spermatozoa can be measured for nuclear length, width and vacuoles with specific digital imaging softwares

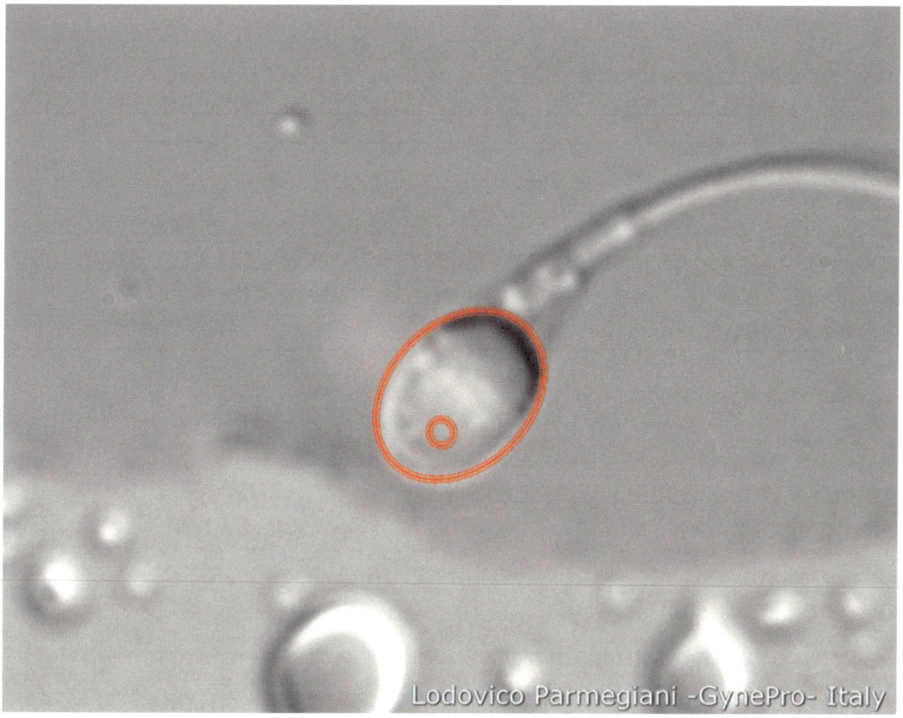

Fig. 4. IMSI procedure. Human Spermatozoa (magnification >10'000 X)

For evaluation of nuclear normalcy, a fixed, transparent, celluloid form of a sperm nucleus fitting MSOME criteria for length and widths is superimposed on the examined cell on the screen: the nuclear shape is considered abnormal if it differs in length or width by 2 standard deviations from the normal mean axes values; vacuoles are examined using a similar celluloid form (Bartoov et al., 2003).

6. Sperm head birefringence

A new tool for sperm selection is the application of polarization microscopy to ICSI (Baccetti, 2004). This method is based on the birefringence characteristics of the sperm protoplasmic texture. In the mature sperm nucleus, there is a strong intrinsic birefringence associated with nucleoprotein filaments that are ordered in rods and longitudinally oriented. An inverted microscope specifically equipped with polarizing lenses allows for the real-time selection of birefringent spermatozoa for ICSI. The localization of the birefringence in the postacrosomial region indicates that the acrosomial reaction has already occurred; the injection of acrosome reacted spermatozoa seems to favour the development of viable ICSI embryos (Gianaroli et al., 2010). The injection of birefringent spermatozoa seems to be useful, especially in cases of oligoasthenoteratozoospermia or testicular spermatozoa (Gianaroli et al., 2008; 2010).

7. Conclusions

The introduction of ICSI (Palermo et al., 1992) has changed in a revolutionary way the world of assisted reproduction technology allowing us to efficiently treat patients with:

- oligoasthenoteratozoospermia
- testicular spermatozoa
- limited number of oocytes
- previous IVF failures

In these situations, suboptimal spermatozoa could by-pass the physiological check-points of natural fertilization and generate embryos, and subsequently babies. Conventional ICSI has the hypothetical risk of injecting immature, DNA damaged, aneuploid, low motile, morphologically abnormal, zona binding deficient, poor acrosome reacted, spermatozoa. Nowadays, we have no real knowledge of the effects of suboptimal sperm selection on ICSI adults in the long term, at least for humans. A potentially worrying aspect of the injection of DNA damaged spermatozoa for example, has been suggested by studies performed on animals which showed not only a negative effect on pregnancy and birth, but also later side effects on the health of adult animals such as aberrant growth, premature ageing, abnormal behaviour, and mesenchymal tumours (Fernandez-Gonzales et al., 2008).

Fortunately, in humans, the risk of injecting DNA damaged spermatozoa seems to be minimized by classical sperm preparation techniques prior to ICSI (Zini et al. 2000; Younglai et al., 2001; Donnelly et al., 2000; Ahmad et al., 2007; Jackson et al., 2010; Marchesi et al., 2010; Castillo et al., 2011: Ebner et al, 2011) and follow-up studies on ICSI children have demonstrated the safety of this technique (Van Steirteghem et al., 2002, Leunens et al., 2008; Belva et al., 2011; Woldringh et al., 2011) although a slight increase of chromosome aberration seems to be caused by the injection of aneuploid spermatozoa (Bonduelle et al., 2002).

The recent refinements of the ICSI procedure described in this chapter, are reliable, easy-to-do, non-invasive and in some cases "closest to the nature" than the conventional procedure. For example, selecting spermatozoa prior to ICSI by their maturation markers such as HA-ZP receptors (Huszar et al., 2003; Paes de Almeida Ferreira Braga et al., 2009) it is possible at very least to mimic nature in order to restore physiological selection and prevent hypothetical fertilization by DNA damaged and chromosomal unbalanced spermatozoa. In addition, non-invasive imaging sperm selection techniques such as IMSI (Bartoov et al., 2003) or sperm head birefringence (Gianaroli et al., 2008) can be valid tools for helping in selection of the ideal spermatozoa.

In fact, sperm selection based on non invasive morphology or maturity markers helps the embryologist in selection of the "ideal" spermatozoa to inject. These new advances in ICSI may allow the selection of the spermatozoa contributing to the improve:

- fertilization
- embryo quality
- blastocyst formation
- pregnancy
- reduction in abortion.

Furthermore, some of these new technologies also help the standardization of ICSI, reducing intra-operator and inter-operator variability in choosing the spermatozoon to inject. For example, HA-ICSI offers to the embryologist the possibility to recognize the spermatozoa which have completed the maturation process. On the other hand, IMSI allows a precise sperm evaluation and measurement. In particular, these two techniques may also be merged together, pre-selecting HA-bound spermatozoa before High -magnification evaluation. This combined procedure (Physiologic IMSI) speeds up the "time consuming" sperm selection according to MSOME criteria (Parmegiani et al, 2010 a)

The easy reproducibility of these new advances in ICSI should encourage the embryologists and clinicians to automatically offer these technical improvements to all ICSI patients, not only to optimize clinical results but most of all to restore some basic check-points of natural fertilization which are bypassed in the conventional ICSI.

8. Acknowledgment

The authors wish to thank Ms Maggie Baigent for revising the manuscript.

9. References

Ahmad L, Jalali S, Shami SA, Akram Z. (2007) Sperm preparation: DNA damage by comet assay in normo- and teratozoospermics. *Arch. Androl* 53, 325-338.

Antinori M, Licata E, Dani G, Cerusico F, Versaci C, D'angelo D, Antinori S. (2008) Intracytoplasmic morphologically selected sperm injection: a prospective randomized trial. *Reprod Biomed Online* 16, 835-841.

Baccetti B. (2004) Microscopical advances in assisted reproduction. *J Submicrosc Cytol Pathol* 36, 333-339.

Balaban B, Lundin K, Morrell JM, Tjellström H, Urman B, Holmes PV. (2003) An alternative to PVP for slowing sperm prior to ICSI. *Hum Reprod* 18, 1887-1889.

Balaban B, Yakin K, Alatas C, Oktem O, Isiklar A, Urman B. (2011) Clinical outcome of intracytoplasmic injection of spermatozoa morphologically selected under high magnification: a prospective randomized study. *Reprod Biomed Online* 22, 472-476

Barak Y, Menezo Y, Veiga A, Elder K. (2001) A physiological replacement for polyvinylpyrrolidone (PVP) in assisted reproductive technology. *Hum Fert* 4, 99-103.

Bartoov B, Eltes F, Pansky M, Langzam J, Reichart M, Soffer Y. (1994) Improved diagnosis of male fertility potential via a combination of quantitative ultramorphology and routine semen analyses. *Hum Reprod* 9, 2069-2075.

Bartoov B, Berkovitz A, Eltes F. (2001) Selection of spermatozoa with normal nuclei to improve the pregnancy rate with intracytoplasmic sperm injection. *N Engl J Med* 345, 1067-1068.

Bartoov B, Berkovitz A, Eltes F, Kogosowski A, Menezo Y, Barak Y. (2002) Real-time fine morphology of motile human sperm cells is associated with IVF-ICSI outcome. *J Androl* 23, 1-8.

Bartoov B, Berkovitz A, Eltes F, Kogosovsky A, Yagoda A, Lederman H, Artzi S, Gross M, Barak Y. (2003) Pregnancy rates are higher with intracytoplasmic morphologically selected sperm injection than with conventional intracytoplasmic injection. *Fertil Steril* 80, 1413-1419

Belva F, De Schrijver F, Tournaye H, Liebaers I, Devroey P, Haentjens P, Bonduelle M. (2011) Neonatal outcome of 724 children born after ICSI using non-ejaculated sperm. *Hum Reprod* 7, 1752-1758.

Berkovitz A, Eltes F, Yaari S, Katz N, Barr I, Fishman A, Bartoov B. (2005) The morphological normalcy of the sperm nucleus and pregnancy rate of intracytoplasmic injection with morphologically selected sperm. *Hum Reprod* 20, 185-190.

Berkovitz A, Eltes F, Ellenbogen A, Peer S, Feldberg D, Bartoov B. (2006a) Does the presence of nuclear vacuoles in human sperm selected for ICSI affect pregnancy outcome? *Hum Reprod* 21, 1787-1790.

Berkovitz A, Eltes F, Lederman H, Peer S, Ellenbogen A, Feldberg B, Bartoov B. (2006b) How to improve IVF-ICSI outcome by sperm selection. *Reprod Biomed Online* 12, 634-638.

Black M, Liu de Y, Bourne H, Baker HW. (2010) Comparison of outcomes of conventional intracytoplasmic sperm injection and intracytoplasmic sperm injection using sperm bound to the zona pellucida of immature oocytes. *Fertil Steril* 93, 672-674.

Boitrelle F, Ferfouri F, Petit JM, Segretain D, Tourain C, Bergere M, Bailly M, Vialard F. Albert M. Selva J. (2011) Large human sperm vacuoles observed in motile spermatozoa under high magnification: nuclear thumbprints linked to failure of chromatin condensation. *Hum Reprod* 7,1650-1658.

Bonduelle M, Van Assche.E, Joris H, Keymolen K, Devroey P, Van Steriteghem A, Liebaers I. (2002) Prenatal testing in ICSI pregnancies: incidence of chromosomal anomalies in 1586 karyotypes and relation to sperm parameters. *Hum Reprod* 17, 2600-2614.

Castillo J, Simon L, de Mateo S, Lewis S, Oliva R.(2011) Protamine/DNA ratios and DNA damage in native and density gradient centrifugated sperm from infertile patients. J Androl 32, 324-32.

Cassuto NG, Bouret D, Plouchart JM, Jellad S, Vanderzwalmen P, Balet R, Larue L, Barak Y. (2009) A new real-time morphology classification for human spermatozoa: a link for fertilization and improved embryo quality. *Fertil Steril* 92, 1616-1625.

Cayli S, Jakab A, Ovari L, Delpiano E, Celik-Ozenci C, Sakkas D, Ward D, Huszar G. (2003) Biochemical markers of sperm function: male fertility and sperm selection for ICSI. *Reprod Biomed Online* 7, 462-468.

Celik-Ozenci C, Jakab A, Kovacs T, Catalanotti J, Demir R, Bray-Ward P, Ward D, Huszar G. (2004) Sperm selection for ICSI: shape properties do not predict the absence or presence of numerical chromosomal aberrations. *Hum Reprod* 19, 2052-2059.

Donnelly ET, O'Connell M, McClure N, Lewis SE. (2000) Differences in nuclear DNA fragmentation and mitochondrial integrity of semen and prepared human spermatozoa. *Hum Reprod* 15, 1552-1561.

Dozortsev D, Rybouchkin A, De Sutter P, Dhont M. (1995) Sperm plasma membrane damage prior to intracytoplasmic sperm injection: a necessary condition for sperm nucleus decondensation. *Hum Reprod* 10, 2960-2964.

Ebner T, Shebl O, Moser M, Mayer RB, Arzt W, Tews G. (2011) Easy sperm processing technique allowing exclusive accumulation and later usage of DNA-strandbreak-free spermatozoa. *Reprod Biomed Online* 22, 37-43.

Fernandez-Gonzalez R, Moreira PN, Perez-Crespo M, Sanchez-Martin M, Ramirez MA, Pericuesta E, Bilbao A, Bermejo-Alvarez P, de Dios HJ, De Fonseca FR, Gutiérrez-Adán A. (2008) Long-term effects of mouse intracytoplasmic sperm injection with DNA-fragmented sperm on health and behavior of adult offspring. *Biol Reprod* 78, 761-772.

Figueira R de C, Braga DP, Setti AS, Iaconelli A Jr, Borges E Jr. (2011). Morphological nuclear integrity of sperm cells is associated with preimplantation genetic aneuploidy screening cycle outcomes. *Fertil Steril* 95, 990-993.

Franco JG Jr, Baruffi RL, Mauri AL, Petersen CG, Oliveira JB, Vagnini L. (2008) Significance of large nuclear vacuoles in human spermatozoa: implications for ICSI. *Reprod Biomed Online* 17, 42-45.

French DB, Sabanegh ES Jr, Goldfarb J, Desai N. (2010) Does severe teratozoospermia affect blastocyst formation, live birth rate, and other clinical outcome parameters in ICSI cycles? *Fertil Steril* 93, 1097-1103.

Garolla A, Fortini D, Menegazzo M, De Toni L, Nicoletti V, Moretti A, Selice R, Engl B, Foresta C. (2008) High-power microscopy for selecting spermatozoa for ICSI by physiological status. *Reprod Biomed Online* 17, 610-616.

Gianaroli L, Magli MC, Collodel G, Moretti E, Ferraretti AP, Baccetti B. (2008) Sperm head's birefringence: a new criterion for sperm selection. *Fertil Steril* 90, 104-112.

Gianaroli L, Magli MC, Ferraretti AP, Crippa A, Lappi M, Capitani S, Baccetti B. (2010) Birefringence characteristics in sperm heads allow for the selection of reacted spermatozoa for intracytoplasmic sperm injection. *Fertil Steril* 93, 807-813.

Hazout A, Dumont-Hassan M, Junca AM, Cohen BP, Tesarik J. (2006) High-magnification ICSI overcomes paternal effect resistant to conventional ICSI. *Reprod Biomed Online* 12, 19-25.

Heytens E, Parrington J, Coward K, Young C, Lambrecht S, Yoon SY, Fissore RA, Hamer R, Deane CM, Ruas M, Grasa P, Soleimani R, Cuvelier CA, Gerris J, Dhont M, Deforce D, Leybaert L, De Sutter P. (2009) Reduced amounts and abnormal forms of phospholipase C zeta (PLCζ) in spermatozoa from infertile men. *Hum Reprod* 24, 2417-2428.

Hunnicutt GR, Primakoff P, Myles DG. (1996) Sperm surface protein PH-20 is bifunctional: one activity is a hyaluronidase and a second, distinct activity is required in secondary sperm-zona binding. *Biol Reprod* 55, 80-86.

Huszar G & Vigue L. (1993) Incomplete development of human spermatozoa is associated with increased creatine phosphokinase concentration and abnormal head morphology. *Mol Reprod Dev* 34, 292-298.

Huszar G, Stone K, Dix D, Vigue L. (2000) Putative creatine kinase M-isoform in human sperm is identified as the 70-kilodalton heat shock protein HspA2. *Biol Reprod* 63, 925-932.

Huszar G, Ozenci CC, Cayli S, Zavaczki Z, Hansch E, Vigue L. (2003) Hyaluronic acid binding by human sperm indicates cellular maturity, viability, and unreacted acrosomal status. *Fertil Steril* 79 (Suppl 3), 1616-1624.

Huszar G, Jakab A, Sakkas D, Ozenci CC, Cayli S, Delpiano E, Ozkavukcu S. (2007). Fertility testing and ICSI sperm selection by hyaluronic acid binding: clinical and genetic aspects. *Reprod Biomed Online* 14, 650-663.

Jackson RE, Bormann CL, Hassun PA, Rocha AM, Motta EL, Serafini PC, Smith GD.(2010) Effects of semen storage and separation techniques on sperm DNA fragmentation. *Fertil Steril* 94, 2626-2630.

Jakab A, Sakkas D, Delpiano E, Cayli S, Kovanci E, Ward D, Revelli A, Huszar G. (2005) Intracytoplasmic sperm injection: a novel selection method for sperm with normal frequency of chromosomal aneuploidies. *Fertil Steril* 84, 1665-1673.

Jean M, Barriere P and Mirallie S. (1996) Intracytoplasmic sperm injection without polyvinylpyrrolidone: an essential precaution? *Hum Reprod* 11,2332.

Jean M, Mirallie S, Boudineau M, Tatin C and Barriere P. (2001) Intracytoplasmic sperm injection with polyvinylpyrrolidone: a potential risk. Fertil Steril, 76,419-420.

Kruger TF, Menkveld R, Stander FS, Lombard CJ, Van der Merwe JP, van Zyl JA, Smith K. (1986) Sperm morphologic features as a prognostic factor in in vitro fertilization. *Fertil Steril* 46, 1118-1123.

Kruger TF, Acosta AA, Simmons KF, Swanson RJ, Matta JF, Oehninger S. (1988) Predictive value of abnormal sperm morphology in in vitro fertilization. *Fertil Steril* 49, 112-117.

Leunens L, Celestin-Westreich S, Bonduelle M, Liebaers I, Ponjaert-Kristoffersen I. (2008) Follow-up of cognitive and motor development of 10-year-old singleton children born after ICSI compared with spontaneously conceived children. *Hum Reprod* 23,105-111.

Liu F, Qiu Y, Zou Y, Deng ZH, Yang H, Liu DY. (2010). Use of zona pellucida-bound sperm for intracytoplasmic sperm injection produces higher embryo quality and implantation than conventional intracytoplasmic sperm injection. *Fertil Steril* 95, 815-818.

Marchesi DE, Biederman H, Ferrara S, Hershlag A, Feng HL. (2010) The effect of semen processing on sperm DNA integrity: comparison of two techniques using the novel Toluidine Blue Assay. *Eur J Obstet Gynecol Reprod Biol* 151, 176-180.

Markoulaki S, Kurokawa M, Yoon SY, Matson S, Ducibella T, Fissore R (2007) Comparison of Ca2+ and CaMKII responses in IVF and ICSI in the mouse. *Mol Hum Reprod* 13, 265-272.

Mauri AL, Petersen CG, Oliveire JB, Massaro FC, Baruffi LR, Franco JG Jr. (2010) Comparison of day 2 embryo quality after conventional ICSI versus intracytoplasmic morphologically selected sperm injection (IMSI) using sibling oocytes. *Eur J Obstet Gynecol Reprod Biol* 150, 42-46.

Menezo Y & Nicollet B. (2004) Replacement of PVP by Hyaluronate (SpermSlow™) in ICSI - Impact on outcome. Abstract of 18th World Congress on Fertility and Sterility IFFS.

Menezo Y, Junca AM, Dumont-Hassan M, De Mouzon J, Cohen-Bacrie P, Ben Khalifa M. (2010) "Physiologic" (hyaluronic acid-carried) icsi results in the same embryo quality and pregnancy rates as with the use of potentially toxic polyvinylpyrrolidone (PVP). *Fertil Steril* 94 (Supp 1): 232.

Navarro-Costa P, Nogueira P, Carvalho M, Leal F, Cordeiro I, Calhaz-Jorge C, Gonçalves J, Plancha CE (2010) Incorrect DNA methylation of the DAZL promoter CpG island associates with defective human sperm. *Hum Reprod* 25, 2647-2654.

Nadalini M, Tarozzi N, Distratis V, Scaravelli G, Borini A (2009) Impact of intracytoplasmic morphologically selected sperm injection on assisted reproduction outcome: a review. *Reprod Biomed Online* 19 (Supp l3), 45-55

Nasr-Esfahani MH, Razavi S, Vahdati AA, Fathi F, Tavalaee M (2008) Evaluation of sperm selection procedure based on hyaluronic acid binding ability on ICSI outcome. *J Assist Reprod Genet* 25, 197-203.

Oehninger S. (2011) Clinical management of male infertility in assisted reproduction: ICSI and beyond. Int J Androl, 34:e319-329

Paes Almeida Ferreira de Braga D, Iaconelli A Jr, Cassia Savio de FR, Madaschi C, Semiao-Francisco L, Borges E Jr. (2009) Outcome of ICSI using zona pellucida-bound spermatozoa and conventionally selected spermatozoa. *Reprod Biomed Online* 19, 802-807.

Palermo G, Joris H, Devroey P, Van Steirteghem AC. (1992) Pregnancies after intracytoplasmic injection of single spermatozoon into an oocyte. *Lancet* 340(8810),17-18.

Parmegiani L, Cognigni GE, Bernardi S, Troilo E, Ciampaglia W, Filicori M (2010a) "Physiologic ICSI": hyaluronic acid (HA) favors selection of spermatozoa without DNA fragmentation and with normal nucleus, resulting in improvement of embryo quality. *Fertil Steril* 93, 598-604.

Parmegiani L, Cognigni GE, Ciampaglia W, Pocognoli P, Marchi F, Filicori M. (2010b) Efficiency of hyaluronic acid (HA) sperm selection. *J Assist Reprod Genet* 27, 13-16.

Parmegiani L, Cognigni GE, Filicori M. (2010c) Risks in injecting hyaluronic acid non-bound spermatozoa. *Reprod Biomed Online* 20,437-438.

Peer S, Eltes F, Berkovitz A, Yehuda R, Itsykson P, Bartoov B. (2007) Is fine morphology of the human sperm nuclei affected by in vitro incubation at 37 degrees C? *Fertil Steril* 88, 1589-1594.

Prinosilova P, Kruger T, Sati L, Ozkavukcu S, Vigue L, Kovanci E, Huszar G. (2009) Selectivity of hyaluronic acid binding for spermatozoa with normal Tygerberg strict morphology. *Reprod Biomed Online* 18, 177-183.

Sakkas D, Bianchi PG, Manicardi GC. (1997) Chromatin packaging anomalies and DNA damage in human sperm: their possible implications in the treatment of male factor infertility. In: *Genetics of human male infertility* (eds Barratt C, De Jonge C, Mortimer D, Parinaud J), pp 205-221. Editions EDK, Paris, UK.

Sanchez M, Aran B, Blanco J, Vidal F, Veiga A, Barri PN, Huszar G. (2005) Preliminary clinical and FISH results on hyaluronic acid sperm selection to improve ICSI. *Hum Reprod* 20 (Suppl1), i200.

Schatten H & Sun QY. (2007) The role of centrosomes in mammalian fertilization and its significance for ICSI. *Mol Hum Reprod* 15, 531-538.

Souza Setti A, Ferreira RC, Paes de Almeida Ferreira Braga D, de Cássia Sávio Figueira R, Iaconelli A Jr, Borges E J. (2010) Intracytoplasmic sperm injection outcome versus intracytoplasmic morphologically selected sperm injection outcome: a meta-analysis. *Reprod Biomed Online* 21, 450-455

Sousa Setti A, Figueira RD, Paes de Almeida Ferreira Braga D, Iaconelli A Jr, Borges E Jr. (2011) Intracytoplasmic morphologically selected sperm injection benefits for patients with oligoasthenozoospermia according to the 2010 World Health Organization reference values. *Fertil Steril* 95, 2711-2714.

Svalander P, Jakobsson AH, Forsberg AS, Bengtsson AC, Wikland M. (1996) The outcome of intracytoplasmic sperm injection is unrelated to 'strict criteria' sperm morphology. *Hum Reprod* 11, 1019-1022.

Van Den Bergh M. Fahy-Deshe M. Hohl M.K. (2009) Pronuclear zygote score following intracytoplasmic injection of hyaluronan-bound spermatozoa: a prospective randomized study. *Reprod Biomed Online* 19, 796-801.

Vanderzwalmen P, Hiemer A, Rubner P, Bach M, Neyer A, Stecher A, Uher P, Zintz M, Lejeune B, Vanderzwalmen S, Cassuto C, Zech NH. (2008) Blastocyst development after sperm selection at high magnification is associated with size and number of nuclear vacuoles. *Reprod Biomed Online* 17, 617-627.

Van Steirteghem AC, Nagy Z, Joris H, Liu J, Staessen C, Smitz J, Wisanto A, Devroey P. (1993) High fertilization and implantation rates after intracytoplasmic sperm injection. *Hum Reprod* 8, 1061-1066.

Van Steirteghem AC, Bonduelle M, Devroey P, Liebaers I. (2002) Follow-up of children born after ICSI. *Hum Reprod Update* 8, 111-116.

Wilding M, Coppola G, di Matteo L, Palagiano A, Fusco E, Dale B. (2011) Intracytoplasmic injection of morphologically selected spermatozoa (IMSI) improves outcome after assisted reproduction by deselecting physiologically poor quality spermatozoa. *J Assist Reprod Genet* 28, 253-262.

Woldringh GH, Horvers M, Janssen AJ, Reuser JJ, de Groot SA, Steiner K, D'Hauwers KW, Wetzels AM, Kremer JA (2011) Follow-up of children born after ICSI with epididymal spermatozoa. Hum Reprod 7: 1759-1767.

Worrilow KC, Huynh HT, Bower JB, Anderson AR, Schillings W, Crain JL. (2007) PICSI vs. ICSI: statistically significant improvement in clinical outcomes in 240 in vitro fertilization (IVF) patients. *Fertil Steril* 88 (Suppl1), s37.

Worrilow KC, Eid S, Matthews J, Pelts E, Khoury C, Liebermann J. (2010) Multi-site clinical trial evaluating PICSI, a method for selection of hyaluronan bound sperm (HBS) for use in ICSI: improved clinical outcomes. *Hum Reprod* 25 (Suppl1), i7.

Yagci A, Murk W, Stronk J, Huszar G. (2010) Spermatozoa bound to solid state hyaluronic acid show chromatin structure with high DNA chain integrity: an acridine orange fluorescence study. *J Androl* 31,566-572.

Yanagimachi R. (1994) Mammalian Fertilization. In: *The Physiology of Reproduction.*(eds: Knobil E & Neill JD), pp. 189-317. Raven Press Ltd, New York,.

Younglai EV, Holt D, Brown P, Jurisicova A, Casper RF. (2001) Sperm swim-up techniques and DNA fragmentation. *Hum Reprod* 16, 1950-1953.

Zini A, Finelli A, Phang D, Jarvi K. (2000) Influence of semen processing technique on human sperm DNA integrity. *Urology* 56, 1081-1084.

8

Advances in Fertility Options of Azoospermic Men

Bin Wu[1], Timothy J. Gelety[1] and Juanzi Shi[2]
[1]*Arizona Center for Reproductive Endocrinology and Infertility*
Tucson, Arizona
[2]*Shaanxi Province Hospital for Women and Children Health Care*
Xi'an, Shaanxi
[1]*USA*
[2]*People's Republic of China*

1. Introduction

Infertility is defined as the failure of a couple to become pregnant after one year of regular, unprotected, sexual intercourse. Misconceptions about infertility are very common. Infertility affects roughly 15% of all couples during their reproductive lives. Infertility is not "just a female problem" as there is a male infertility component in approximately 50% of couples. A couple experiencing infertility should not underestimate the significance of the problems that can exist in the male. Male infertility may be the sole contributing reason for the couple's failure to conceive and should be best identified by a male infertility specialist. According to the 2009 national summary report of the American Society for Assisted Reproductive Technology, nearly 35% of infertility is attributed to the male factor. In the late last century, treatment for severe male factor infertility was limited to inseminations or *in vitro* fertilization using donor sperm. However, most infertile couples, and particularly men, are reluctant to use donor sperm because of bias maintained across cultural and ethnic boundaries. Today, exciting advances in male infertility have introduced innovative therapeutic options, in particular, intracytoplasmic sperm injection (ICSI), which offers men, including those with no sperm (azoospermia) in their ejaculate due to genetic conditions, a greatly improved chance to conceive their own biological offspring (Palermo, et al.. 1992). Currently, despite severe male factor infertility, pregnancy may still be achieved. This is mainly attributed to the success of the ICSI technique and advanced surgical testicular sperm retrieval techniques. In recent years, the ICSI technique has evolved into intracytoplasmic morphologically selected sperm injection (IMSI) and a method for selection of hyaluronan bound sperm for use in ICSI (PICSI) (Parmegiani et al., 2010a,b; Said & Land 2011; Berger et al., 2011), resulting in significantly increased fertilization and pregnancy rates over the world IVF clinics. Because the advanced ICSI technique in human IVF is covered in depth by other chapters of this book, the main emphasis here will be on the application of testicular biopsy sperm, round or elongated spermatids from azoospermic men to human IVF as well as explore new technologies to produce artificial sperm from stem cells and somatic cells.

2. Evaluation of male infertility-definition of azoospermia

There are a variety of conditions that may lead to male infertility. An important component in the treatment of men with infertility is establishing the correct diagnosis through a thorough clinical evaluation of each couple. The cornerstone of the male fertility evaluation is the semen analysis, which is also the simplest evaluation for a male fertility. Complete evaluation of the infertile male involves a comprehensive medical history, physical examination and two and more semen analyses.

In addition to semen analysis, specialized sperm function testing are available, including measurement of sperm capacitation and the acrosome reaction, computer assisted sperm motion analysis (CASA), sperm antibody testing, and leukocyte quantitation. According to the World Health Organization (WHO, 2010), the lower reference limit for semen characteristics should include a semen volume (1.4-1.7ml), sperm concentration (12-16 million/ml), motility (38-42%), and morphology (3.0-4.0), as an integral screen of sperm fertilization potential. A persistently abnormal finding outside of the normal range often indicates male infertility. An abnormal semen analysis may be the first sign of significant pathology that may be life threatening in up to 1-2% of cases. The diagnosis of infertility may not only indicate a problem with the husband but also may put the health of his offspring at risk. With a growing understanding about the genetics of male infertility, a genetic cause may exist in up to 20% of patients. The primary goal of the evaluation is to determine the cause of the problem and to exclude life threatening pathology. Thus, genetic diagnosis of male infertility plays an important role in the application of assisted reproductive technology. Today, genetic testing for cystic fibrosis, Karyotyping and Y microdeletion analysis are important male infertility diagnostic tests for couples who are at risk of inherited genetic diseases.

After detailed semen analysis, potential causes of male infertility may present (Comhaire & Vermenlen, 1995) as (1) complete absence of sperm (azoospermia), (2) low sperm count (oligozoospermia), (3) abnormal sperm shape (teratozoospermia), (4) problems with sperm movement (asthenozoospermia), (5) completely immobile sperm (necrozoospermia), where the sperm may be alive and not moving, or they may be dead (6) problems with sperm delivery, due to sexual dysfunction, an obstruction, previous vasectomy, or retrograde ejaculation. In an earlier generation of investigations, the most common cause of male infertility was reported to be the presence of a varicocele, which is the presence of a varicose vein found in the scrotum. The extra heat caused by the vein was suggested to lead to low sperm counts and impaired sperm movement. However, some clinical studies have failed to demonstrate a significant increase in pregnancy following varicocele repair. It is likely that genetic abnormalities noted in the modern studies of Y chromosomal micro-deletions account for abnormal parameters. With the development of intracytoplasmic sperm injection (ICSI) technology, a laboratory specialist uses microscopic tools to isolate a single sperm and then injects it directly into an egg. This technique, used in conjunction with *in vitro* fertilization (IVF), has been especially successful as a treatment for men who have a low sperm count (oligozoospermia), asthenozoospermia and women who have a small number of mature eggs. Also, oligozoospermic men often carry seminal populations demonstrating increased chromosomal aberrations and compromised DNA integrity. Therefore, the *in vitro* selection of sperm for ICSI is critical and directly influences the paternal contribution to preimplantation embryogenesis. Hyaluronan (H), a major constituent of the cumulus matrix, may play a critical role in the selection of functionally competent sperm during *in vivo* fertilization (Parmegiani et al., 2010a). Hyaluronan bound sperm (HBS) exhibit decreased levels of cytoplasmic inclusions and residual histones, an increased expression of the HspA2 chaperone protein and a marked reduction in the incidence of chromosomal aneuploidy. The relationship between HBS and enhanced levels of developmental competence led to the current clinical trial (Worrilow et al., 2010). Thus, as a HBS test, a PCISI technique, a method for selection of hyaluronan bound sperm for use in ICSI, has been developed to treat oligozoospermic and asthenozoospermic man infertility problem. Additionally, recently advanced IMSI technique has been used to treat sperm morphology problems (teratozoospermia). In cases of necrozoospermia, motile spermatozoa may be found by adding pentoxifylline or other chemicals such as 2-deoxyadenosine to treat semen and sperm (Angelopoulos et al., 1999), or live sperm will be determined by hypo-osmotic swelling test (Takahashi et al., 1990).

The most sever cases of male infertility are those presenting with no sperm in the ejaculate (azoospermia). Some men have a condition where their reproductive ducts may be absent or blocked (obstructive azoospermia or OA), where others may have no sperm production with normal reproductive anatomy (non-obstructive azoospermia or NOA). Azoospermia is found in 10% of male infertility cases. Patients with OA due to congenital bilateral absence of the vas deferens or those in whom reconstructive surgery fails have historically been considered infertile. Men who can not produce sperm in their testes with apparent absence of spermatogenesis diagnosed by testicular biopsy are classified as NOA. Once testicular and epidiymal function can be verified, surgery may be justified to correct or remove the blockage. Alternatively, the current optimal method for treatment of azoospermic men is to acquire sperm from the testis or epididymis by either non-surgical or surgical means.

3. Acquiring sperm from azoospermic men

For men with no sperm at all in their semen, sperm may be obtained by non-surgical or surgical techniques based on the complete evaluation and diagnosis of male factor infertility.

3.1 Non-surgical sperm retrieval techniques

3.1.1 Electro-ejaculation (EEJ)

Many factors may predispose spinal cord injured men to infertility. Ejaculatory dysfunction, abnormalities of sperm production, chronic infections and blockage of sperm within the male reproductive tract are all potential factors. Currently a number of different methods have been used to obtain sperm from azoospermic men. For example, sperm can often be obtained through vibratory stimulation to the head and shaft of the penis. Men with ejaculatory failure due to nerve damage caused by spinal injury, and occasionally by other conditions, can produce sperm by electrical stimulation of the ejaculatory ducts internally. Electro-ejaculation or sperm harvesting along the ejaculatory path from the vas deferens, epididymis, and directly from the testis is a very successful form of therapy for men who have normal sperm production but can not ejaculate because of a short circuit in the nervous system. Though sperm quality is often poor due to remaining too long in the body, the sperm are usually suitable for ICSI treatment. EEJ has also proven effective for loss of ejaculation in patients with other conditions such as diabetes, retroperitoneal lymph node dissection, pelvic surgery, multiple sclerosis, or unexplained loss of orgasm. EEJ is non-invasive and patients routinely return back to desk type work that day after a pain-free procedure of 30 minutes with local anesthesia at an outpatient surgery center. Electro-ejaculation allows the retrieval of sperm in more than 90% of patients, but in most of cases, sperm concentration and sperm motility is relatively low. Combining EEJ with current ICSI techniques, this may yield up to a 50% pregnancy rate. Overall, the chances for pregnancy in the informed and motivated patient are similar to those of a healthy male. However, electro-ejaculation must be performed under satisfactory anesthesia in men with spinal cord injuries with sensation in or below the abdomen. To avoid the complication of autonomic dysreflexia, a complete urologic examination must be performed prior to the procedure to detect and treat any urinary tract infections. Often during this procedure retrograde ejaculation occurs, which is a backwards ejaculation into the bladder, and sperm must be collected from the urine.

3.1.2 Testicular sperm aspiration (TESA) and percutaneous epididymal sperm aspiration (PESA)

TESA and PESA have been used as minimally invasive or non-surgical sperm aspiration techniques for use in conjuncture with assisted reproductive technology. This technique is a quick and painless procedure performed under sedation. A tiny percutaneous needle is used to extract sperm directly from the testis or epididymis. Using these minimally invasive techniques, sperm can be obtained from men with vasectomy, failed vasectomy reversal, absence of the vas deferens, or uncorrectable blockages anywhere along the seminal tract (obstructive azoospermia). In addition, individual sperm occasionally may be obtained in some cases of non-obstructive azoospermia (NOA). Sperm retrieval procedures are typically done at an outpatient surgery and last about one hour. The advantages of percutaneous aspiration techniques are that they can be performed with local anesthesia, without open scrotal exploration and its attendant postoperative discomfort, and without microsurgical expertise. Also it does not require hospitalization, and recovery is virtually immediate. Patients return back to desk type work in one or two days. It should be noted that for some men, a single percutaneous aspiration procedure may yield enough sperm to permit sperm freezing for several subsequent ICSI attempts. While the ejaculate normally contains 100 to 300 million sperm, aspiration of as few as 100-200 sperm by this technique have been enough to achieve pregnancy when it is combined with ICSI.

3.2 Surgical sperm retrieval techniques

In cases where sperm production is low or there is some atrophy of testes or epididymis, microsurgical techniques known as Microscopic Epididymal Sperm Aspiration (MESA) and Testicular Sperm Extraction (TESE) can be used to obtain sperm from the epididymis, the sperm rich tube at the back of the testis, or removing small samples of testis tissue for processing and eventual extraction of sperm. These two techniques are more aggressive ways of recovering sperm. Microscopic TESE (MicroTESE) is a very exacting search for sperm under high magnification in cases of extremely low sperm production. MESA and TESE procedures are the most popular because the goal is retrieval of sufficient sperm for freezing and use in future ICSI cycles. MESA involves direct retrieval of spermatozoa from epididymal tubuli, thus it minimizes contamination of the epididymal fluid by blood cells, which may affect spermatozoa fertilizing capacity during IVF (Cornell Physicians, 2010). However, in the most clinical situations, the results of MESA are often poor and unpredictable. Thus, testicular sperm extraction (TESE) is an effective method and a well accepted technique for sperm retrieval from men with non-obstructive azoospermia or obstructive azoospermia for ICSI. However, the conventional TESE technique requires multiple blind testis biopsies, with excision of large volumes (>700 mg) of testicular tissue and risks permanent damage to the testis. Recent research ((Pühse et al., 2011) has suggested that testicular biopsy is not necessary for diagnosis of OA because they have normal FSH and glucoside levels and normal testicular volumes. However, normal spermatogenesis often appears in the larger testis. Thus, the use of unilateral therapeutic biopsy in men with OA is feasible and the large side testicle should be operated on when there is a significant size difference between two testicles. Using optical magnification, a relatively avascular region of the testis is located for an incision. Currently, because many urology clinics do not have advanced micro-surgical instruments, testicular tissue is often removed from testis or epididymis by routine surgical biopsy. The testis is exposed and a long incision is made in the tunica to expose the testicular parenchyma. The seminiferous tubules are gently separated and examined under an operating microscope. Testicular sperm may be found within testicular tissue of many men with non-obstructive azoospermia. The optimal technique of sperm extraction would be minimally invasive and avoid destruction of testicular function without compromising the chance of retrieval adequate numbers of spermatozoa to perform ICSI. Since testicular biopsy is an invasive procedure, the efficient use of TESE would reduce surgical aspiration to single sperm retrieval by including cryopreservation.

4. Optimal use of testicular biopsy sperm

Surgical retrieval of testicular sperm for ICSI is now a widely practiced technique in the treatment of azoospermic men, but testicular biopsy is an invasive procedure. Thus, the optimal use of testicular biopsy tissue for patient treatment would reduce surgical extractions to retrieval of a single sample. In the last decade, many groups have suggested methods to optimize the use of testicular biopsy specimens. Several strategies have been developed to optimally manage a testicular biopsy, including improvement of sperm motility and increasing the motile sperm recovery rate after freezing (Wu et al., 2005). In most cases, only few spermatozoa can be obtained from minced testicular tissue and many of these free spermatozoa display complete immotility and occasionally only an individual sperm shows a slowly "twitching" movement. The goal of therapy is to obtain sufficient motile sperm from testicular biopsy tissue for use with ICSI to treat male infertility. In our clinical practice, we use the following three methods to optimize use of a single testicular biopsy specimen.

4.1 Motile or non-motile sperm recovery from testicular biopsy tissue

The surgical biopsy of testicular tissue is often carried out by an urologist under local anesthesia. After obtaining the testicular biopsy tissue (TESE), an examination for the presence of sperm and their motility should be immediately performed, but the TESE samples often contain a lot of tissue, red blood cells and debris. In our laboratory, after mincing and cutting the specimen into small pieces, all tissue and medium are transferred into a centrifuge tube and washed with modified modified human tubal fluid (mHTF) medium (Irvine scientific, CA) by centrifuge. After removing supernatant, the pellet is suspended again with 1-2 ml mHTF medium and mixed. After that, a slide with a small piece tissue is made to check for the presence of sperm under the microscope.

4.2 *In vitro* maturation of testicular biopsy tissue

The only requirement for ICSI is one living spermatozoon per oocyte (Nagy et al., 1995). Sperm movement itself is not necessary for successful fertilization but it is the most reliable marker of viability. Although testicular sperm extraction is used frequently to obtain sufficient sperm for ICSI, very few spermatozoa demonstrate twitching motility or are completely immotile in the initial testicular biopsy samples. Our research observed less than 3% motile sperm (slight twitching) during the initial collection of testicular biopsy samples (Wu et al., 2005). In most cases, it is very difficult to find sufficient motile sperm in the initial or frozen-thawed TESE samples. Thus, our study indicated that culturing testicular biopsy tissue for a period has been a reliable method to obtain motile sperm with ICSI. In order to get more motile sperm from fresh or frozen-thawing testicular biopsy tissue, we conducted a comparative experiment with two culture medium, mHTF and HTF (Figure 1).

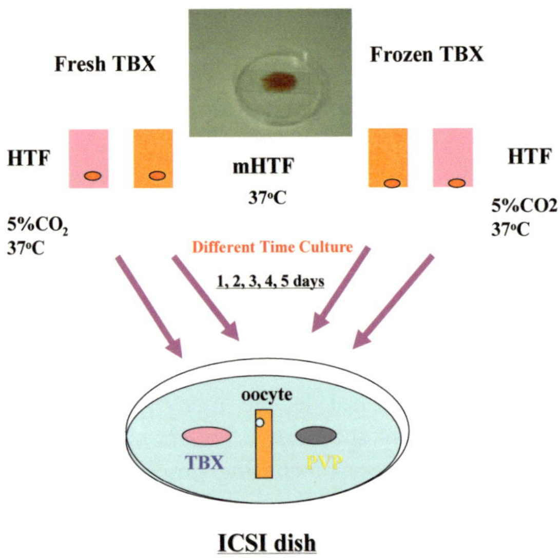

Fig. 1. Procedure for culture of testicular biopsy tissue in two media (mHTF and HTF). Minced tissues were divided into two parts and were cultured in HTF with CO2 incubation or mHTF without CO2 incubation. After one to 5 days of culture, motile sperm numbers were compared.

Our result indicates that either fresh or frozen-thawing testicular biopsy tissue is cultured slightly better in HTF medium under 5% CO_2 at 37°C than in mHTF medium at 37°C, but there was no significant difference (Table 1). Our further experiment showed that after 24 hour *in vitro* culture, the number of motile sperm increases remarkably, with a maximum motility rate seen between 48-72 hours of culture (Figure 2). Motile spermatozoa still are observed up to 120 hours in culture (Wu et al., 2005). Based on our research and clinical practice, it appears that the optimal time for ICSI using testicular sperm is after 24-48 hours of culture. This may allow the testicular biopsy procedure to be performed 1 or 2 days before oocyte retrieval and provides flexibility in scheduling these procedures in clinical practice.

Culture Time	0 hr	24 hrs	48 hrs	72 hrs	96 hrs	120 hrs
HTF medium	2.1 ±2	9.0±7.2	15.0±6.5	35.0±15.3	25.4 ±11	15.0±9.3
mHTF medium	2.0±2	7.5±6.5	12.0±7.6	31.0 ±17.2	23.0±12	13.0 ±9.9

Note: At 0 hour, the initial motile sperm from collecting biopsy tissue just display twitching tail. After culture, some movement sperm were observed at different time. Motile sperm numbers in HTF medium are slightly higher than in mHTF medium, but there is no significant statistic difference (P>0.05).

Table 1. Effect of *in vitro* culture of testicular tissue in two media on sperm motility

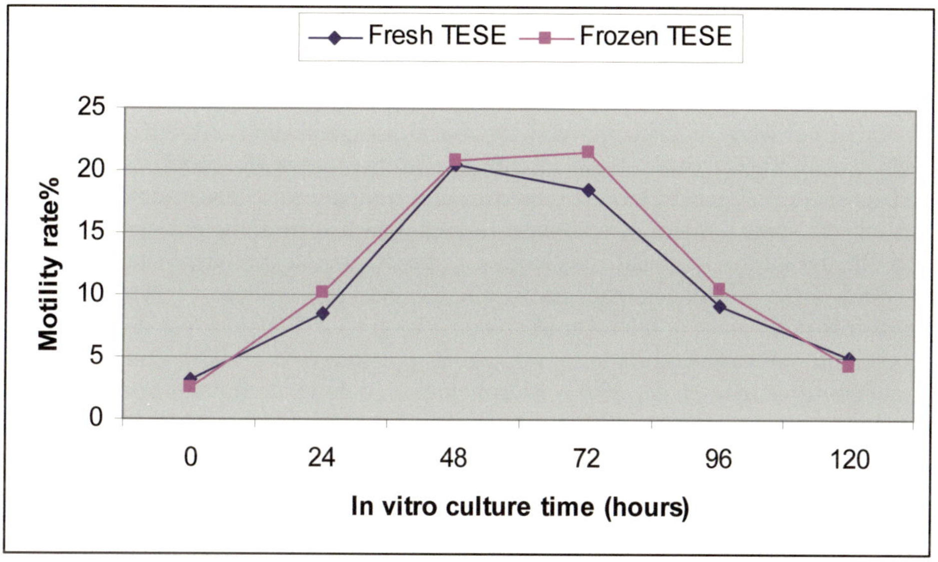

Fig. 2. Effect of *in vitro* culture time of TESE on sperm motility.

4.3 Cryopreservation of testicular biopsy tissue

Open surgical testicular biopsy is an invasive intervention. Cryopreservation of the testicular biopsy specimen can avoid repeated testicular biopsies in azoospermic patients in whom the only source of spermatozoa is the biopsy. Cryopreservation of testicular sperm using a simple freezing protocol is promising in patients with obstructive and non-obstructive azoospermia augmenting the overall success achieved after surgical sperm retrieval (Friedle et al., 1997). Also, when the frozen-thawed testicular spermatozoa were cultured for 48 hours, sperm motility showed a significant improvement (Figure 2). Our studies indicate that frozen-thawed TESE specimen displayed similar motility to fresh TESE samples during *in vitro* culture. After 24 hours of culture, frozen-thawed TESE samples also showed an increased number of motile sperm. We did not observed a significant detrimental effect of freezing on testicular sperm survival in most specimens. However, we did observe freezing damage to other cells including spermatids and germ cells. The freezing protocol using test yolk buffer containing glycerol (Irvine Scientific, Santa Ana, CA) is simple, practical and provides reliable sperm survival. We therefore would recommend cryopreservation of all testicular biopsy specimens routinely in IVF clinical practice.

In summary, freezing and *in vitro* maturation culture of testicular biopsy specimens are useful approaches to the management of testicular biopsy samples from both obstructive and non-obstructive azoospermic patients. These techniques offer the possibility of several attempts at IVF/ICSI from single testicular biopsy sample. One to three days of *in vitro* culture for fresh and frozen samples before an oocyte retrieval may increase the availability of motile spermatozoa for ICSI. Testicular biopsy freezing and subsequent culture may be a reliable alternative for patients to undergo testicular biopsy surgery prior to oocyte retrieval, allowing for flexibility in scheduling patients for clinical procedures.

5. Treatment for globozoospermia

Globozoospermia, found in <0.1% of infertile male patients, results in the inability of the sperm to fertilize an oocyte. Globozoospermia is an uncommon sperm disorder associated with infertility and is also a severe form of teratozoospermia, characterized by round-headed sperm with an absence of acrosome vesicles and a disorganization of the midpiece and tail (Holstein *et al.* 1973). Sigh et al., (1992) described different types of globozoospermia with 100% affected sperm or only partial teratozoospermia and complete lack of acrosome and spherical nucleus or with some remains of acrosome vesicles detached from the nucleus. Transmission electron micrographs of spermatozoon from a globozoospermic man demonstrate the typical round head, large vacuolated regions within the nucleus, absence of acrosome and an abnormal mid-piece and tail (Stone et al., 2000, Dam et al., 2007). Nuclear damage was also described with abnormal chromatin packaging (Larson *et al.*, 2001) and mitochondria abnormalities (Battaglia *et al.*, 1997). Morphological defects in human sperm cells raise suspicion for further anomalies within the sperm cell and could have implications in clinical practice. Recently, Dam et al., (2007) reviewed and summarized the phenotypic manifestations, and possible causes of the condition as well as implications for clinical practice of globozoospermia, as a prerequisite for genetic analysis. In globozoospermia, there is an absence of acrosomal structures leading to absence of spermatozoa binding to the zone pellucida. Thus, ICSI is an only treatment option for these patients, but poor fertilization and only few baby births have been reported since the first live-birth from globozoospermia was reported in 1995 (Trokoudes et al., 1995). This poor fertilization rate can probably be explained by abnormal oocyte activation (Battaglia *et al.*, 1997; Nardo *et al.*, 2002). Low fertilization rates after ICSI indicate that these sperm do not have an ability to activate the oocyte. Thus, various oocyte activation methods including conventional ICSI sucking ooplasm or calcium ionophore have been used with some pregnancies and live births have been reported (Rybouchkin et al., 1996; Eldar-Geva, et al., 2003). However, some cases have reported normal live-births after intracytoplasmic sperm injection for globozoospermia without assisted oocyte activation (Stone et al., 2000; Banker et al., 2009). Generally speaking, the use of the ICSI technique in conjuncture oocyte activation may allow the globozoospermic patient to realize their dream to have a baby, however low fertilization and pregnancy rates seriously influence the overall success. Also, the use of these sperm does not appear to increase abortion, miscarriage rates or aneuploid / birth defects in the offspring of such men (Dam et al. 2007). Currently in clinical IVF practice, the only treatment option in these cases is ICSI, although repeated treatment cycles can be performed and no apparent predictors of success have been identified.

6. Selection of spermatids

In some azoospermic men, even though extensive surgical techniques such as microepididymal sperm aspiration (MESA), fine needle aspiration (FNA), testicular sperm extraction (TESE) and testicular sperm aspiration (TESA) have been used, no spermatozoa can be found. Thus, many attempts have been made to develop new techniques of assisted fertilization using immature male germ cells. Some studies have showed that spermatids can be efficiently used as substitute gametes because of their high fertilizing ability comparable with that of mature sperm (Al-Hasani et al, 1999; Mansour et al., 2003). This technique is an exciting breakthrough in treatment of the infertile man with azoospermia. Spermatids are immature haploid germ cells that have not yet undergone the biochemical and morphological changes that accompany spermiogenesis through to the formation of spermatozoa. Morphologically, the shaping of the mammalian sperm involves the elongation and condensation of the spermatid nucleus, the development of the acrosome, and the transient appearance of the microtubular manchette, thus spermatids may display round or elongate shapes (Kierszenbaum et al., 2007). The elongating and elongated spermatids seem to have an advanced development compared with round spermatids. At this developmental stage, the elongating spermatids are easy to recognize among the other cell types in a wet preparation (Figure 3). Men with non-obstructive azoospermia can be treated by using intra-oocyte round spermatid injection (ROSI) or elongated spermatid injection (ELSI). It has been suggested that spermatids should be injected intact and that elongated spermatids are preferred to round spermatids where possible (Fishel, 1995). Spermatids can be retrieved from semen or from testis biopsy tissue before the final stage of spermatogenesis and the formation of sperm (Figure 3). The nucleus of these cells contains half the number of the chromosomes, thus may be injected directly into oocytes. The fertilization rate was not different between round and elongated spermatids, although the fertilization rates for round and elongated spermatids in the ejaculate were 33 and 18% respectively, compared with 22 and 38% respectively when testicular spermatids were utilized (Fishel et al., 1997). However, multiple comparisons have shown that spermatozoa and elongated spermatids gave better implantation and birth rates than did round spermatids, while spermatozoa and elongated spermatozoa were indistinguishable in their ability to support embryonic development (Ogonuki et al., 2010). Since the first baby was born as a result of spermatid injection (Tesarik et al., 1995), many healthy babies have been born using spermatid injection. In the past few years, our IVF center has injected round spermatids to five patients' oocytes and a health boy was born in 2007. A typical case was that 6 oocytes were retrieved from a 23 age woman and only 4 matured oocytes were injected with her husband's round spermatids from fresh testicular biopsy tissue in April 2006. One egg displayed normal two pronuclei and another egg was abnormal three pronuclei. Other two were unfertilized oocytes. On day 3, only normal fertilized embryo at 6-cell stage was transferred and finally a boy was born in February of 2007. Our clinical practice provides experienced diagnosis that when normal living spermatozoa or elongated spermatids cannot be found in the testicular biopsy specimen, round spermatids can be used successfully and result in the delivery of healthy offspring. However, the fertilization rate with round spermatid injection is relative low and only young couples may be good candidates successful for pregnancy.

Although spermatids may be used in azoospermic patients as a treatment option for their infertility, its efficiency is questionable because low fertilization and pregnancy rates influence seriously its success (Sousa et al., 1998; Akhondi et al., 2003). One major question facing spermatid use may be associated with problems related to incomplete nuclear protein maturation. Accordingly, many investigators are interested in spermatid *in vitro* culture and

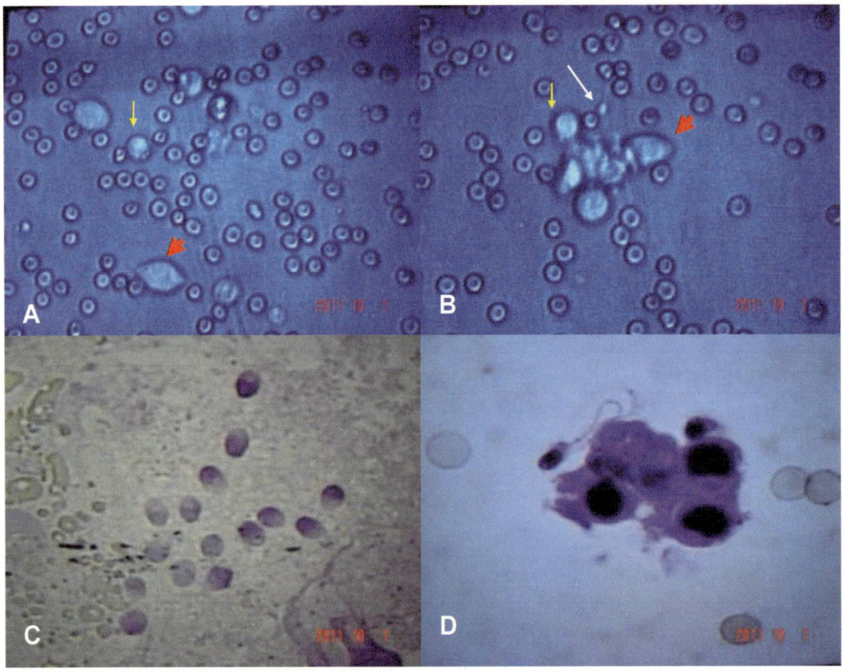

Fig. 3. Spermatids and global sperm in the testicular biopsy tissue. Figure A and B indicate unstained testicular biopsy tissue and red and yellow arrows indicate elongated and round spermatids, respectively. White arrow indicates a spermatozoon. The round cells are blood cells. Figure C and D are stained slides with Testsimplets®. Global sperm without tail could be observed (C) and spermatids and a spermatozoon were seen in D.

an attempt to find the appropriate medium that could successfully mature round spermatids up to the elongated stage *in vitro* or even to mature spermatozoa at a reasonable rate (Cremades et al., 1999). Also, the research on *in vitro* culturing of round spermatids should study the optimum temperature for maturation, the reason why spermatogenesis *in vitro* seems accelerated, and whether the whole spermatogenic population can be used instead of isolated cells (Tesarik et al., 2000; Amarin et al, 2002). In our TESE culture experiments, a few round spermatids displayed a slight shape changes after 24 to 48 hour culture, but we can not determine whether this culture may promote round spermatids to become elongated spermatids because we did not track individual spermatid growth. Although some reports indicated that round spermatids can develop flagellum and elongate after *in vitro* culture under special media (Aslam and Fishel, 1999), we suggest that selecting optimally shaped spermatids without membrane damage for oocyte injection seems to be an important factor in achieving fertilization. In spite of the fact that *in vitro* culture of round spermatids is a promising approach, we recommend that before using *in vitro* matured spermatids for clinical trials, these cells should be firstly examined to verify if they are viable (Trypan Blue exclusion staining), if they contain normal chromosomal [fluorescent in-situ hybridization (FISH)], if they are able to fertilize oocytes (experimental injections and determination of normal fertilization and cleavage rates), and if the embryos produced are genetically normal by FISH. Injection of a live spermatid into an oocyte will increase the fertilization opportunity, but identification of a live spermatid is difficult. Thus, choosing optimally shaped cells may be helpful in distinguishing live spermatids from most cells in testicular biopsy specimens by simply respecting the criteria of cell size and detecting the presence of a round nucleus surrounded by a rim of cytoplasm in wet preparations with Hoffman optics (Figure 3; Silber et al., 2000).

As described above, spermatids have a nuclear protein immature statue, but activated oocyte cytoplasm may induce nuclear protein maturation after injecting spermatid to oocyte intracytoplasm. Thus, oocyte activation is very important for spermatid injection. Oocytes can be activated before or during injection in order to destroy maturation promoting factor (MPF) by various artificial treatments such as physically vigorous ooplasmic aspiration during injection, electrical pulses and injection of oscillin, and chemically calcium ionophores or ethanol stimulation. In fact, treatment of spermatid injected oocytes with inophore A 23187 has been shown the increase of the fertilization rate and has resulted in the birth of a healthy child with ROSI (Ahmady & Michael 2007). Based on our clinic practice, we suggest that the spermatid membrane should be broken by injection pipette when it is placed in oocyte cytoplasm without other oocyte activation. A round spermatid is 7-8μm in diameter and has a round shape with smooth outlines. When these spermatids are selected for injection into an oocyte, a same size (7-8μm) pipette in inner diameter may be used. Using this technique, the spermatid is aspirated into the pipette and the spermatid membrane can be broken by pipette squeezing when it is pushed out of the pipette. This simple technique may greatly increase spermatid fertilization.

7. Use of secondary spermatocytes

Round or elongated cytoplasmic spermatid injection can result in the delivery of normal offspring in human IVF, but it is sometimes difficult to distinguish Hoffman optics whether they are haploid round spermatids, diploid spermatocytes, spermatogonia, or even somatic cells like Sertoli cell nuclei or Leydig cells. Can we consider the use of immature spermatogenic germ cells for fertilization? Based on our understanding of the oocyte maturation mechanism, oocyte maturation arrests at the meiosis II stage because the mammalian oocyte contains two key factors: metaphase-promoting factor (MPF) and cytostatic factor (CSF), in which the c-Mos proto-oncoprotein is a major component (Wu et al, 1997a,b). These two key factors are active in the oocyte cytoplasm and maintain the chromosomes of mature oocytes in metaphase of the second meiotic division. When the oocyte is activated by the above-mentioned methods, the degradation of c-Mos onco-protein causes CSF and MPF inactivity in the cytoplasm and the chromosomes of injected spermatid or spermatozoon as well as the oocyte begin condensation, which leads to halploidization of both chromosome sets and forms formal fertilized zygotes. However, when immature diploid spermatocytes are injected into oocytes, oocyte activation should be absent. Thus, the injected cell nucleus is exposed to MPF and CSF environment in which MPF and CSF may induce injected cell nucleus to enter metaphase stage as the same way as does the oocyte nucleus. (Tesarik, 1996). If the oocyte is activated, the disappearance of MPF and CSF activity will lead the injected cell nucleus to undergo condensation and to complete meiosis and form a haploid chromosome set. Thus, the premature chromosome condensation of injected cells occurring in the absence of oocyte activation is essential for achieving fertilization with secondary spermataocytes (Kimura and Yanagimachi 1995).

8. Adult somatic cell induction

Using the same theory and technique, somatic cells also may be induced into a haploid chromosome set by immature or mature oocytes (Tesarik 2002; Keefer 2007; Neri et al., 2009) because some important materials of germinal vesicle oocyte is essential for cell nucleus remodeling (Gao et al., 2002). In our preliminary animal experiments, a bovine cumulus cell from ovary follicular fluid was injected into an enucleated oocyte. After 24 hour *in vitro* culture, injected cell nuclei were stained by Hoechst 33258 and two separated chromosome sets were observed using fluorescence microscopy (Figure 4A). After two sets of chromosome were taken out by manipulation, their chromosome numbers were counted. Adult cattle have 60 diploid chromosomes. After induction, each set contains 30 chromosomes (Figure 4B and 4C). Thus, the immature oocyte can induce successfully somatic cells to become haploid. When the haploid nucleus is moved out of the induced matured oocyte and transferred into a normal female oocyte, using electro-fusion activation, both the oocyte nucleus and the injected male nucleus begin condensation to form a similar zygote which develops into an embryo for transfer (Figure 5).

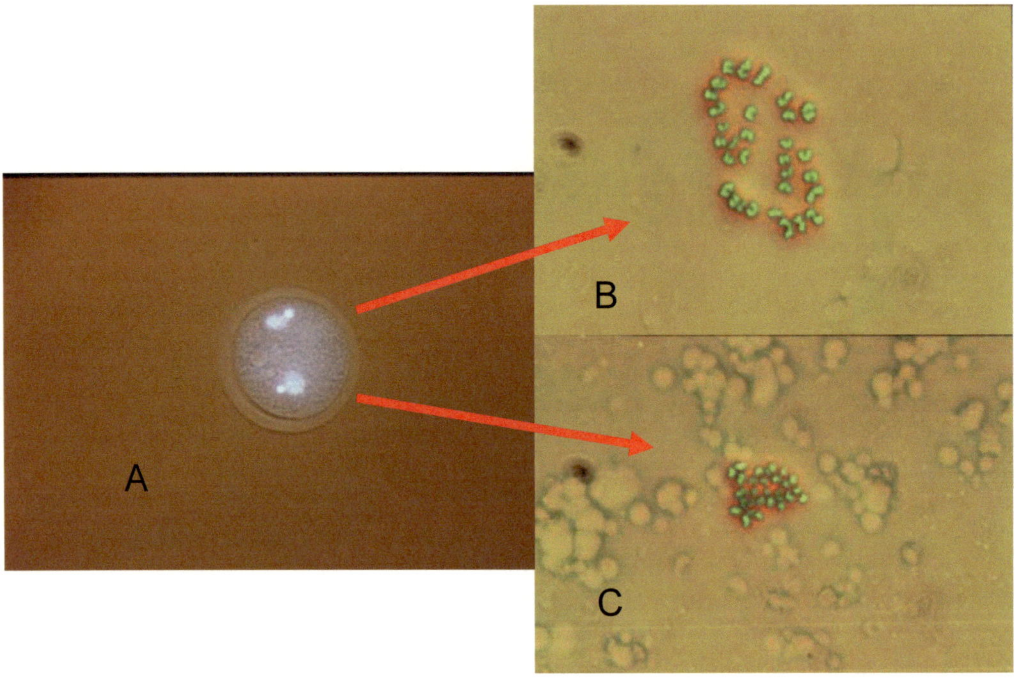

Fig. 4. Preliminary experiments of using an oocyte to induce somatic cell chromosomes into a haploid chromosome set. A single bovine cumulus cell was injected into an enucleated immature oocyte. After 24 hour *in vitro* culture, injected cell nuclei were stained by Hoechst 33258 and two chromosome sets were observed using fluorescence microscopy (blue color, A). After each chromosome set was separated by manipulation, 30 chromosomes were counted in each set (green color, B and C). Authors greatly appreciate Dr. Bin Wang's courtesy unpublished photos.

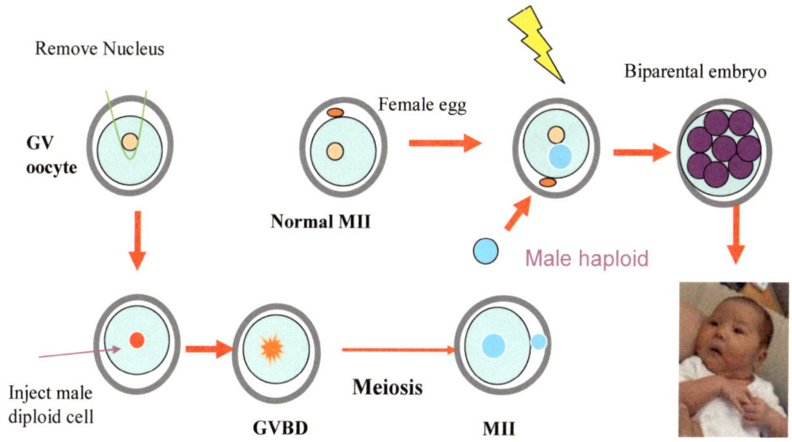

Fig. 5. Scenario for using immature oocytes to induce male somatic cell complete meiosis. The nucleus of the immature oocyte is removed and a male diploid cell was injected into the enucleated oocyte. After completing meiotic division, the induced haploid nucleus was transferred into a normal female mature oocyte to form a biparental embryo for transfer.

9. Sperm cell cloning

In some men with oligozoospermia and azoospermia, occasionally a single viable sperm may be found in their semen and/or testicular biopsy tissue. Therefore, such a sperm is precious to couples wishing to conceive. How can this single sperm be utilized to help patients realize their dream of having a baby? If only one sperm is found, we must be reluctant to use it for anything but fertilization. As described above, because the cytoplasm of oocyte may induce heterogonous cell nucleus condensation, we may try to inject a sperm into an enucleated oocyte to observe sperm nucleus kinetics (Jones et al., 2010; Ogonuki et al., 2010). Recent studies demonstrated possibility of artificially replicating a single sperm genome, which could help men with very low sperm counts become fathers. This is called "cloning of sperm cells or male genome cloning" (Figure 6). With this technique it should be possible to create enough sperm nuclei to ensure that produced and implanted embryo is healthy. The cloning of sperm cells has been practiced on mice by injecting a mouse sperm into a mouse oocyte which had its nucleus removed (Hopkin, 2007). The sperm may form a single male pronucleus in this enucleated oocyte by egg activation and electrofused. The haploid zygote may become cleaved embryos. When the resulting embryo develops to 4 to 8 cells, each blastomere may be separated by a specific solution (Figure 6). The process worked well in almost all cases and the produced blastomere from original sperm was found to be chromosomally identical to its originator in over 80% of the clones analyzed. Then, the resulting cells were fused with a normal egg that had been previously chemically activated. Based on this technique, Dr. Palermo's research group created 64 blastocyst embryos and implanted them into 6 host mother mice resulting in only 4 developed into normal baby mice (Takeuchi et al., 2008). This offspring born as a result of such replication had shown a level of abnormalities consistent with that shown in cloned animals. This technique provides a new hope for azoospermic men to have a child, but we are a long way from the time when this will be able to be used in humans (Takeuchi et al., 2008). There is much work still needed to be done to understand why impaired development and abnormalities in the embryo occur, and to take steps to avoid that occurrence (Neri et al., 2009).

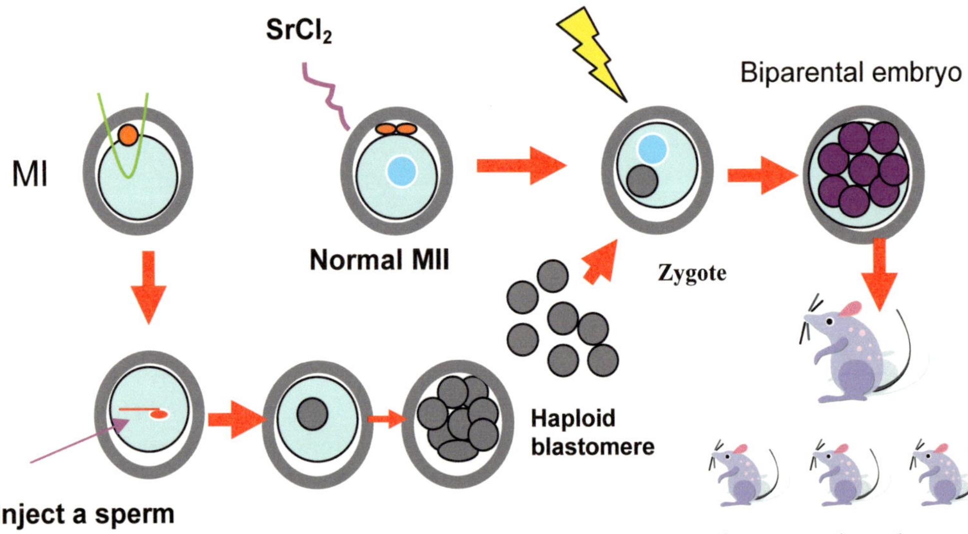

Fig. 6. Scenario for sperm genome cloning. A single sperm is injected into enucleated oocyte and this oocyte goes through a parthenogenesis process to become a 4-8 cell haploid embryo. A single blastomere is transferred into a normal mature oocyte to form a zygote. The developed embryos are transferred to recipient mice to deliver offspring.

10. Artificial sperm production

Development of embryo stem cell technology has resulted in a breakthrough for artificial sperm production (Ogawa, 2008). In the last decade, many research groups have attempted to re-create the process of sperm production in the laboratory using stem cells as the starting material, especially using mice as an animal model. In 2003, American scientists successfully coaxed embryonic stem cells from mice to mature into primitive sperm, which were then injected into eggs to form normal embryos. This "artificial sperm" capable of fertilizing an egg has been created in the laboratory for the first time in an experiment that could bring an end to male infertility. In 2005, British scientists took a step towards showing that the human egg and sperm could be created from stem cells and in 2009, this human sperm have been created from stem cells in world first from British university (Alleyne, 2009). This is the first time human sperm has been created anywhere in the world in a laboratory. However, the experiment has proved controversial, threatening to reopen the fierce debate over embryo research. Recently, Japanese researchers were able to turn mouse embryonic stem cells into early sperm cells called primordial germ cells (PGCs) and successfully implanted early sperm cells which were made from the stem cells into infertile mice, which after the treatment were able to produce healthy offspring (Hayashi et al., 2011).

The procedure of artificial sperm production was successfully repeated using another type of embryonic cell that was manipulated into a stem cell state. These stem cells are known as induced pluripotent stem (iPS) cells and have previously been created from a variety of different starting cells, including skin cells. Male embryonic stem cells with green protein makers may be selected and extracted from mouse embryos. These embryonic stem cells are a type of cell that has the ability to differentiate into any of the specialized cell types that make up the body. Under a given condition, the embryonic stem cells are induced to develop into a particular type of cell, called "primordial germ cell-like cells or PGCs". Primordial germ cells go on to form germ cells, which then produce sperm. Then the primordial germ cell-like cells were transplanted into the testes of mice that lacked their own germ cells. When these cells develop into sperm, they may be extracted from testes and injected into normal mouse oocytes. The embryos produced were transferred into female mice so that healthy offspring were born. This study has huge implications for furthering our understanding of how sperm are made, but may also one day lead to a clinical application whereby we could make sperm for infertile men. In next ten years, we believe that this technique could also be used to allow infertile couples without any sperm and spermatids to have children that are genetically their own. It could even be possible to create sperm from female stem cells, which would ultimately mean a woman having a baby without a man.

11. Conclusions

Exciting advances in male infertility have introduced innovative therapeutic options. This is mainly attributed to the success of the ICSI technique rapidly gaining popularity among infertile couples and advanced surgical testicular sperm retrieval techniques in azoospermic men, which offer infertile couples, including those with no sperm (azoospermia) in their ejaculate due to genetic conditions, a greatly improved chance to conceive their own biological offspring. Currently, despite severe male factor infertility, pregnancy may still be achieved by current developed technology. As the ICSI technique further improves, a single good morphologic and functional spermatozoon may be selected by IMSI or PICSI methods and an improved embryo implantation and pregnancy rate will be obtained. Testicular biopsy seems to be one of the most feasible techniques obtaining spermatozoa for azoospermic men because a single biopsy of testis may provide either spermatozoa if the specimen contains sperm or spermatids if biopsy tissues do not contain any sperm for ICSI. Using testis biopsy sperm for azoospermia may gain the same high pregnancy rate as the normal ejaculation sperm, but efficiency of spermatid application is doubted because low fertilization and pregnancy rates influence seriously its success. As cell cloning technology develops, other options for treatment of azoospermic men include use of secondary spermataocytes, sperm cell cloning, and artificial sperm production by inducing stem cells and adult somatic cells into sperm cells. Although these technologies still remain at animal research stage and demonstrate a low efficiency, we believe that application of these novel techniques will greatly improve chance for infertile couples (particular azoospermic men) to conceive their own biological offspring in the next decade.

12. References

Ahmady A, Michael E (2007) Successful pregnancy and delivery following intracytoplasmic injection of frozen-thawed non-viable testicular sperm and oocyte activation with calcium ionosphere. *J Androl* 28:13-14.

Akhondi MA, Sedighi MA, Amirjannati N, Sadri-Ardekani H (2003) Use of spermatide for treatment of non-obstructive azoospermic patients. *J Reprod Infertil* 4(3):177-183.

Al-Hasani S, Ludwig M, Palermo I, Küpker W, Sandmann J, Johannisson R, Fornara P, Sturm R, Bals-Pratsch M, Bauer O, Diedrich K (1999) Intracytoplasmic injection of round and elongated spermatids from azoospermic patients: results and review. *Hum Reprod* Suppl 1:97-107

Alleyne R, Science Correspondent 7:01AM BST 08 Jul 2009 Human sperm created from stem cells in world first, claims British university *The Telgraph* 08 Jul 2009.

Amarin ZO, Jamal HS, Rouzi AA (2002) Successful pregnancy after round spermatid microinjection. *Saudi Medical Journal* 23 (1): 113-114.

Angelopoulos T, Adler A, Krey L, Licciardi f, Noyes, McCullough A (1999) Enhancement or initiation of testicular sperm motility by in vitro culture of testicular tissue. *Fertil Steril* 71(2): 240-243.

Arakil Y, Ogawa S, Ohnol M, Moshizawa m, Araki S, Aslam I, Fishel S. (1999) Successful metaphase chromosome analysis of human elongated spermatids using mouse oocytes. *Mol Hum Reprod* 5 (8): 784-787.

Aslam I, Fishel S (1999) Evaluation of the fertilization potential of freshly isolated, in-vitro cultured and cryopreserved human spermatids by injection into hamster oocytes. *Hum Reprod* 14 (6): 1528-1533.

Banker MR, Patel PM, Joshi BV, Shah PB, Goyal B. Successful pregnancies and a live birth after intracytoplasmic sperm injection in globozoospermia *J Hum Reprod Sci* 2009, 2: 81-82.

Battaglia DE, Koehler JK, Klein NA and Tucker MJ (1997): Failure of oocyte activation after intracytoplasmic sperm injection using round-headed sperm. *Fertil Steril* 68,118–122.

Berger DS, AbdelHafez F, Russell H, Goldfarb J, Desai N (2011) Severe teratozoospermia and its influence on pronuclear morphology, embryonic cleavage and compaction. *Reprod Biol Endocrinol* 9: 37

Comhaire F, Vermenlen L (1995) Human semen analysis. *Hum Reprod Update* 1:343-362.

Cornell Physicians (2011) Male infertility/sperm retrieval techniques. www.cornellurology.com/infertility/srt/icsi.shtml

Cremades N, Bernabeu R, Barros A, Sousa (1999) In-vitro maturation of round spermatids using co-culture on Vero cells. *Hum Reprod* 14 (5): 1287-1293.

Dam AH, Feenstra I, Westphal JR, Ramos L, van Golde RJ, Kremer JA (2007) Globozoospermia revisited. *Hum Reprod Update* 13:63-75.

Eldar-Geva, T, Brooks B, Margalioth EJ, Zylber-Haran E, Gal M, Silber, SJ (2003). Successful pregnancy and delivery after calcium ionophore oocyte activation in a normozoospermic patient with previous repeated failed fertilization after intracytoplasmic sperm injection *Fertil Steril* 79(suppl. 3):1656-1658

Fishel S, Green S, Hunter A, Lisi F, Rinaldi L, Lisi R, McDermott H (1997) Human fertilization with round and elongated spermatids. *Hum Reprod* 12 (2): 336-340.

Friedler S, Raziel A, Soffer Y, Strassburger D, Komarovsky D, Ron-EI R (1997) Introcytoplamic injection of fresh and cryopreserved testicular spermatozoa in patients with non-obstructive azoospermia: A comparative study. *Fertil Steril* 68:892-897.

Gao S, Gasperrini B, Mcgarry M, Ferrier T, Fletcher J, Harkness L, De Sousa P, Wilmut I (2002) Germinal Vesicle Material Is Essential for Nucleus Remodeling after Nuclear Transfer. *Biol Reprod* 67(3):928-934.

Girardi SK, Schlegel PN (1996) Microsurgical epididymal sperm aspiration: Review of techniques, preoperative considerations, and results. *J Androl* 1:5-9.

Hayashi K, Ohta H, Kurimoto K, Aramaki S, Saitoou M (2011) Reconstitution of the mouse germ cell specification pathway in culture by pluripotent stem cells. *Cell* 146:519-532.

Holstein AF, Schirren CG, Schirren C, Mauss J (1973) Round headed spermatozoa: A cause of male infertility. *Dtsch Med Wochenschr* 98:61-2.

Hopkin M (2007) Mice born from cloned sperm Technique raises hopes for infertile men. Published online 3 July 2007 | *Nature* | doi:10.1038/news070702-8 http://www.nature.com/news/2007/070702/full/news070702-8.html

Jones EL, Mudrak O, Zalensky AO (2010) Kinetics of human male pronuclear development in a heterologous ICSI model. *J Assist Reprod Genet* 27(6): 277–283.

Jow WW, Steckel J, Schlegel PN, Magid MS, Goldstein M (1993) Motile sperm in human testis biopsy specimens. *J Androl* 14:194-198.

Keefer Cl, (2008) Lessons learned from nuclear transfer (cloning). Theriogenology 69(1):48-54.

Kierszenbaum AL, Rivkin E, Tres LL (2007) Molecular biology of sperm head shaping. *Soc Reprod Fertil* Suppl. 65:33-43.

Kimura Y, Yanagimachi R (1995) Development of normal mice from injected with secondary spermatocytes nuclei. *Biol Reprod* 53:855-852.

Larson KL, Brannian JD, Singh NP, Burbach JA, Jost LK, Hansen KP, Kreger DO, Evenson DP (2001) Chromatin structure in globozoospermia: a case report. *J Androl* 22,424–431

Maggiulli R, Neri QV, Monahan D, Hu J, Takeuchi T, Rosenwaks Z, Palermo GD (2010) What to do when ICSI fails. *Syst Biol Reprod Med* 6(5):376-87.

Mansour RT, Fahmy IM, Taha AK, Tawab NA, Serour HI, Aboulghar MA (2003) Intracytoplasmic spermatid injection can result in the delivery of normal offspring. *J Andrology* 24(5):

Matthews GJ, Goldstein M (1996) A simplified method of epididymal sperm aspiration. *Urology* 47:123-125.

Nagy Z, Liu J, Cecile J, Silber s, Devroey P, Van Steirteghem A (1995) Using ejaculated, fresh and frozen-thawed epididymal and testicular spermatozoa gives rise to comparable results after intracytoplasmic sperm injection. *Fertil Steril* 63:808-815.

Nardo LG, Sinatra F, Bartoloni G, Zafarana S and Nardo F (2002) Ultrastructural features and ICSI treatment of severe teratozoospermia: report of two human cases of globozoospermia. *Eur J Obstet Gynecol Reprod Biol* 104:40–42.

Neri QV, Takeuchi T, Rosenwaks Z, Palermo GD (2009): Treatment options for impaired spermatogenesis: germ cell transplantation and stem-cell based therapy. *Minerva Ginecol* 61(4):253-9

Ogawa T (2008) Reproductive stem cell research and its application to urology. *International Journal of Urology* 15(2):121–127.

Ogonuki N, Mori M, Shinmen A, Inoue K, Mochida K (2010) The effect on intracytoplasmic sperm injection outcome of genotype, male germ cell stage and freeze-thawing in mice. *PLoS ONE* 5(6): e11062. doi:10.1371/journal.pone.0011062

Palermo G, Joris H, Devroey P, Van Steirteghem AC (1992) Pregnancies after intracytoplasmic injection of a single spermatozoon into an oocyte. *Lancet* 340:17-18.

Parmegiani L, Cognigni GE, Bernardi S, Troilo E, Ciampaglia W, Filicori M (2010a) "Physiologic ICSI": Hyaluronic acid (HA) favors selection of spermatozoa without DNA fragmentation and with normal nucleus, resulting in improvement of embryo quality. *Fertil Steril* 93: 598-604

Parmegiani L, Cognigni GE, Ciampaglia W, Pocognoli P, Marchi F, Filicori M (2010b) Efficiency of hyaluronic acid (HA) sperm selection. *J Assist Reprod Genet* 27(1):13-6

Pühse G, Hense J, Bergmann M, Kliesch S (2011): Bilateral histological evaluation of exocrine testicular function in men with obstructive azoospermia: condition of spermatogenesis and andrological implications? *Human Reprod* 26(10):2606-2612

Rybouchkin A, Dozortsev D, Pelinck MJ, De Sutter P, Dhont M (1996) Analysis of the oocyte activating capacity and chromosomal complement of round-headed human spermatozoa by their injection into mouse oocytes. *Hum Reprod* 11:2170-5.

Said TM, Land JA (2011) Effects of advanced selection methods on sperm quality and ART outcome: a systematic review. *Hum Reprod Update* doi: 10.1093/humupd/dmr032 First published online: August 25, 2011

Schlegel PN, Palermo GD, Goldstein M (1997) Testicular sperm extraction with ICSI for non-obstructive azoospermia. *Urology* 49:435-440.

Sheynkin YR, Schlegel PN (1997) Sperm retrieval for assisted reproductive technologies. *Contemporary OB/GYN* 15:113-129.

Silber S, Johnson L, Verheyen G, Van Steirteghem A (2000) Round spermatid injection. *Fert Sterit* 73:897-900.

Silber SJ, Nagy ZP, Liu J et al. (1994) Conventional in-vitro fertilization versus intracytoplamic sperm injection for patients requiring microsurgical sperm aspiration. *Hum Reprod* 9:1705-1709

Singh G (1992) Ultrastructural features of round-headed human spermatozoa. *Int J Fertil* 37:99–102.

Sousa M, Barros A, Tesarik J (1998) Current problems with spermatid conception. *Human Reprod* 13(2):255-258.

Stone S, O'Mahony F, Khalaf Y, Taylor A and Braude P (2000) A normal livebirth after intracytoplasmic sperm injection for globozoospermia without assisted oocyte activation: case report. *Hum Reprod* 15,139–141.

Takahashi K, Uchida A, Kitao M (1990) Hypoosmotic swelling test of sperm. *Arch Androl* 25(3):225-42.

Takeuchi T, Neri QV, Palermo GD (2008) Male gamete empowerment. *Ann NY Acad Sci* 1127:64-6

Tesarik J (1996) Fertilization of oocytes by injecting spermatozoa, spermatids and spermatocytes. *Review of Reproduction* 1:149-152.

Tesarik J (2002) Reproductive semi-cloning respecting biparental embryo origin: Embryos from syngamy between a gamete and a haploidized somatic cell. *Hum Reprod* 17 (8): 1933-1937.

Tesarik J, Mendoza C, GrecoE (2000) Immature germ cell conception ± in vitro germ cell manipulation. *BaillieÁre's Clinical Endocrinology and Metabolism* 14(3):437-452.

Tesarik J, Mendoza C, Testart J (1995) Viable embryos from injection of round spermatids into oocytes. *New England Journal of Medicine* 333:525.

Trokoudes KM, Danos N, Kalogirou L, Vlachou R, Lysiotis T, Georghiades N, Lerios S and Kyriacou K (1995) Pregnancy with spermatozoa from a globozoospermic man after intracytoplasmic sperm injection treatment. *Hum Reprod* 10,880–882.

WHO (2010) WHO laboratory manual for the examination and processing of human semen. Fifth Edition, World Health Organization, Switzerland, Page 223.

Worrilow KC, Eid S, Matthews J, Pelts E, Khoury C, Liebermann J (2010) Multi-site clinical trial evaluating PICSI®, a method for selection of hyaluronan bound sperm (HBS) for use in ICSI: improved clinical outcomes. *Human Reprod* 25(suppl 1): 6-9.

Wu B, Ignotz G, Currie WB, Yang X(1997a) Dynamics of maturation-promoting factor and its constituent protein during in vitro maturation of bovine oocytes. *Boil Reprod* 56:253-259.

Wu B, Ignotz G, Currie WB, Yang X(1997b) Expression of Mos proto-oncoprotein in bovine oocytes during maturation in vitro. *Biol Reprod* 56: 260-265.

Wu B, Wong D, Lu S, Dickstein S, Silver M, Gelety T (2005) Optimal use of fresh and frozen-thawed testicular sperm for intracytoplasmic sperm injection in azoospermic patients. *J Assist Reprod Genet* 22: 389-394.

Part 4

Embryo Transfer Technology

9

Increasing Pregnancy by Improving Embryo Transfer Techniques

Tahereh Madani and Nadia Jahangiri
Endocrinology and Female Infertility Department, Reproductive Biomedicine Research Center, Royan Institute for Reproductive Biomedicine, ACECR, Tehran
Iran

1. Introduction

Embryo transfer (ET) is universally recognized as the final and most critical stage in an in vitro fertilization (IVF) outcome (Neithardt et al., 2005; Ghazzawi et al., 1999). The majority of couples (approximately 80%) who undergo IVF reach the embryo transfer stage, yet few pregnancies occur (Mansour & Aboulghar, 2002; Adamson et al., 2006). Although embryo genetic abnormalities (Munne et al., 1995) and imperfections in uterine receptivity are some important factors which influence implantation, embryo transfer technique may be directly responsible for a lot of unsuccessful embryo implantations. Embryo transfer necessitates the joint attempts of the reproductive biologist and the clinician. Without healthy embryos, embryo transfer will fail. On the other hand, a poor embryo transfer technique often results in embryo implantation failure (Schoolcraft et al., 2001). However, comparatively less attention has been paid to ET techniques than IVF technique (Mansour & Aboulghar, 2002; Schoolcraft et al., 2001). This might be due to misconception of some clinicians in which the type of transfer does not affect the outcome (Schoolcraft et al., 2001). The early researchers recommended that a careful embryo transfer technique is necessary for successful IVF (Meldrum et al., 1987). Recently, many investigators have identified the relationship between IVF outcome and different techniques and they have noted a pregnancy rate of 33.3% for "excellent" transfers, and 10.5% for "poor" transfers (Englert et al., 1986, as cited in Schoolcraft et al., 2001). In this chapter we attempt to review the variables and, techniques that may refine the embryo transfer technique and divide them to the following three stages: before, during, and after embryo transfer.

2. First stage: The preparation before embryo transfer

Variables affecting the pregnancy rate include: evaluation of the cervico-uterine axis, the performance of a dummy or mock transfer, and appropriate evaluation of the uterine cavity (Derks et al., 2009).

2.1 Evaluating the cervico-uterine axis

This evaluation is necessary to ensure suitable embryos placement. It can be undertaken by both dummy embryo transfer and ultrasonography. Both procedures are important for evaluating the direction and length of the uterine cavity and cervical canal. To improve the outcome, it has been suggested that a dummy embryo transfer should be performed prior to the stimulation cycle (Mansour et al., 1990), or just before the actual embryo transfer (Sharif et al., 1995). If this technique is performed close to the time of embryo transfer for example at the time of oocyte retrieval, the pregnancy rate will decrease significantly due to late uterine contractions (Madani et al., 2009a). We previously assessed the appropriate time for evaluation of the cervical axis and uterine measurement. A total of 124 women who underwent IVF treatment were included in our study and divided equally into two groups. Measurement of the uterine cavity length from the external cervical os to the fundus, as well as determination of the cervico-uterine axis, was performed on days 2 or 3 of the menstrual cycle or at the time of oocyte retrieval. Our results indicated a statistically significant difference in clinical pregnancy rates between the two groups (64.2% vs. 35.8%, $P<0.005$). Also, our results showed that the time of measurement affected clinical pregnancy rates in IVF cycles and the best time for uterine measurement is probably on days 2 or 3 of menstruation (Madani et al., 2009a).

2.2 Performing a dummy or mock transfer

Many unexpected agents make entering the uterine cavity difficult, such as cervical polyps or fibroids, a pin-point external os, and cervical deformation due to congenital anomalies or resulting from a previous surgery, all of which can be discovered by a 'dummy' or 'mock' transfer. In the case of cervical stenosis, cervical dilatation should be performed before ovarian stimulation (Mansour & Aboulghar, 2002).

2.3 Appropriate evaluation of the uterine cavity

Assessment of the uterine cavity by ultrasonography prior to the IVF cycle is essential for detecting uterine polyps as well as any fibroids that may be invading the uterine cavity or deformities to the cervical canal (Mansour & Aboulghar, 2002; Niknejadi et al., 2010). Polyps are the most common structural pathologies in the uterine cavity (Isikoglu et al., 2006) which it's incidental finding during ovarian stimulation, in either IVF or intracytoplasmic sperm injection (ICSI) cycles, is a challenge.

Polyp size (Lass et al., 1999; Isikoglu et al., 2006) and location (Yanaihara et al., 2008) may influence the success of embryo implantation during assisted reproductive treatment cycles. According to some research studies, endometrial polyps less than 1.5cm do not negatively influence the pregnancy outcome, whereas increased loss of pregnancy has been reported in others (Lass et al., 1999; Isikoglu et al., 2006). Endometrial damage by endometrial sampling (Barash et al., 2003) or hysteroscopic polypectomy (Varasteh et al., 1999; Spiewankiewicz et al., 2003; Stamatellos et al., 2008) may significantly improve the pregnancy rates. Recently, we reported the outcome of nine women with endometrial polyps less than 1.5 cm after hysteroscopic polypectomy (Madani et al., 2009b). Polypectomy was performed during ovarian stimulation (in eight patients with the standard long protocol) or during hormone replacement therapy (in one donor egg recipient). The interval between polyp resection and embryo transfer was 2-16 days. A relatively high pregnancy rate was noted in our study. One possible mechanism that has been proposed for the improvement of endometrial receptivity following endometrial damage by hysteroscopic polypectomy could be the events related to wound healing. During this process, there is a massive secretion of different cytokines and growth factors, known to play important roles in implantation (Basak et al., 2002). Although several studies have reported good outcomes following hysteroscopic polypectomy during ovarian stimulation in IVF cycles (Batioglu & Kaymak, 2005; Madani et al., 2009b), due to debates over this topic, it is advisable to evaluate the uterine cavity prior to stimulation in order to determine the presence of an existing endometrial pathology.

3. Second stage: Measures during embryo transfer

A great attention has been paid to the embryo transfer technique during IVF. To ensure success, the crucial technique is to deposit embryos in the uterine cavity in the least traumatic manner possible (Mansour et al., 1990). Factors of influencing the pregnancy rate during this stage include (Derks et al., 2009; Schoolcraft et al., 2001) 1) cervical preparation, removal of mucus or blood on the catheter; 2) straightening the utero-cervical angle; 3) ultrasound use; 4) type of catheter; 5) Loading the embryo medium; 6) Embryo load method for transfer; 7) time of embryo transfer with regard to uterine contractions problem; 8) air injection before withdrawal of the embryo transfer catheter (Madani et al., 2010).

3.1 Cervical preparation, and removing the mucus or blood on the catheter

Cervical mucus seems to interfere with embryo entry into the uterus from the transfer catheter. This interference can be caused by excess cervical mucus that cover the transfer catheter and make the injection of the embryos effortless (Visschers et al., 2007). The presence of blood or mucus on the catheter, from tissues trauma, may also reduce implantation rates (Schoolcraft et al., 2001). It has been reported that, while drawing the catheter, cervical mucus may surround the embryos and dislodge them from their original place (Eskandar et al., 2007). Contamination of the catheter tip and uterus by cervical flora is another risk that has been reported to correlate with a lower pregnancy rate (Eskandar et al., 2007; Derks et al., 2009). The endometrial cavity may also be contaminated by cervical mucus. In a study performed by Egbase and colleagues (Egbase et al., 1996), positive cultures of the cervical mucus (70.9%) and catheter tip (49.1%) have been reported. The researchers noted improved clinical pregnancy rates for catheter tip-negative (57.1%) women compared with catheter-tip positive (29.6%) women. Similarly, another investigator has shown that the positive culture has a significant negative impact on transfer outcome (Fanchin et al., 1998a). Also better results may be obtained when vigorous cervical lavage was used prior to embryo transfer to remove all visible mucus (McNamee et al., 1998). Since bacterial contamination from the cervix and pelvic infections (such as pelvic abscesses) has been reported after embryo transfer (Sauer & Paulson, 1992), we cannot give prominence to the careful cleaning of the cervix prior to embryo transfer.

3.2 Straightening the utero-cervical angle

The smooth introduction of the transfer catheter into the uterine cavity can be compromised by the common anteverted uterus, which is found in most women (Sundstrom et al., 1984, as cited in Derks et al., 2009). By straightening the uteru-cervical angle, uterine contractions and insertion trauma will be avoided, thus the embryo transfer success will be much higher. The utero-cervical angle can be straightened by means of following techniques (Derks et al., 2009) 1) distended bladder: a full bladder acts as a useful adjunct for transfer, particularly in cases of retroverted and anteflaxus uterus

(Abou-Setta, 2007; Lewin et al., 1997); 2) gripping the cervix with a tenaculum 3) using an inner metal guide; 4) changing the patient position during embryo transfer.

3.3 Use of ultrasound guidance

Embryos are generally deposited in the uterine cavity by means of a transcervical transfer catheter. Traditionally, the "clinical touch" method has been used to guide catheter placement approximately 1 cm from the uterine fundus. This is a blind technique and clinicians must rely on their sense of touch to judge whether the transfer catheter has been introduced in its proper place (Brown et al., 2010). Therefore this method is often unreliable for evaluating the correct catheter location. Woolcott and Stanger (Woolcott & Stanger, 1997) used transvaginal ultrasound for embryo transfer so that catheter insertion to endometrial surface and uterine fundus was observed. They reported optimal catheter insertion in less than half of the cases because of the catheter either indenting or becoming embedded in the endometrium. It has been demonstrated that ultrasound-guided embryo transfer is helpful for women who have previously had difficult transfers (Kan et al., 1999), and that the rates of implantation and pregnancy have a significantly improvement (Coroleu et al., 2000). Other important benefits of ultrasound guided embryo transfer include providing an opportunity to observe the transfer catheter, the air bubble, the endometrial cavity and the endometrial feature (Strickler et al., 1985). The transferred air bubbles are often considered a marker for the embryo's position in the uterus. By performing the transfer under ultrasonographic guidance, the catheter and air bubble can be precisely located (Lambers et al., 2007). Based on some studies, catheter insertion at 1.5 or 2 cm from the fundus is better than insertion at 1 cm from the fundus (Coroleu et al., 2002). The air bubble position at embryo transfer is relevant to the pregnancy rate (Lambers et al., 2007).

3.4 Type of catheter

A Soft, flexible embryo transfer catheter is the best choice for minimizing the risk of trauma to the endocervix or endometrium, facilitating smooth insertion. Earlier studies have reported the benefit of using a soft catheter for embryo transfer. Many studies have evaluated various types of embryo transfer catheters and have confirmed a significantly better pregnancy rate with the use of soft catheters (Wood et al., 2000; Wisanto et al., 1989; Mansour et al., 1994; Ghazzawi et al., 1999; Mansour & Aboulghar, 2002). It is important to point out that in order to benefits from the catheter's softness; the outer rigid sheath should be stopped just at the internal cervical os, and not pushed beyond it. Stimulation due to passage of the embryo transfer catheter through the internal cervical os, can start contractions, which are caused by the release of prostaglandins (Fraser, 1992). Therefore, the idea of performing an embryo transfer without cervical manipulation seems wise (Dorn et al., 1999; Lesny et al., 1999b; Mansour & Aboulghar, 2002). In all, it is highly recommended to use agents that can facilitate a smooth embryo transfer and reduce unintended stimulation of the fundus, for example the application of soft-tipped catheters, which can improve pregnancy rate (Neithardt et al., 2005).

3.5 Loading the embryo medium

The composition of the medium that surrounds the embryo during embryo transfer is believed to be important at this critical stage. To enhance the chances of pregnancy by increasing the probability of the embryo adhering to the uterus, adherence compounds have been developed which are added to the embryo transfer medium. One natural and most important adherent macromolecule recommended to be introduced into transfer media is hyaluronic acid which is known as an implantation enhancing-molecule (Bontekoe et al., 2010). Despite the lack of evidence, an exact mechanism by which hyaluronic acid improves implantation has led to the speculation that it increases cell-to-cell adhesion and cell-to-matrix adhesion (Turley & Moore, 1984 as cited in Bontekoe et al., 2010). Hyaluronic acid generates a viscous solution that might improve the embryo transfer process, preventing embryo expulsion (Simon et al., 2003).

Albumin is a macromolecule traditionally used as the main macromolecule in most culture media. Serum albumin, which is derived from blood, is an impure substance and there is a risk of contamination through the transmission of viruses. Studies have demonstrated that hyaluronic acid has a positive effect on pregnancy rates and can successfully replace albumin as a transfer medium (Simon et al., 2003; Mahani & Davar, 2007). The results of mouse studies have revealed significantly higher implantation and embryo development following addition of hyaluronic acid to the transfer medium when compared to transfer medium with no hyaluronic acid (Gardner 1999). EmbryoGlue ® is a useful and available embryo transfer medium with a high concentration of hyaluronic acid which in some infertile patients it can improve clinical implantation and ongoing pregnancy rates. We have previously evaluated the efficacy of Embryo-Glue® as a human embryo transfer medium in IVF/ICSI cycles on 815 patients who were randomly divided into study (n=417) and control (n=398) groups. In both groups, the embryo culture medium was G-1TMver 3, supplemented with 10% recombinant human albumin. On the day of embryo transfer (day 3), excellent or good quality embryos were selected for transfer and then were placed in either Embryo-Glue® (study group) or fresh culture medium (control group) prior to transfer. According to our results, a significantly higher rates of clinical pregnancy and implantation in the tubal factors, a significantly better implantation rate in recurrent implantation failures were observed with Embryo-Glue® than G-1TMver3 (Valojerdi et al., 2006).

3.6 Embryo load method for transfer

The final aim of embryo transfer is to transport the embryo close to the fundal wall to create optimal conditions for implantation in the endometrium. Although there are different methods of catheter loading in IVF centers, similarities are observed in using the transfer of small volumes which are compositions of a sequence of air and liquid contents. It has been postulated that if the contents of the catheter load consist of liquid alone, the distribution of the embryos may occur throughout a larger area. On the other hand, since the uterine tissue can absorb air faster than liquid, the use of air in the transferred liquid can be beneficial (Eytan et al., 2004). The method of embryo transfer at our fertility center and in the majority of centers is the three-drop procedure (Friedman et al., 2011), with air bubbles separating the drop of medium that contains the embryo from two drops of Embryo-Glue® before and after the embryo drop (Figure. 1).

The advantage of using the air and liquid content for catheter loading is to prevent the embryo from adhering to the wall of the catheter at the time of injection (Eytan et al., 2004). The presence of two air bubbles on both sides of the medium that contains the embryo prevents the transfer of the embryo within the catheter (Eytan et al., 2004) and beside, in the transfer under ultrasonographic guidance, the air bubbles are often considered a marker for the embryo's position in the uterus (Lambers et al., 2007). Finally by loading 1 μl of medium on the catheter tip, the probability of embryo expulsion will be stopped. It has been reported that larger volumes of fluid transferred (60 μl) correlate with retained embryos, yet it is advisable that a certain amount of media be loaded to assist with expelling the embryo (Hearns-Stokes et al., 2000). On the other hand, the transferred air volumes should be small enough to prevent the transport of the embryos into the cervix (Eytan et al., 2004). Based on the fact that a low speed of injection upon the catheter load into the uterus produces bubbles, which assist with transporting more transferred media into the fundus, it is advisable to transfer the embryo gently with minimal ejection speed. However, the speed of injection has not been studied clinically (L. Bungum & M. Bungum, 2009). It is proposed that to minimize the risk of retained embryos, the transfer catheter should be slowly withdrawn (Mansour & Aboulghar, 2002; Eytan et al., 2007).

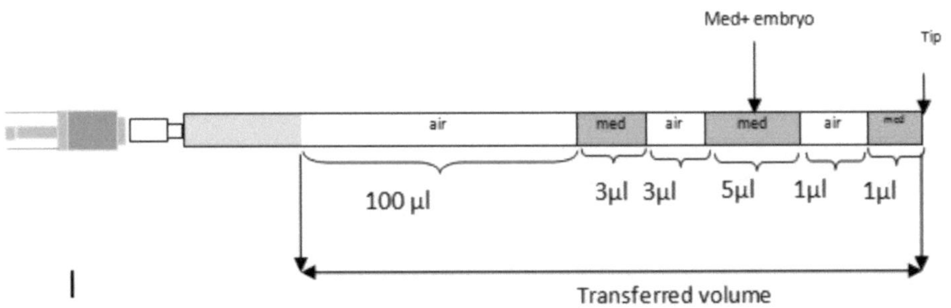

Fig. 1. The catheter load with a sequence of air and transfer medium

3.7 Time of embryo transfer with regard to uterine contraction problem

Studies in animals have demonstrated that uterine contractions have an effect on the implantation of embryos (Adams, 1980; Schoolcraft et al., 2001). In a study by Fanchin and colleagues (Fanchin et al., 1998b), the 5 minute ultrasound scans of the uterus were digitized for counting the occurrence of myometrial contractile activity. Their result showed an overall mean uterine contraction frequency of 4.3 per minute. They also noted that with increased frequency of the uterine contractions, the rates of implantation and pregnancy were reduced. The variables correlated with the frequency of uterine contractions are (Schoolcraft et al., 2001) 1) serum progesterone levels on the day of embryo transfer: By increasing progesterone levels, uterine contractions decrease; 2) difficulty of embryo transfer: the occurrence of uterine contractions depends on the difficulty of the embryo transfer. An investigation that used 30 μL of an opaque medium in 14 oocyte donors showed that, with easy mock embryo transfer, the frequency of uterine contractions were not altered and the opaque contrast medium remained for 45 minutes in the upper part of the uterine cavity. Conversely, forceful, random and fundocervical uterine contractions have been shown to occur following a difficult embryo transfer (Lesny et al., 1998); 3) applying a tenaculum: Uterine contractility increases when a tenaculum is used to grasp the cervix (Lesny et al., 1999b); 4) progression into the luteal phase: Uterine contractility lessens with progression into the luteal phase. This can be a causal factor for success of the embryo transfer in the blastocyst stage after five days of culture (Lesny et al., 1999a).

3.8 Injection of air before embryo transfer catheter withdrawal

A higher occurrence of immediate or delayed embryo expulsion is correlated with capillary action or the negative force created by moving the catheter back (Schoolcraft et al., 2001; Woolcott & Stanger, 1997). Some researchers have indicated that 15% of the transferred embryos are pushed out after embryo transfer and are found in the catheter tip, cervix and on the vaginal speculum (Mansour, 2005, Poindexter et al., 1986). This can be a reason for IVF failure (Ghazzawi et al., 1999; Mansour et al., 1994).

Pushing 0.2 mL of air into the catheter immediately following embryo transfer is an easy and low-cost addition to standard embryo transfer techniques (Madani et al., 2010). This appears to improve pregnancy rates. Recently we used this improved technique to perform 110 infertile women embryo transfers, and obtained a significant higher implantation and clinical pregnancy rates than controls. In this research, our purpose was to prevent embryo expulsion. By pushing air gently after driving out the embryos into the uterine cavity, we have tried to generate a positive air pressure in order to stop embryos from back-tracking with the catheter removal, or the creation of a force against the waves generated by uterine contractions, thus finally reducing the rate of embryo expulsion. However, we recommend further randomized clinical studies to confirm better treatment outcomes and clarify the exact mechanism of this simple, modified embryo transfer technique (Madani et al., 2010).

4. Third stage: Measures after embryo transfer

Recently, the use of evidence-based guidelines has been emphasized in order to optimize and standardize the embryo transfer protocol. However, there is debate on the post-transfer aspects of the embryo transfer. There are three main approaches for post embryo transfer intervention (Abou-Setta et al., 2009): 1) prevention of the expulsion of fluids and embryos from the cervix; 2) the use of a fibrin sealant (Bar-Hava et al., 1999, Feichtinger et al., 1992); 3) bed rest after embryo transfer (Sharif et al., 1998)

4.1 Prevention of the expulsion of fluids and embryos from the cervix

Closing the cervix following embryo transfer is one method proposed for preventing embryo expulsion. A recent prospective, randomized study has suggested mechanical closure of the cervix (Mansour, 2005) by loosening the screw of the vaginal speculum, following the introduction of the embryo transfer catheter. In this study, the cervical portio-vaginalis was closed by the two lips of the speculum. After gently withdrawing the embryo transfer catheter, the vaginal speculum was left for 5-7 minutes to put pressure on the cervix. Suprapubic heaviness and mild discomfort were the only complications reported in this study. To better confirm the usefulness of this intervention as a post-embryo transfer strategy, more well-designed and powered randomized controlled trials are needed (Abou-Setta et al., 2009).

4.2 Fibrin sealant

In the investigation by Ben-Rafael et al. (Ben-Rafael et al., 1995), "two step" technique (Feichtinger et al., 1992) has been applied for using a fibrin sealant. In this method, the application of multiple columns of air or medium cause splitting of the fibrin sealant and embryo sections. Initially, the sealant ingredients, followed by either an air or medium column are loaded into the embryo transfer catheter. This method ends with the loading of a medium column containing the embryos into the transfer catheter. The proximity of the embryos to the uterine cavity and the creation of a layer between the embryos and the uterine cavity (by columns of media and fibrin sealant) are the basis of this technique. According to the theory which states that when embryos are next to the endometrium, the relationship between embryos and the mother tissue becomes easier, thus facilitating the adhesion process, and increasing the pregnancy rate (Abou-Setta et al., 2009). Movement of the fluid from the uterine cavity is an unwanted event after embryo transfer and usually observed in clinical practice (Schulman, 1986; Ghazzawi et al., 1999; Mansour, 2005). Of note, sometimes this fluid contains the transferred embryo (Ghazzawi et al., 1999) and this causes movement of the embryo away from its deposition place (Ghazzawi et al., 1999; Mansour, 2005; Schulman, 1986).

4.3 Bed rest

It has been speculated that embryo movement after transfer happens with instant mobilization following embryo transfer. A linear relationship between the success rates of embryo transfer and the time spent in a lying position has been seen. Since, limited numbers of embryos are transferred; embryo expulsion usually leads to transfer failure. Any interference that could stop this unintended exclusion would increase pregnancy rate (Abou-Setta et al., 2009). In the past, as a guarantee of success, complete bed rest was prescribed after embryo transfer for at least 24 hours with the aim of stopping the expulsion of fluids that contain the embryo due to gravity. With the intention of making the procedure easier and more patient-friendly, clinicians decided to reduce the time of resting (Sharif et al., 1998). Recent guidelines have considered 15 minutes as the time needed for bed rest (Abou-Setta et al., 2009). According to the research by Purcell and colleagues (Purcell et al., 2007), the bed rest period did not affect clinical pregnancy rate.

5. Single embryo transfer (SET)

Regardless of many advances in assisted reproductive technologies (ART), the live birth rate is still unsatisfactory; however, the success rate of ART has increased during the past 10-15 years (Gerris, 2009). In accordance with the report of the Society for Assisted Reproductive Technology, the live birth rate has increased by 4% in 6 years (28% in 1996 to 32% in 2002) (Neithardt et al., 2005). It is also important to note that in multiple embryo transfers, although the success rate of the pregnancy will increase, the live birth rate will not raise (Gerris, 2009). Over the past decade, the first study in 2003 indicated a similar pregnancy rate between single embryo transfer and double embryo transfer (Poikkeus & Tiitinen, 2008). Furthermore, on the base of several studies, pregnancy rates equaling double embryo transfer rates have been achieved by utilizing the combination of single embryo transfer and a later frozen embryo transfer (Thurin et al., 2004; Milliez & Dickens, 2009), decreasing the twin birth rate from 25 to 1%. The major benefit of single embryo transfer is the decrease in all known increased risks of obstetric and neonatal complications that are four times higher in twins than in singletons (Davis, 2004; Poikkeus & Tiitinen, 2008; Milliez & Dickens, 2009). Several investigators have proposed that careful patient selection and good quality embryos transfer (elective embryo transfer) reduces the risk of multiple pregnancies while maintaining a comparable live birth rate (Gerris, 2009).

Some others analyze single embryo transfer from an economic point of view (Bergh, 2005; Fiddelers et al., 2007). From a societal perspective, these studies show that savings in health costs related to twin pregnancies may equal the direct additional costs of the repeat SET cycles needed to achieve the same take-home baby rate. In many cases, the direct costs of treatment are the responsibility of the patients, whereas the costs related to multiple pregnancies are imposed on both patients and the government (Roberts et al., 2010). Finally, a more cost-effective and safer procedure may be offered by elective single embryo transfer for patients who undergo assisted reproductive technology.

6. Conclusion

Despite transferring one or two good quality embryos, there is still a question as to why the transfer is inefficient. The mechanisms underlying the implantation phenomenon are unknown and the clinical implications remain poorly understood. After embryo transfer, the control of the transferred embryos will be lost and we cannot distinguish which embryos reach the endometrial cavity and whether all of them have the same chance of implantation. There are numerous variables involved in embryo implantation and pregnancy, while embryo transfer technique is one of key factors which affect embryo transfer success. For this purpose, embryo transfer must be performed in a gentle and non-traumatic manner. Minimizing blood on the catheter tip (cervical trauma), the cervical mucus, the risk of embryo expulsion or retained embryos, the frequency and severity of uterine contractions, and performing a trial embryo transfer before the actual transfer all seems to be useful for embryo transfer. Additionally, the use of ultrasonographic guidance and soft catheters appears to enhance the chances of a successful outcome. Due to insufficient evidence from clinical trials, it is not clear which factors are crucial. Great attention should be paid to all these factors, which could optimize the embryo transfer. There are a number of questions to be answered by current and future research, in which a better outcome may be achieved. For example, enhanced knowledge about the conditions for implantation can be guidance for providing various types of media that are more compatible with normal embryo development. An improved catheter design perhaps by microcamera, may lead to the efficiency of embryo transfer by minimizing the damage to the uterine cavity, and finally determination of the exact mechanism of uterine contractions (mechanical, chemical or hormonal), may result in the use of materials and new techniques for decreasing the deleterious effects that occur during embryo transfer.

7. Acknowledgment

The authors wish to express their gratitude to Royan Institute and the staff.

8. References

Abou-Setta, A. M. (2007). Effect of passive uterine straightening during embryo transfer: a systematic review and meta-analysis. *Acta obstetricia et gynecologica Scandinavica*, Vol.86, No.5, PP. 516-22, ISSN 0001-6349

Abou-Setta, A. M., D'angelo, A., Sallam, H. N., Hart, R. J. & Al-Inany, H. G. (2009). Post-embryo transfer interventions for in vitro fertilization and intracytoplasmic sperm injection patients. *Cochrane database of systematic reviews,* No.4, PP. CD006567, ISSN 1469-493X

Adams, C. E. (1980). Retention and development of eggs transferred to the uterus at various times after ovulation in the rabbit. *Journal of reproduction and fertility,* Vol.60, No.2, PP. 309-15, ISSN 0022-4251

Adamson, G. D., DE Mouzon, J., Lancaster, P., Nygren, K. G., Sullivan, E. & Zegers-Hochschild, F. (2006). World collaborative report on in vitro fertilization, 2000. *Fertility and sterility,* Vol.85, No.6, PP. 1586-622, ISSN 0015-0282

Bar-Hava, I., Krissi, H., Ashkenazi, J., Orvieto, R., Shelef, M. & Ben-Rafael, Z. (1999). Fibrin glue improves pregnancy rates in women of advanced reproductive age and in patients in whom in vitro fertilization attempts repeatedly fail. *Fertility and sterility,* Vol.71, No.5, PP. 821-4, ISSN 0015-0282

Barash, A., Dekel, N., Fieldust, S., Segal, I., Schechtman, E. & Granot, I. (2003). Local injury to the endometrium doubles the incidence of successful pregnancies in patients undergoing in vitro fertilization. *Fertility and sterility,* Vol.79, No.6, PP. 1317-22, ISSN 0015-0282

Basak, S., Dubanchet, S., Zourbas, S., Chaouat, G. & Das, C. (2002). Expression of pro-inflammatory cytokines in mouse blastocysts during implantation: modulation by steroid hormones. *American journal of reproductive immunolog ,* Vol.47, No.1, PP. 2-11, ISSN 1046-7408

Batioglu, S. & Kaymak, O. (2005). Does hysteroscopic polypectomy without cycle cancellation affect IVF? *Reproductive biomedicine online,* Vol.10, No.6, PP. 767-9, ISSN 1472-6483

Ben-Rafael, Z., Ashkenazi, J., Shelef, M., Farhi, J., Voliovitch, I., Feldberg, D. & Orvieto, R. (1995). The use of fibrin sealant in in vitro fertilization and embryo transfer. *International journal of fertility and menopausal studies,* Vol.40, No.6, PP. 303-6, ISSN 1069-3130

Bergh, C. (2005). Single embryo transfer: a mini-review. *Human reproduction,* Vol.20, No.2, PP. 323-7, ISSN 0268-1161

Bontekoe, S., Blake, D., Heineman, M. J., Williams, E. C. & Johnson, N. (2010). Adherence compounds in embryo transfer media for assisted reproductive technologies. *Cochrane database of systematic reviews,* No.7, PP. CD007421, ISSN 1469-493X

Brown, J., Buckingham, K., Abou-Setta, A. M. & Buckett, W. (2010). Ultrasound versus 'clinical touch' for catheter guidance during embryo transfer in women. *Cochrane database of systematic reviews,* No.1, PP. CD006107, ISSN 1469-493X

Bungum, L. & Bungum, M. (2009). Embryo transfer, In: *Texbook of assisted reproductive technologies: Laboratory and clinical perspectives.* Gardner, D. K., Weissman, A., Howles, C. M., Shoham, Z, PP.693-701, Informa Healthcare, 978-0415448949, United kingdom

Coroleu, B., Carreras, O., Veiga, A., Martell, A., Martinez, F., Belil, I., Hereter, L. & Barri, P. N. (2000). Embryo transfer under ultrasound guidance improves pregnancy rates after in-vitro fertilization. *Human reproduction,* Vol.15, No.3, PP. 616-20, ISSN 0268-1161

Coroleu, B., Barri, P. N., Carreras, O., Martinez, F., Parriego, M., Hereter, L., Parera, N., Veiga, A. & Balasch, J. (2002). The influence of the depth of embryo replacement into the uterine cavity on implantation rates after IVF: a controlled, ultrasound-guided study. *Human reproduction,* Vol.17, No.2, PP. 341-6, ISSN 0268-1161

Davis, O. K. (2004). Elective single-embryo transfer--has its time arrived? *The New England journal of medicine,* Vol.351, No.23, PP. 2440-2, ISSN 0028-4793

Derks, R. S., Farquhar, C., Mol, B. W., Buckingham, K. & Heineman, M. J. (2009). Techniques for preparation prior to embryo transfer. *Cochrane database of systematic reviews,* No.4, PP. CD007682, ISSN 1469-493X

Dorn, C., Reinsberg, J., Schlebusch, H., Prietl, G., Van Der Ven, H. & Krebs, D. (1999). Serum oxytocin concentration during embryo transfer procedure. *European journal of obstetrics, gynecology, and reproductive biology*, Vol.87, No.1, PP. 77-80, ISSN 0301-2115

Egbase, P. E., Al-Sharhan, M., Al-Othman, S., Al-Mutawa, M., Udo, E. E. & Grudzinskas, J. G. (1996). Incidence of microbial growth from the tip of the embryo transfer catheter after embryo transfer in relation to clinical pregnancy rate following in-vitro fertilization and embryo transfer. *Human reproduction*, Vol.11, No.8, PP. 1687-9, ISSN 0268-1161

Englert, Y., Puissant, F., Camus, M., Van Hoeck, J. & Leroy, F. (1986). Clinical study on embryo transfer after human in vitro fertilization. *Journal of in vitro fertilization and embryo transfer*, Vol.3, No.4, PP. 243-6, ISSN 0740-7769

Eskandar, M. A., Abou-Setta, A. M., El-Amin, M., Almushait, M. A. & Sobande, A. A. (2007). Removal of cervical mucus prior to embryo transfer improves pregnancy rates in women undergoing assisted reproduction. *Reproductive biomedicine online*, Vol.14, No.3, PP. 308-13, ISSN 1472-6483

Eytan, O., Elad, D., Zaretsky, U. & Jaffa, A. J. (2004). A glance into the uterus during in vitro simulation of embryo transfer. *Human reproduction*, Vol.19, No.3, PP. 562-9, ISSN 0268-1161

Eytan, O., Elad, D. & Jaffa, A. J. (2007). Evaluation of the embryo transfer protocol by a laboratory model of the uterus. *Fertility and sterility*, Vol.88, No.2, PP. 485-93, ISSN 0015-0282

Fanchin, R., Harmas, A., Benaoudia, F., Lundkvist, U., Olivennes, F. & Frydman, R. (1998a). Microbial flora of the cervix assessed at the time of embryo transfer adversely affects in vitro fertilization outcome. *Fertility and sterility*, Vol.70, No.5, PP. 866-70, ISSN 0015-0282

Fanchin, R., Righini, C., Ayoubi, J. M., Olivennes, F., De Ziegler, D. & Frydman, R. (1998b). [Uterine contractions at the time of embryo transfer: a hindrance to implantation?]. *Contraception, fertilité, sexualité*, Vol.26, No.7-8, PP. 498-505, ISSN 1165-1083

Feichtinger, W., Strohmer, H., Radner, K. M. & Goldin, M. (1992). The use of fibrin sealant for embryo transfer: development and clinical studies. *Human reproduction*, Vol.7, No.6, PP. 890-3, ISSN 0268-1161

Fiddelers, A. A., Severens, J. L., Dirksen, C. D., Dumoulin, J. C., Land, J. A. & Evers, J. L. (2007). Economic evaluations of single- versus double-embryo transfer in IVF. *Human reproduction Update*, Vol.13, No.1, PP. 5-13, ISSN 1355-4786

Fraser, I. S. (1992). Prostaglandins, prostaglandin inhibitors and their roles in gynaecological disorders. *Baillieres Clin Obstet Gynaecol*, Vol.6, No.4, PP. 829-57, ISSN 0950-3552

Friedman, B. E., Lathi, R. B., Henne, M. B., Fisher, S. L. & Milki, A. A. (2011). The effect of air bubble position after blastocyst transfer on pregnancy rates in IVF cycles. *Fertility and sterility*, Vol.95, No. 3, PP. 944-7, ISSN 0015-0282

Gardner, D. K., Rodriegez-Martinez, H. & Lane, M. (1999). Fetal development after transfer is increased by replacing protein with the glycosaminoglycan hyaluronan for mouse embryo culture and transfer. *Human reproduction*, Vol.14, No.10, PP. 2575-80, ISSN 0268-1161

Gerris, J. (2009). Single-embryo transfer versus multiple-embryo transfer. *Reproductive biomedicine online*, Vol.18 Suppl 2, PP. 63-70, ISSN 1472-6483

Ghazzawi, I. M., Al-Hasani, S., Karaki, R. & Souso, S. (1999). Transfer technique and catheter choice influence the incidence of transcervical embryo expulsion and the outcome of IVF. *Human reproduction*, Vol.14, No.3, PP. 677-82, ISSN 0268-1161

Hearns-Stokes, R. M., Miller, B. T., Scott, L., Creuss, D., Chakraborty, P. K. & Segars, J. H. (2000). Pregnancy rates after embryo transfer depend on the provider at embryo transfer. Fertility and sterility, Vol.74, No.1, PP. 80-6, ISSN 0015-0282

Isikoglu, M., Berkkanoglu, M., Senturk, Z., Coetzee, K. & Ozgur, K. (2006). Endometrial polyps smaller than 1.5 cm do not affect ICSI outcome. *Reproductive biomedicine online,* Vol.12, No.2, PP. 199-204, ISSN 1472-6483

Kan, A. K., Abdalla, H. I., Gafar, A. H., Nappi, L., Ogunyemi, B. O., Thomas, A. & Ola-Ojo, O. O. (1999). Embryo transfer: ultrasound-guided versus clinical touch. *Human reproduction,* Vol.14, No.5, PP. 1259-61, ISSN 0268-1161

Lambers, M. J., Dogan, E., Lens, J. W., Schats, R. & Hompes, P. G. (2007). The position of transferred air bubbles after embryo transfer is related to pregnancy rate. *Fertility and sterility,* Vol.88, No.1, PP. 68-73, ISSN 0015-0282

Lass, A., Williams, G., Abusheikha, N. & Brinsden, P. (1999). The effect of endometrial polyps on outcomes of in vitro fertilization (IVF) cycles. *Journal of assisted reproduction and genetics,* Vol.16, No.8, PP. 410-5, ISSN 1058-0468

Lesny, P., Killick, S. R., Tetlow, R. L., Robinson, J. & Maguiness, S. D. (1998). Embryo transfer--can we learn anything new from the observation of junctional zone contractions? *Human reproduction,* Vol.13, No.6, PP. 1540-6, ISSN 0268-1161

Lesny, P., Killick, S. R., Robinson, J. & Maguiness, S. D. (1999a). Transcervical embryo transfer as a risk factor for ectopic pregnancy. *Fertility and sterility,* Vol.72, No.2, PP. 305-9, ISSN 0015-0282

Lesny, P., Killick, S. R., Robinson, J., Raven, G. & Maguiness, S. D. (1999b). Junctional zone contractions and embryo transfer: is it safe to use a tenaculum? *Human reproduction,* Vol.14, No.9, PP. 2367-70, ISSN 0268-1161

Lewin, A., Schenker, J. G., Avrech, O., Shapira, S., Safran, A. & Friedler, S. (1997). The role of uterine straightening by passive bladder distension before embryo transfer in IVF cycles. *Journal of assisted reproduction and genetics,* Vol.14, No.1, PP. 32-4, ISSN 1058-0468

Madani, T., Ashrafi, M., Abadi, A. B. & Kiani, K. (2009a). Appropriate timing of uterine cavity length measurement positively affects assisted reproduction cycle outcome. *Reproductive biomedicine online,* Vol.19, No.5, PP. 734-6, ISSN 1472-6483

Madani, T., Ghaffari, F., Kiani, K. & Hosseini, F. (2009b). Hysteroscopic polypectomy without cycle cancellation in IVF cycles. *Reproductive biomedicine online,* Vol.18, No.3, PP. 412-5, ISSN 1472-6483

Madani, T., Ashrafi, M., Jahangiri, N., Abadi, A. B. & Lankarani, N. (2010). Improvement of pregnancy rate by modification of embryo transfer technique: a randomized clinical trial. *Fertility and sterility,* Vol.94, No.6, PP. 2424-6, ISSN 0015-0282

Mansour, R., Aboulghar, M. & Serour, G. (1990). Dummy embryo transfer: a technique that minimizes the problems of embryo transfer and improves the pregnancy rate in human in vitro fertilization. *Fertility and sterility,* Vol.54, No.4, PP. 678-81, ISSN 0015-0282

Mansour, R. T., Aboulghar, M. A., Serour, G. I. & Amin, Y. M. (1994). Dummy embryo transfer using methylene blue dye. *Human reproduction,* Vol.9, No.7, PP. 1257-9, ISSN 0268-1161

Mansour, R. T. & Aboulghar, M. A. (2002). Optimizing the embryo transfer technique. *Human reproduction,* Vol.17, No.5, PP. 1149-53, ISSN 0268-1161

Mansour, R. (2005). Minimizing embryo expulsion after embryo transfer: a randomized controlled study. *Human reproduction,* Vol.20, No.1, PP. 170-4, ISSN 0268-1161

Mcnamee, P., Huang, T. & Carwile, A. (1998). Significant increase in pregnancy rates achieved by vigorous irrigation of endocervical mucus prior to embryo transfer with a Wallace catheter in an IVF-ET program. *Fertility and sterility,* Vol.70 No.Suppl PP. 1:S228,

Meldrum, D. R., Chetkowski, R., Steingold, K. A., De Ziegler, D., Cedars, M. I. & Hamilton, M. (1987). Evolution of a highly successful in vitro fertilization-embryo transfer program. *Fertility and sterility,* Vol.48, No.1, PP. 86-93, ISSN 0015-0282

Milliez, J. & Dickens, B. (2009). Legal Aspects of Iatrogenic Multiple Pregnancy. *International journal of Fertility and sterility,* Vol.3, No.2, PP. 84-86, ISSN 2008-0778

Munne, S., Alikani, M., Tomkin, G., Grifo, J. & Cohen, J. (1995). Embryo morphology, developmental rates, and maternal age are correlated with chromosome abnormalities. *Fertility and sterility,* Vol.64, No.2, PP. 382-91, ISSN 0015-0282

Neithardt, A. B., Segars, J. H., Hennessy, S., James, A. N. & Mckeeby, J. L. (2005). Embryo afterloading: a refinement in embryo transfer technique that may increase clinical pregnancy. *Fertility and sterility,* Vol.83, No.3, PP. 710-4, ISSN 0015-0282

Niknejadi, M., Ahmadi, F., Zafarani, F., Khalili, G., Ghaderi, F. & Rashidi, Z. (2010). Diagnostic Accuracy of Transvaginal Sonography in Infertile Patients with Endometrial Polyps. *International journal of Fertility and sterility,* Vol.3, No.4, PP. 157-160, ISSN 2008-0778

Poikkeus, P. & Tiitinen, A. (2008). Does single embryo transfer improve the obstetric and neonatal outcome of singleton pregnancy? *Acta obstetricia et gynecologica Scandinavica,* Vol.87, No.9, PP. 888-92, ISSN 0001-6349

Poindexter, A. N., 3rd, Thompson, D. J., Gibbons, W. E., Findley, W. E., Dodson, M. G. & Young, R. L. (1986). Residual embryos in failed embryo transfer. *Fertility and sterility,* Vol.46, No.2, PP. 262-7, ISSN 0015-0282

Purcell, K. J., Schembri, M., Telles, T. L., Fujimoto, V. Y. & Cedars, M. I. (2007). Bed rest after embryo transfer: a randomized controlled trial. *Fertility and sterility,* Vol.87, No.6, PP. 1322-6, ISSN 0015-0282

Roberts, S., Mcgowan, L., Hirst, W., Brison, D., Vail, A. & Lieberman, B. (2010). Towards single embryo transfer? Modelling clinical outcomes of potential treatment choices using multiple data sources: predictive models and patient perspectives. *Health technology assessment,* Vol.14, No.38, PP. 1-237, ISSN 1366-5278

Sauer, M. V. & Paulson, R. J. (1992). Pelvic abscess complicating transcervical embryo transfer. American *journal of obstetrics and gynecology,* Vol.166, No.1 Pt 1, PP. 148-9, ISSN 0002-9378

Schoolcraft, W. B., Surrey, E. S. & Gardner, D. K. (2001). Embryo transfer: techniques and variables affecting success. *Fertility and sterility,* Vol.76, No.5, PP. 863-70, ISSN 0015-0282

Schulman, J. D. (1986). Delayed expulsion of transfer fluid after IVF/ET. *Lancet,* Vol.1, No.8471, PP. 44, ISSN 0140-6736

Sharif, K., Afnan, M. & Lenton, W. (1995). Mock embryo transfer with a full bladder immediately before the real transfer for in-vitro fertilization treatment: the Birmingham experience of 113 cases. *Human reproduction,* Vol.10, No.7, PP. 1715-8, ISSN 0268-1161

Sharif, K., Afnan, M., Lashen, H., Elgendy, M., Morgan, C. & Sinclair, L. (1998). Is bed rest following embryo transfer necessary? *Fertility and sterility,* Vol.69, No.3, PP. 478-81, ISSN 0015-0282

Simon, A., Safran, A., Revel, A., Aizenman, E., Reubinoff, B., Porat-Katz, A., Lewin, A. & Laufer, N. (2003). Hyaluronic acid can successfully replace albumin as the sole macromolecule in a human embryo transfer medium. *Fertility and sterility,* Vol.79, No.6, PP. 1434-8, ISSN 0015-0282

Spiewankiewicz, B., Stelmachow, J., Sawicki, W., Cendrowski, K., Wypych, P. & Swiderska, K. (2003). The effectiveness of hysteroscopic polypectomy in cases of female infertility. *Clinical and experimental obstetrics & gynecology,* Vol.30, No.1, PP. 23-5, ISSN 0390-6663

Stamatellos, I., Apostolides, A., Stamatopoulos, P. & Bontis, J. (2008). Pregnancy rates after hysteroscopic polypectomy depending on the size or number of the polyps. *Archives of gynecology and obstetrics,* Vol.277, No.5, PP. 395-9, ISSN 0932-0067

Strickler, R. C., Christianson, C., Crane, J. P., Curato, A., Knight, A. B. & YANG, V. (1985). Ultrasound guidance for human embryo transfer. *Fertility and sterility,* Vol.43, No.1, PP. 54-61, ISSN 0015-0282

Sundstrom, P., Wramsby, H., Persson, P. H. & Liedholm, P. (1984). Filled bladder simplifies human embryo transfer. *British journal of obstetrics and gynaecology,* Vol.91, No.5, PP. 506-7, ISSN 0306-5456

Thurin, A., Hausken, J., Hillensjo, T., Jablonowska, B., Pinborg, A., Strandell, A. & Bergh, C. (2004). Elective single-embryo transfer versus double-embryo transfer in in vitro fertilization. *New England journal of medicine,* Vol.351, No.23, PP. 2392-402, ISSN 0028-4793

Turley, E. & Moore, D. (1984). Hyaluronate binding proteins also bind to fibronectin, laminin and collagen. *Biochemical and biophysical research communications,* Vol.121, No.3, PP. 808-14, ISSN 0006-291X

Valojerdi, M. R., Karimian, L., Yazdi, P. E., Gilani, M. A., Madani, T. & Baghestani, A. R. (2006). Efficacy of a human embryo transfer medium: a prospective, randomized clinical trial study. *Journal of assisted reproduction and genetics,* Vol.23, No.5, PP. 207-12, ISSN 1058-0468

Varasteh, N. N., Neuwirth, R. S., Levin, B. & Keltz, M. D. (1999). Pregnancy rates after hysteroscopic polypectomy and myomectomy in infertile women. *Obstetrics and gynecology,* Vol.94, No.2, PP. 168-71, ISSN 0029-7844

Visschers, B. A., Bots, R. S., Peeters, M. F., Mol, B. W. & Van Dessel, H. J. (2007). Removal of cervical mucus: effect on pregnancy rates in IVF/ICSI. *Reproductive biomedicine online,* Vol.15, No.3, PP. 310-5, ISSN 1472-6483

Wisanto, A., Janssens, R., Deschacht, J., Camus, M., Devroey, P. & Van Steirteghem, A. C. (1989). Performance of different embryo transfer catheters in a human in vitro fertilization program. *Fertility and sterility,* Vol.52, No.1, PP. 79-84, ISSN 0015-0282

Wood, E. G., Batzer, F. R., Go, K. J., Gutmann, J. N. & Corson, S. L. (2000). Ultrasound-guided soft catheter embryo transfers will improve pregnancy rates in in-vitro fertilization. *Human reproduction,* Vol.15, No.1, PP. 107-12, ISSN 0268-1161

Woolcott, R. & Stanger, J. (1997). Potentially important variables identified by transvaginal ultrasound-guided embryo transfer. *Human reproduction,* Vol.12, No.5, PP. 963-6, ISSN 0268-1161

Yanaihara, A., Yorimitsu, T., Motoyama, H., Iwasaki, S. & Kawamura, T. (2008). Location of endometrial polyp and pregnancy rate in infertility patients. *Fertility and sterility,* Vol.90, No.1, PP. 180-2, ISSN 0015-0282

10

Optimizing Embryo Transfer Outcomes: Determinants for Improved Outcomes Using the Oocyte Donation Model

Alan M. Martinez and Steven R. Lindheim
University of Cincinnati College of Medicine, Cincinnati, OH
USA

1. Introduction

The past decade has seen increased success rates with assisted reproductive technologies (ART), however, the overall pregnancy and implantation rates have remained relatively low. These low rates continue even though we now have improved stimulation protocols and laboratory techniques. Three areas that have gained specific attention include 1) identification of the optimal uterine environment; 2) extended embryo culture to the blastocyst stage; and 3) the embryo transfer (ET) technique, which has historically been viewed as an unimportant variable in the success of an ART treatment cycle.

Discerning the impact on folliculogenesis and the endometrial level is difficult in conventional IVF cycles. Moreover, due to ethical quandaries, any study as complex as embryo and endometrial synchrony and receptivity is difficult to perform and thus reported studies in humans are more suggestive than conclusive. In contrast, the ovum donation model, which has been successfully used in treating infertility for over 25 years (Trounson et al., 1983), allows for the study of isolated parameters that may affect outcome by standardizing for embryo quality and endometrial receptivity and by optimizing the recruitment of high quality oocytes from the egg donor and eliminates the possible adverse effects of ovarian hyperstimulation (Acosta, 2000; Garcia, 1984; Oehninger, 2008).

In this chapter we will review the clinical variables that have gained increasing importance as prognostic determinants of implantation and variables to maximize ET outcomes of oocyte donation in an attempt to control for confounding variables seen in other clinical studies.

2. Endometrial thickness and pregnancy outcome in oocyte donation cycles

To date, significant research has been done to directly assess uterine receptivity including histologic dating, measurement of endometrial sex steroid receptor concentrations using immuno-histochemical methods, assessing pinopod expression through scanning electron microscopy, and more recently the role of cytokines, growth factors, and integrin molecules have been studied (Castelbaum, 1997; Noci, 1995; Noyes, 1950; Paulson, 1997). Although these methods are important in furthering our understanding of uterine receptivity, they are not practical in actual ET cycles.

The measurement of endometrial thickness and its echogenic pattern, however, is an easy, non-invasive technique that has been used to assess endometrial receptivity prior to the embryo transfer. It is generally accepted that a thin endometrial stripe on transvaginal ultrasound is associated with a reduced embryo implantation potential (McWilliams, 2007; Rashidi, 2005; Schild, 2001; Zang, 2005; Zenke, 2004), while others have even reported an adverse effect of an increased endometrial thickness (Amir et al., 2007; Kovacs, 2003; Richter, 2007). The echogenic pattern of the endometrium has also been suggested to be a predictor of pregnancy outcome (Noyes, 2001; Sharara, 1999; Sher, 1991). Conversely, other studies have not shown sonographic assessment of the endometrium to be of any benefit in the characterization of uterine receptivity in IVF patients (Barufi, 2002; Dietterich, 2002; Garcia-Velasco, 2003; Sundstrom, 1998; Yuval, 1999). Nonetheless, despite these reports, the value of endometrial thickness and echogenic pattern are still undetermined as prognostic factors of implantation.

Oocyte donation cycles provide a unique model to eliminate confounding variables that typically occur when comparing groups of patients undergoing autologous IVF, where embryo quality and possible adverse effects of ovarian hyperstimulation on endometrial receptivity cannot be controlled. Endometrial proliferation strongly correlates with ovarian estradiol production, and therefore depends on ovarian function. Since age has an impact on ovarian function, embryo quality, estradiol production, endometrial thickness and pregnancy outcome often change in the same direction. In autologous cycles, poor endometrial development could be the sign of poor ovarian function (reduced estradiol production) and therefore is not independently responsible for lower implantation and pregnancy rates. Using an oocyte donation model, the endometrium can be developed by administration of exogenous sex steroids, with dose adjustment based on response (measured by serum estradiol level or endometrial thickness). Therefore endometrial proliferation becomes independent of ovarian function. In addition, oocyte donors are typically young women with normal ovarian reserve, thus embryos should characteristically be healthy with good implantation potential.

Few studies have evaluated the association between endometrial thickness pattern and pregnancy outcome using an oocyte donation model. Noyes et al., retrospectively analyzed 343 oocyte recipient cycles, in which endometrial thickness and pattern was evaluated on cycle day 12. They found that clinical pregnancy rate and live birth rate were significantly lower when endometrial thickness was less then 8mm than when endometrial thickness was greater than 9mm (Noyes et al., 2001). Zenke and Chetkowski reported in 41 recipient pairs with discordant outcomes that endometrial thickness less than 8 mm one week prior to oocyte retrieval was found in failed cycles (Zenke & Chetkowski, 2004).

In contrast, Remohi et al., performed a retrospective review of 465 oocyte donor cycles and found that there was no correlation between ultrasound appearance of the endometrium the day before embryo transfer and pregnancy rates (Remohi et al., 1997). Garcia-Velasco performed a matched pair analysis of 365 recipients with discordant outcome and found that endometrial thickness measured on cycle day 15 or 16 was not a significant finding (Garcia-Velasco et al., 2003). Barker et al. retrospectively examined endometrial thickness (in both the late follicular and mid-luteal phase) and treatment outcome in 132 oocyte donor IVF-ET cycles, using only blastocyst stage embryos which was thought to provide the best opportunity to assess the effect of these parameters on treatment outcome independent of other confounding variables (Barker et al., 2009). Other studies using cleavage stage embryo transfer or a mixture of cleavage and blastocyst stage transfer therefore did not maximally control for the embryo factor (Abdalla, 1994; Check, 1993; Garcia-Velasco, 2003; Noyes, 2001; Remohi, 1997; Zenke, 2004). While this study was limited due to its retrospective design and limited power, it suggests that endometrial thickness in both the late-follicular and mid-luteal phase is not predictive of pregnancy outcomes. Moreover, thin endometrium and thickened endometrium (<7 mm, and >13 mm respectively), as well as pattern did not appear to be useful indicators of adverse endometrial receptivity (i.e. clinical outcomes).

In summary, research suggests that endometrial thickness may not be as helpful in predicting success as previously thought. Nonetheless, despite the many reports (some conflicting), the endometrial thickness and endometrial pattern are reassuring as a marker of endometrial receptivity and pregnancy outcomes. Further larger studies should confirm the present observations and what appears to be critical is the need for a uniform agreement by investigators to assess endometrial thickness and pattern in a more rigorous and standardized fashion to gain further insight into their relative importance.

3. Blastocyst embryo transfer is the primary determinant for improved outcomes in oocyte donation cycles

Another area that has drawn considerable attention is the blastocyst ET. Embryo culture has been extended from cleavage to the blastocyst stage transfer secondary to the introduction of sequential media allowing embryos to undergo cell compaction and genomic activation (Braude, 1988; Gardner, 1998). Two large randomized clinical trials and a recent Cochrane meta-analysis (Blake, 2007; Papnikolaou, 2005, 2006) suggest that blastocyst embryo transfers (ET) in good prognosis patients result in overall higher pregnancy and live-birth rates per ET, and has allowed for a reduction in the mean number of embryos transferred. Implantation rates have been reported to be as high as 60 to 65% per embryo transfer (Schoolcraft, 2001; Schillaci, 2002) with some in-vitro fertilization (IVF) programs advocating elective single ET in good prognosis patients (women <36 years of age) (Papnikolaou et al., 2006).

While our understanding of the developmental biology of pre-implantation stage embryos has substantially increased, overall implantation rates have remained relatively low with day-3 cleavage embryo transfers. Many IVF failures of seemingly normal embryos may occur as evidence suggests that extended blastocyst stage transfers result in significantly improved live-birth rates, including a Cochrane review by Blake et al (Blake et al., 2007).

The higher implantation and pregnancy rates appear to have a twofold explanation. First, it is principally thought to be the result of self selection and that only the most viable embryos develop into blastocysts, allowing these embryos to be transferred or cryopreserved (Schoolcraft, 2001; Schillaci, 2002). Studies suggest that a significant proportion of morphologically normal cleavage stage embryos are chromosomally abnormal and not destined to reach the blastocyst stage (Magli, 1998; Staessen, 2004), which appears to account for the high implantation failures seen in most cleavage stage ET cycles. This is despite the use of embryo classification systems including cell number and morphologic features of the fertilized oocyte, and cleavage stage embryos including pronuclei morphology, fragmentation, and blastomere uniformity (De Placido, 2002;

Gamiz, 2003; Gianarolo, 2003; Hnida, 2004; Nagy, 2003; Nikas, 1999; Montag, 2001; Rienzi, 2005; Van Royen, 1999; Ziebe, 1997).

The second factor appears to be related to the contribution of the uterine environment, where endometrial receptivity occurs within a short window of <48 hours and is precisely timed with exposure to progesterone secretion (Nikas, 1999; Valbuena, 2001). However, unlike in-vivo embryos that normally travel through the fallopian tube and do not reach the uterus before the morula stage (four days post-ovulation), in-vitro cultured embryos that are transferred to the uterine cavity at the cleavage stage may be subjected to stress that normally would not occur. Some have argued that this environmental milieu and possible higher uterine contractility during cleavage stage ET results in expulsion of earlier transferred embryos and may account for the exceedingly high implantation failures seen in most IVF programs (Croxatto, 1972; Fanchin, 2001; Valbuena, 2001).

It is apparent that the uterine environment remains a critical component of embryo implantation. A variety of factors from both the blastocyst and endometrium appear to be critical to implantation including apposition, attachment, and invasion during a defined window, however, the blastocyst-endometrial interaction remains the least explored embryonic event (Garcia et al.,) and its role in implantation is not completely understood.

Clearly due to ethical quandaries, any study as complex as embryo and endometrial synchrony and receptivity is difficult to perform, and thus more suggestive than conclusive. Shapiro et al. demonstrated higher implantation and pregnancy rates occurring in day-5 compared to day-6 fresh autologous cycles, yet cryopreserved day-6 embryos in frozen transfer cycles outperformed day-6 fresh autologous cycles, while day-5 and day-6 cryopreserved embryos in frozen transfer cycles resulted in similar outcomes (Shapiro et al., 2008). These findings suggest the presence of different endometrial receptivities, and it is hypothesized that this may be due to better uterine synchrony. The egg donation model also shows that endometrial receptivity clearly plays a significant role, as evidenced by studies looking at discordant outcomes between autologous IVF patients who share half their oocytes to recipients. The recipient group was found to have both higher implantation and pregnancy rates, suggesting the importance of endometrial receptivity and the tenuous nature of the uterine environment (Check, 1999).

Using oocyte donation cycles (n=93), Porat et al. retrospectively evaluated the pregnancy and implantation rates in cleavage stage (day-3) versus blastocyst stage (day-6) embryo transfers (ET); and assessed 1) the predictive value of blastocyst formation rates based on objective cleavage cell stage and morphology grade and 2) evaluate the subjective ability (4 blinded reviewers) to predict formation of high quality blastocysts (fully expanded or hatching, with at least a fair inner cell mass and trophoectoderm, scored ≥4BB using Gardner's scoring system)in 546 normally fertilized embryos (n=546) that were cultured in sequential media (Porat et al., 2010). Cleavage stage cycles resulted in significantly lower pregnancy per ET, clinical pregnancy per ET, and implantation rates (47%; 40%; and 27% compared to blastocyst cleavage stage ET 82%; 73%; and 64%), despite significantly reduced numbers of embryos transferred compared to day-3 cleavage stage ET. In total, HQ blastocysts more likely resulted from HQ day-3 embryos (>6 cells, grades 1 and 1.5 [uniform cells, slight or no fragmentation]) (59%) compared to either good quality (43%) or fair-to poor quality day-3 embryos (55%), respectively. In a Cochrane review published in 2010, a comparison of cleavage versus blastocyst stage embryo transfer in ART (including 9 randomized controlled studies with 1144 patients) provided evidence of a significant difference in live-birth rate per couple favoring blastocyst culture, with an odds ratio of 1.35 (Blake et al., 2010). Also, clinical pregnancy rate per couple in this review included 17 studies, 2557 patients, with the odds ratio of 1.17 again favoring blastocyst culture.

With respect to the ability to select HQ blastocysts, in cases where ≥6 good and high quality day-3 embryos were available, retrospective-blinded selection of one, two, and three embryo(s) was accurately selected more than 95% of the time and two embryos were correctly selected close to 70% of the time. Given the high likelihood of correctly identifying embryo(s) that would have been picked on day-6 and the increase in implantation rates from day-3 cleavage stage to day-6 blastocyst ET, the data suggest that the improved clinical pregnancy and implantation rates are not only the result of the extended embryo culture (thus allowing for the selection and transfer of the highest quality embryos), but also the more physiologic timing of the ET. Appropriate timing appears to play a significant and underestimated role in optimizing outcomes.

4. The ultrasound guided embryo transfer

Historically, ET has been viewed as an unimportant variable in the success of an ART treatment cycle (Stafford-Bell, 1999) and the technique has typically been performed in a blinded fashion without the use of ultrasound guidance. Recent studies have specifically addressed the technique of ET as being critical for optimizing outcome success, including factors such as the technique itself, the type of catheter, and the use of ultrasound (US) guidance (Abou-Setta, 2005, 2006; Bucket, 2003; Sallam & Sadek, 2003). The application of ultrasound guidance (two-dimensional transabdominal, as well as three-dimensional and four dimensional ultrasound-guided) to ET (Baba et al., 2000) has been described in more than 150 clinical trials including 20 randomized clinical trials and four meta-analyses including a Cochrane review (Abou-Setta, 2007; Brown, 2007; Buckett, 2003; Sallam & Sadek, 2003). These studies suggest that ultrasound-guided ET provides a benefit with respect to increases in clinical pregnancy and implantation rates, compared to the blind, "clinical touch" method and is a critical factor in optimizing pregnancy outcomes. However, other studies including a randomized controlled trial of 2295 embryo transfers by Drakeley et al failed to demonstrate any differences in ultrasound-guided ET compared to the blind, clinical touch which has not been included in any of the meta-analysis (Drakeley et al., 2008).

To date, only two studies have assessed US guided ET using the ovum donation model to eliminate confounding variables. In a retrospective study, Lindheim et al. assessed the impact of US guided easy or difficult ET on pregnancy rates, implantation rates, and multiple gestation rates in 137 cycles with and without US guidance using transvaginal or transabdominal US. US guidance significantly improved implantation and pregnancy rates in cycles with easy ET (29% vs. 18% and 63% vs. 36%, respectively $p<0.05$), without impacting multiple pregnancy rates. Similar trends for pregnancy, implantation, and multiple rates were seen for difficult ET, although statistical significance was not seen.

The only randomized clinical trail in patients undergoing oocyte donation was performed by Garcia-Velasco et al. They attempted to determine whether transabdominal ultrasound guidance during embryo transfer (ET) was a useful tool for increasing pregnancy rates. In this prospective, randomized, controlled trial that was powered to see a 15% increase chance of pregnancy, 374 patients undergoing oocyte donation were assigned to a transabdominal ultrasound-guided ET or the blind clinical touch.

Comparable pregnancy rates (60% ultrasound vs. 55% control); implantation rates (31% ultrasound vs. 26% control); miscarriage rates (11% ultrasound vs. 9% control); and multiple pregnancy rates (21% ultrasound vs. 23% control) were seen between groups. The authors concluded that that US guided ET did not provide any benefit in terms of pregnancy rate in oocyte recipients for whom ET was performed under direct transabdominal ultrasound visualization of the endometrial cavity.

Though these two studies are limited by their study design and adequate power, the overwhelming data suggest that US guided ET are associated with improved outcomes after IVF compared to the blind, clinical touch method and is a critical factor in optimizing pregnancy outcomes dispelling the historical notion that ET is an unimportant variable in the success of an ART treatment cycle (Brown, Mains & Van Voorhis, 2010). Moreover, it has been suggested that the ultrasound confirms the position of the tip of ET catheter and site of embryo deposition within the uterine cavity, increases the frequency of easy ET's, and avoids endometrial indentation. Most importantly, others argue that it allows for standardization of the transfer technique between physicians thus minimizing variation.

It is known that ease of the ET is strongly correlated to pregnancy outcome, and a difficult transfer, specifically with use of a more rigid catheter or the use of additional instrumentation may lower success rates. Soft catheters (Cook, Wallace) are preferred to the firm catheters (TDT, Frydman, Tomcat, Tefcat, Rocket) because of less cervical and endometrial trauma during the ET procedure, and easier transfer along the uterine axis (Mains, 2010; McDonald, 2002; Sallam, 2003). In comparisons between various soft catheters, pregnancy rates have not been shown to be significantly different (Saldeen et al., 2008).

5. Conclusion

While improved stimulation protocols and laboratory techniques are given the most attention to optimizing outcomes in ART cycles, an increasing awareness to the importance ET has come into focus. Continued research in the area of the ET including endometrial receptivity (endometrial thickness as a surrogate marker), optimal embryo selection and replacement (using the blastocyst transfer), and ET technique (with ultrasound guidance) play significant factors in improving ART outcomes. The oocyte donation model provides a unique environment while eliminating many confounding variables seen in autologous cycles allowing the study of these important variables involved in IVF/ET success.

Current literature supports the notion that an endometrial thickness >7mm increases overall pregnancy outcomes Therefore, consideration of this variable should be noted in the treatment and counseling of patients undergoing IVF/ET. With respect to the timing of embryo transfer, there is clear evidence that blastocyst ET in good prognosis patients results in overall higher pregnancy and live-birth rates per ET. In addition, these enhanced rates have allowed for a reduction in the mean number of embryos transferred. Extending culture to the blastocyst stage, particularly in high quality cleavage-stage embryos, allows for selection of viable chromosomally normal embryos that may have an implantation advantage due to the timing of transfer on day 5 or 6. Therefore, selection of high quality embryos remain paramount, and if possible delay of transfer to the blastocyst stage can allow for enhanced outcomes and an overall movement towards single embryo transfers. Lastly, US guided ET provides evidence for a standardized approach, minimizing operator variability in technique, and is likely an important asset in the embryo transfer process. There is overwhelming data suggesting that US guided ET are associated with improved outcomes compared to the blind, clinical touch method, and is another critical factor in optimizing pregnancy outcomes.

As reviewed in this chapter, the oocyte donation model has allowed for more precise control of many confounding variables seen in autologous IVF cycles, and should continue to play a vital role in our pursuit for optimizing outcomes. The variables discussed in this chapter, specifically the role of endometrial thickness and pattern, advent of blastocyst embryo transfer, and the assistance of embryo transfer with ultrasound guidance will no doubt continue to be evaluated as important determinants of IVF outcomes.

6. References

Abdalla, HI., Brooks, AA., Johnson, MR., Kirkland, A., Thomas, A., & Studd, JW. (1994). Endometrial thickness: a predictor of implantation in ovum recipients? *Human Reproduction*, Vol.9, No.2, (Feburary 1994), pp.363-5, ISSN 0268-1161

Abou-Setta, AM., Al-Inany, HG., Mansour, RT., Serour, GI., & ABoulghar, MA. (2005). Soft versus firm embryo transfer catheters for assisted reproduction: a systematic review and meta-analysis. *Human Reproduction*, Vol.20, No.11, (November 2005), pp.114-21, ISSN 0268-1161

Abou-Setta, AM. (2006). Firm embryo transfer catheters for assisted reproduction: a systematic review and meta analysis using direct and adjusted indirect comparisons. *Reproductive Biomedicine Online*, Vol.12, No.2, (February 2006), pp.191-8, ISSN 1472-6483

Abou-Setta, AM., Mansour, RT., Al-Inany, HG., Aboulghar, MM., Aboulghar, MA., & Serour, GI. (2007). Among women undergoing embryo transfer, is the probability of pregnancy and live birth improved with ultrasound guidance over clinical touch alone? A systemic review and meta-analysis of prospective randomized trials. *Fertility and Sterility*, Vol.88, No.2, (August 2007), pp.333-41, ISSN 0015-0282

Acosta, AA., Elberger, L., Borghi, M., Calamera, JC., Chemes, H., Doncel, GF, Kliman, H., Lema, B., Lustig, L., & Papier, S. (2000). Endometrial dating and determination of the window of implantation in healthy fertile women. *Fertility and Sterility*, Vol.73, No.4, (April 2000), pp.788-9, ISSN 0015-0282

Amir, W., Micha, B., Ariel, H., Liat, LG., Jehoshua, D., & Adrian, S. (2007). Predicting factors for endometrial thickness during treatment with assisted reproductive technology. *Fertility and Sterility*, Vol.87, No.4, (April 2007), pp.799-804, ISSN 0015-0282

Baba, K., Ishihara, N., Saitoh, M., Taya, J., & Kinoshita, K. (2007). Three-dimensional ultrasound in embryo transfer. *Ultrasound In Obstetrics & Gynecology*, Vol.16, No.4, (September 2000), pp.372-3, ISSN 1469-0705

Barker, MA., Boehnlein, LM., Christianson, MS., Kovacs, P., & Lindheim, SR. (2009). Relationship of Follicular and Luteal Phase Endometrial Thickness plus Echogenic

Pattern and Pregnancy Outcome in Oocyte Donation Cycles. *Journal of Assisted Reproduction and Genetics*, Vol.26, No.5, (May 2009), pp.243-9, ISSN 1573-7330

Baruffi, RLR., Contart, P., Mauri, AL., Peterson, C., Felipe, V., Garbellini, E., & Franco, JG. Jr. (2002). A uterine ultrasonographic scoring system as a method for the prognosis of embryo implantation. *Journal of Assisted Reproduction and Genetics*, Vol.19, No.3, (March 2002), pp.99-102, ISSN 1573-7330

Blake, DA., Farquhar, CM., Johnson, N., & Proctor, M. (2007). Cleavage stage versus blastocyst stage embryo transfer in assisted conception (Review). *Cochrane Database of Systematic Reviews*, Vol. 17, No.4, (October 2007), pp.1-79, ISSN 1469-493X

Braude, P., Bolton, V., & Moore, S. (1988). Human gene expression first occurs between the four and eight-cell stages of pre-implantation development. *Nature*, Vol.332, No.6163, (March 1988), pp.459-61, ISSN 0028-0836

Brown, JA., Buckingham, K., Abou-Setta, A., & Buckett, W. (2007). Ultrasound versus 'clinical touch' for catheter guidance during embryo transfer in women. *Cochrane Database of Systematic Reviews* , Vol.24, No.1, (January 2007), ISSN 1469-493X

Buckett, WM. (2003). A meta-analysis of ultrasound-guided versus clinical touch embryo transfer. *Fertility and Sterility*, Vol.80, No.4, (October 2003), pp.1037-41, ISSN 0015-0282

Castelbaum, AJ., Ying, L., Somkuti, SG., Sun, J., Ilesanni, AO., & Lessey, BA. (1997). Characterization of integrin expression in well differentiated endometrial a endometrial adenocarcinoma cell line (Ishikawa). *The Journal of Clinical Endocrinology and Metabolism*, Vol.82, No.1, (January 1997), pp.136-142. ISSN 1945-7197

Check, JH., Nowroozi, K., Choe, J., Lurie, D., & Dietterich, C. (1993). The effect of endometrial thickness and echo pattern on in vitro fertilization outcome in donor oocyte-embryo transfer cycle. *Fertility and Sterility*, Vol.59, No.1, (January1993), pp.72-5, ISSN 0015-0282

Check, JH., Choe, JK., Kotsoff, D., Summers-Chase, D., & Wilson, C. (1999). Controlled ovarian hyperstimulation adversely affects implantation following in vitro fertilization-embryo transfer. *Journal of Assisted Reproduction and Genetics*, Vol.16, No.8, (September 1999), pp. 416-20, ISSN 1573-7330

Croxatto, HB., Fuentealba, B., Diaz, S., Patene, L., &Tatum, HJ. (1972). A simple nonsurgical technique to obtain unimplanted eggs from human uteri. *American Journal of Obstetrics and Gynecology*, Vol.112, No.5, (March 1972), pp.662-8, ISSN 0002-9378

De Placido, G., Wilding, M., Strina, I., Alviggi, E., Alviggi, C., Mollo, A., Varicchio, MT., Tolino, A., Schiattarella, C., & Dale, B. (2002). High outcome predictability after IVF using a combined score for zygote and embryo morphology and growth rate. *Human Reproduction*, Vol.17, No.9, (September 2002), pp.2402-09, ISSN 0268-1161

Dietterich, C., Check, JH., Choe, JK., Nazari, A., & Lurie, D. (2002). Increased endometrial thickness on the day of human chorionic gonadotropin injection does not adversely affect pregnancy or implantation rates following in vitro fertilization-embryo transfer. *Fertility and Sterility*, Vol.77, No.4, (April 2002), pp.781-86, ISSN 0015-0282

Drakeley, AJ., Jorgensen, A., Sklavounos, J., Aust, T., Gazvani, R., Williamson, P., & Kingsland, CR. (2005). A randomized controlled clinical trial of 2295 ultrasound. *Human Reproduction*, Vol.23, No.5, (2008), pp.1101-06, ISSN 0268-1161

Fanchin, R., Ayoubi, JM., Righini, C., Olivennes, F., Schonauer, LM., & Frydman, R. (2001). Uterine contractility decreases at the time of blastocyst transfers. *Human Reproduction*, Vol.16, No.6, (June 2001), pp.1115-9, ISSN 0268-1161

Gamiz, P., Rubio, C., de los Santos, MJ., Mercader, A., Simon, C., Remohl, J., & Pellicer, A. (2003). The effect of pronuclear morphology on early development and chromosomal abnormalities in cleavage-stage embryos. *Human Reproduction*, Vol.18, No.11, (November 2003), pp.2413-19, ISSN 0268-1161

Garcia, JE., Acosta, AA., Hsiu, JG., & Jones, HW Jr. (1984). Advanced endometrial maturation after ovulation induction with human menopausal gonadotropin human chorionic gonadotropin for in vitro fertilization. *Fertility and Sterility*, Vol.41, No.1, (January 1984), pp.31-5, ISSN 0015-0282

García-Velasco, JA., Isaza, V., Martinez-Salazar, J., Landazábal, A., Requena, A., Remohí, J., & Simón, C. (2002).Transabdominal ultrasound-guided embryo transfer does not increase pregnancy rates in oocyte recipients. *Fertility and Sterility*, Vol. 78, No.3, (September 2002) , pp.534-9, ISSN 0015-0282

Garcia-Velasco, JA., Isaza, V., Caligara, C., Pellicer, A., Remohí, J., & Simón, C. (2003). Factors that determine discordant outcome from shared oocytes. *Fertility and Sterility*, Vol.80, No.1, (July 2003), pp.54-60, ISSN 0015-0282

Gardner, DK., Schoolcraft, WB., Wagley, L., Schlenker, T., Stevens, J., & Hesla, J. (1998). A randomized trial of blastocyst culture and transfer in in-vitro fertilization. *Human Reproduction*, Vol.13, No.12, (December 1998), pp.3434-40, ISSN 0268-1161

Gianaroli, L., Magli, MC., Ferraretti, AP., Fortini, D., & Griecc, N. (2003). Pronuclear morphology and chromosomal abnormalities as scoring criteria for embryo slection. *Fertility and Sterility*, Vol.80, No.2, (August 2003), pp.341-9, ISSN 0015-0282

Hnida, C., Engenheiro, E., & Ziebe, S. (2004). Computer-controlled, multilevel, morphometric analysis of blastomere size as biomarker of fragmentation and multinuclearity in human embryos. *Human Reproduction*, Vol.19, No.2, (February 2004), pp.288-93, ISSN 0268-1161

Kovacs, P., Matyas, S., Boda, K., & Kaali, SG. (2003). The effect of endometrial thickness on IVF/ICSI outcome. *Human Reproduction*, Vol.18, No.11, (November 2003), pp.2337-41, ISSN 0268-1161

Lindheim, SR., Cohen, MA., & Sauer, MV. (1999). Ultrasound guided embryo transfer significantly improves pregnancy rates in women undergoing oocyte donation. *International Journal of Gynaecology and Obstetrics*, Vol. 66, No.3, (September 1999), pp.281-4, ISSN 0020-7292

Magli, MC., Gianaroli, L., Munne, S., & Ferratetti, AP. (1998). Incidence of chromosomal abnormalities from a morphologically normal cohort of embryos in poor-prognosis patients. *Journal of Assisted Reproduction and Genetics*, Vol.15, No.5, (May 1998), pp.297-301, ISSN 1573-7330

Mains, L., & Van Voorhis, BJ. (2010). Optimizing the technique of embryo transfer. *Fertility and Sterility*, Vol.93, No.3, (August 2010), pp.785-790, ISSN 0015-0282

McDonald JA, Norman RJ. A randomized controlled trial of a soft double lumen embryo transfer catheter versus a firm single lumen catheter: significant improvements in pregnancy rates. Hum Reprod 2002;17:1502–6

McWilliams, GD., & Frattarelli, JL. (2007). Changes in measured endometrial thickness predict in vitro fertilization success. *Fertility and Sterility*, Vol.88, No.1, (July 2007), pp.74-81, ISSN 0015-0282

Montag, M., & van der Ven, H. (2001). Evaluation of pronuclear morphology as the only selection criterion for further embryo culture and transfer: results of a prospective randomized multicentre study. Human *Reproduction*, Vol.16, No.11, (November 2001), pp.2384-89, ISSN 0268-1161

Nagy, ZP., Dozortsev, D., Diamond, M., Rienzi, L., Ubaldi, F., Adelmassih, R., & Greco, E. (2003). Pronuclear morphology evaluation with subsequent evaluation of embryo morphology significantly increases implantation rates. *Fertility and Sterility*, Vol.80, No.1, (July 2003), pp.67-74, ISSN 0015-0282

Nikas, G., Develioglu, OH., Toner, JP., & Jones, HW. Jr. (1999). Endometrial pinopodes indicate a shift in the window of receptivity in IVF cycles. *Human Reproduction*, Vol.14, No.3, (March 1999), pp.787-92, ISSN 0268-1161

Noci, I., Borri, P., Chieffi, O, Scarsselli, G., Biaglotti, R., Moncini, D., Paglierani, M., & Taddei, G. (1995). Aging of the human endometrium: a basic morphological and immunohistochemical study. *European Journal of Obstetrics & Gynecology, and Reproductive Biology*, Vol.63, No.2, (December 1995), pp.181-85, ISSN 0301-2115

Noyes, N., Hampton, BS., Berkeley, A., Licciardi, F., Grifo, J., & Krey, L. (2001). Factors useful in predicting the success of oocyte donation: a 3-year retrospective analysis. *Fertility and Sterility*, Vol.76, No.1, (July 2001), pp.92-97, ISSN 0015-0282

Noyes, RW., Hertig, AT., & Rock, J. (1950). Dating the endometrial biopsy. *Fertility and Sterility*, Vol.1, No.3, (March 1950), pp.1-3, ISSN 0015-0282

Oehninger, S. (1950). Revealing the enigmas of implantation: what is the true impact of ovarian hyperstimulation? *Fertility and Sterility*, Vol.89, No.1, (January 1950), pp27–30, 0015-0282

Papnikolaou, EG., D'haeseleer, E., Verheyen, G., Van de Velde, H., Camus, M., Van Steirteghem, A., Devroey, P., & Tournaye, H. (2005). Live birth rate is significantly higher after blastocyst transfer than after cleavage-stage transfer when at least four embryos are available on day 3 of culture. A randomized prospective study. *Human Reproduction*, Vol.20, No.11, (November 2005), pp.3198-203, ISSN 0268-1161

Papnikolaou, EG., Camus, M., Kolibianakis, EM., Landuyt, LV., Van Steirteghem, A., & Devroey, P. (2006). In vitro fertilization with single blastocyst-stage versus cleavage-stage embryos. *New England Journal of Medicine*, Vol.354, No.11, (March 2006), pp.1139-46., ISSN 00284793

Paulson, RJ., Sauer, MV., & Lobo, RA. (1997). Potential enhancement of endometrial receptivity in cycles using controlled ovarian hyperstimulation with antiprogestins: a hypothesis. *Fertility and Sterility*, Vol.67, No.2, (February 1997), pp.321-25, ISSN 0015-0282

Porat, N., Boehnlein, LM., Barker, MA., Kovacs, P., & Lindheim, SR. (2010). Blastocyst Embryo Transfer is the Primary Determinant for Improved Outcomes in Oocyte Donation Cycles. *Journal of Obstetrics and Gynaecology Research*, Vol.36, No.2, (April 2010), pp.357-63, ISSN 1447-0756

Rashidi, BH., Sadeghi, M., Jafarabadi, M., & Tehrani Nejad, ES. (2005). Relationships between pregnancy rates following in vitro fertilization or intracytoplasmic sperm injection and endometrial thickness and pattern. *European Journal of Obstetrics,*

Gynecology, and Reproductive Biology, Vol.120, No.2, (June 2005), pp.179-184, ISSN 0301-2115

Remohí, J., Ardiles, G., García-Velasco, JA., Gaitán, P., Simón, C., & Pellicer, A. (1997). Endometrial thickness and serum oestradiol concentrations as predictors of outcome in oocyte donation. *Human Reproduction*, Vol.12, No.10, (October 1997), pp.2271-2276, ISSN 0268-1161

Rienzi, L., Ubaldi, F., Iacobelli, M., Romano, S., Minasi, MG., Ferrero, S., Sapienza, F., Baroni ,E., & Greco, E. (2005). Significance of morphological attributes of the early embryo. *Reproductive Biomedicine Online*, Vol.10, No.5, (May 2005), pp.669-681, ISSN 1472-6483

Richter, KS., Bugge, KR., Bromer, JG., & Levy, MJ. (2007). Relationship between endometrial thickness and embryo implantation, based on 1,294 cycles of in vitro fertilization with transfer of two blastocyst-stage embryos. *Fertility and Sterility*, Vol.87, No.1, (January 2007), pp.53-59, ISSN 0015-0282

Sallam HN, Agameya AF, Rahman AF, Ezzeldin F, Sallam AN. Impact of technical difficulties, choice of catheter, and the presence of blood on the success of embryo transfer: experience from a single provider. J Assist Reprod Genet 2003;20:135–42

Sallam, HN., & Sadek, SS. (2003). Ultrasound-guided embryo transfer: a meta-analysis of randomized controlled trials. *Fertility and Sterility*, Vol.80, No.4, (October 2003), pp.1042-6, ISSN 0015-0282

Schild, RL., Knobloch, C., Dorn, C., Fimmers, R., van der Ven, H., & Hansmann, M. (2001). Endometrial receptivity in an in vitro fertilization program as assessed by spiral artery blood flow, endometrial thickness, endometrial volume, and uterine artery blood flow. *Fertility and Sterility*, Vol. 75, No.2, (February 2001), pp.361-66, ISSN 0015-0282

Schillaci, R., Castelli, A., Vassiliadis, A., Venzia, R., Sciacca, GM., Perino, A., & Cittadini, E. (2002). Blastocyst stage versus day 2 embryo transfer in IVF cycles. *Abstracts of the 18th Annual Meeting of ESHRE, Vienna*, 2002, P-418.

Schoolcraft, WB., & Gardner, DK. (2001). Blastocyst versus day 2 or 3 transfer. *Seminars in Reproductive Medicine*, Vol.19, No.3, (September 2001), pp.259-268, ISSN 1526-8004

Shapiro, BS., Daneshmand, ST., Garner, FC., Aguirre, M., & Ross, R. (2008). Contrasting patterns in in vitro fertilization pregnancy rates among fresh autologous, fresh oocyte donor, and cryopreserved cycles with the use of day 5 or day 6 blastocysts may reflect differences in embryo-endometrium synchrony. *Fertility and Sterility*, Vol.89, No.1, (January 2008), pp.20-26, ISSN 0015-0282

Sharara, FI., Lim, J., & McClamrock, HD. (1999). Endometrial pattern on the day of oocyte retrieval is more predictive of implantation success than the pattern or thickness on the day of hCG administration. *Journal of Assisted Reproduction and Genetics*, Vol.16, No.10, (November 1999), pp.523-28, ISSN 1573-7330

Sher, G., Herbert, C., Maassarani, G., & Jacobs, MH. (1991). Assessment of the late proliferative phase endometrium by ultrasonography in patients undergoing in-vitro fertilization and embryo transfer (IVF-ET). *Human Reproduction*, Vol.6, No.2, (February 1991), pp.232-37, ISSN 0268-1161

Staessen, C., Platteau, P., Van Assche, E., Michiels, A., Tournaye, H., Camus, M., Devroey, P., Liebaers, I., & Van Steirteghem, A. (2004). Comparison of blastocyst transfer with or without preimplantation genetic diagnosis for aneuploidy screening in couples with advanced maternal age: a prospective randomized controlled trial. *Human Reproduction*, Vol.19, No.12, (December 2004), pp.2849-58, ISSN 0268-1161

Sundström, P. (1998). Es Stafford-Bell, MA. (1999). Which factors are important for successful embryo transfer after in vitro fertilization? *Human Reproduction*, Vol.14, No.10, (October 1999), pp.2678-9, ISSN 0268-1161tablishment of a successful pregnancy following in-vitro fertilization with an endometrial thickness of no more than 4 mm. *Human Reproduction*, Vol.13, No.6, (June 1998), pp.1550-52, ISSN 0268-1161

Trounson, A., Leeton, J., Besanko, M., Wood, C., & Conti, A. Pregnancy established in an infertile patient after transfer of a donated embryo fertilized in vivo. *British Medical Journal*, Vol.286, No.6368 (March 1983), pp.835-838, ISSN 0959-8138

Valbuena, D., Martin, J., dePablo, J., Remohi, J., Pellicer, A., & Simon, C. (2001). Increasing levels of estradiol are deleterious to embryonic implantation because they directly affect the embryo. *Fertility & Sterility*, Vol.76, No.5, (November 2001), pp.962-8, ISSN 0015-0282

Van Royen, E., Mangelschotrs, K., De Neubourg, D., Valkenburg, M., Van de Meerssche, M., Ryckaert, G., Estermans, W., & Gerris, J. (1999). Characterization of a top quality embryo, a step towards single-embryo transfer. *Human Reproduction*, Vol.14, No.9, (September 1999), pp2345-49, ISSN 0268-1161

Yuval, Y., Lipitz, S., Dor, J., & Achiron, R. (1999). The relationships between endometrial thickness, and blood flow and pregnancy rates in in-vitro fertilization. *Human Reproduction*, Vol.14, No.4, (April 1999), pp.1067-71, ISSN 0268-1161

Zenke, U., & Chetkowski, RJ. (2004). Transfer and uterine factors are the major recipient-related determinants of success with donor eggs. *Fertility and Sterility*, Vol.82, No.4, (October 2004), pp.850-56, ISSN 0015-0282

Zhang, X., Chen, CH., Confino, E., Barnes, R., Milad, M., & Kazer, RR. (2005). Increased endometrial thickness is associated with improved treatment outcome for selected patients undergoing in vitro fertilization-embryo transfer. *Fertility and Sterility*,Vol.83, No.2, (February 2005), pp.336-40, ISSN 0015-0282

Ziebe, S., Peterson, K., Lindenberg, S., Andersen, AG., Gabrielsen, A., & Andersen, NA. (1997). Embryo morphology or cleavage stage: How to select the best embryos fro transfer after in-vitro fertilization. *Human Reproduction*, Vol.12, No.7, (July 1997), pp.545-49, ISSN 0268-1161

11

Importance of Blastocyst Morphology in Selection for Transfer

Borut Kovačič and Veljko Vlaisavljević
University Medical Centre Maribor
Slovenia

1. Introduction

Prolonged cultivation of embryos to the blastocyst stage has become a routine practice in the human in vitro fertilization program (IVF) since 1999, when the first commercial sequential media were developed. The culture systems have been improved many times and today most of the blastocyst culture media enable the embryos to reach the blastocyst stage in more than 50% of cases (Gardner et al., 1998; Kovačič et al., 2004). The advantages of blastocyst culture are in the possibilities for selection of embryos that have an activated genome (Braude et al., 1988), higher predictive values for implantation on the basis of their morphological appearance as compared with earlier embryos (Gardner and Schoolcraft, 1999; Kovačič et al., 2004) and in a reduction in the number of transferred embryos without compromising pregnancy rate (Gardner et al., 2000a). Blastocyst is also a stage that is better synchronized with endometrial receptivity for its implantation (Croxatto et al., 1978; Gardner et al., 2000c). By replacement of embryos in the blastocyst stage, their exposure to hyperstimulated milieu and consequent endometrial contractions, which could be fatal for them, is significantly shortened (Lesny et al., 1998). Blastocysts also contain a larger number of cells than early stage embryos and should therefore have a better possibility of survival of cryopreservation (Veeck, 2003).

2. Blastocyst culture

The first synthetic medium of only 9 components for mammalian embryos was developed 50 years ago. Since then, intensive research has continued to develop the optimum chemically defined media for human embryos (Summers and Biggers, 2003). In various parts of the female reproductive tract, a precise biochemical analysis of uterine and Fallopian tubal fluids was carried out and the metabolism of energy substrates has also been studied (Leese et al., 1993; Conagham et al., 1993; Houghton et al., 2002; Gardner et al., 2001). These investigations lead to the development of sequential media for prolonged cultivation of human embryos (Gardner and Lane, 1997). After that, the media have been modified several times by adding other macromolecules, which enhance embryo development and implantation, e.g. EDTA (Gardner et al., 2000b) and hyaluronan (Stojković et al., 2002). Also, the toxicity of the medium occurring due to the degradation of amino acids was decreased by substituting the heat-sensitive glutamine for the more stable alanyl-glutamine (Lane et al., 2001). By using commercial blastocyst media in the human IVF program, a blastocyst development rate should be at least 50%. The blastulation rate and quality of developed blastocysts can be improved by reducing the oxygen concentration in the incubator atmosphere (Kovačič and Vlaisavljević, 2008; Kovačič et al., 2010).

3. Blastocyst development

3.1 Compaction

An early embryo begins to divide without increasing its volume. After the third mitotic division, a substantial protein biosynthesis is restored and the embryo starts growing. Consequently, the junctions between blastomeres change, leading to the formation of the compact stage. Compaction should normally be completed on the fourth day of its development when the embryo reaches the morula stage (Abe et al., 1999).

The junctions are dynamic and change during mitosis. Compaction represents the beginning of differentiation, followed by polarization of peripheral blastomeres and lost of totipotency. The polarization is induced by junctions with neighbouring blastomeres. Due to embryo growth, the cells lose their oval shape and become more tightly connected to each other. Compaction is therefore a process of forming gap junctions, adherens junctions, tight junctions and desmosomes between blastomeres. Gap junctions are especially important for transport of metabolites and molecules that regulate mitotic divisions (Ducibella et al., 1975). The membranes between the cells are difficult to observe with a light microscope. The abnormally tight junctions lead to exclusion of blastomeres from the formation of a compact embryo (Watson, 1992).

3.2 Cavitation

Approximately 24 hours after compaction, the cells start forming a fluid-filled cavity - blastocoel. During cavitation, the cells differentiate into the trophectoderm (TE) and inner cell mass (ICM). TE cells maintain cell polarity. Accumulation of water within the blastocoel is a result of Na^+ transport into the blastocoel. Na/K ATPase on basolateral membrane of TE cells pumps intracellular Na^+ from TE into the blastocoels (Watson and Kidder, 1988). Trophectodermal cells are connected by a small surface area with frequent tight junctions and desmosomes that form a seal between cells and maintain cell polarity. They prevent blastocoel liquid from pouring out and keep sodium ions within the blastocoel. (Gualtieri et al., 1992; Garrod et al., 1996). These ions cause osmotic gradient, which consequently results in the passive diffusion of water molecules into the blastocoel causing the blastocoel to start to grow (Watson, 1992).

The expansion of the blastocoel plays an important role in differentiation between TE and ICM. The ICM cells are non-differentiated and pluripotent and should form a compact and oval formation. Outer membranes of ICM don't have junctions with other cells and communicate directly with blastocoel fluid. They are under the regulation of specific growth factors from the blastocoel that regulate their differentiation into the primitive endoderm. The blastocoel fluid also functions as a culture medium for ICM (Dardik et al., 1993). Its molecular composition mostly depends on TE cells. One of the functions of TE is also in reducing the oxygen concentration in the blastocoel fluid and enabling hypoxic conditions that are required for normal gene transcription in ICM cells (Houghton, 2006).

4. Blastocyst scoring systems

The introduction of blastocyst culture into an IVF program offers the possibility for reducing the number of transferred embryos. But the replacements of more than one blastocyst still results in a very high proportion of multiple pregnancies (Vlaisavljević et al., 2008). For this reason, the tendency for single blastocyst transfer arises and various methods of selecting the optimal blastocyst with good developmental potential have been published. Numerous biochemical studies showed that selection between the blastocysts can be made by evaluating their metabolic activity (Hardy et al., 1989; Conagham et al., 1993; Gardner et al., 2001; Houghton et al., 2002). These biochemical methods are time consuming and require expensive additional laboratory equipment. Besides this, their values in predicting the implantation ability are not higher than values obtained by morphological assessment. Thus, blastocyst morphology evaluation still remains the most frequently-used selection method.

Over the last 20 years, several blastocyst morphology evaluation systems have developed. Dokras et al. (1993) were the first who attempted to define the optimal blastocyst by differentiating them according to whether the blastocoele originated from early cavitation or from several vacuoles. In the early period of human blastocyst culture, many gave the priority for selecting the embryos for transfer to blastocysts with more expanded blastocoeles (Shoukir et al., 1998) and to hatching blastocysts (Balaban et al., 2000; Yoon et al., 2001). Later, Gardner and Schoolcraft (1999) described the new three part scoring system that took three morphologic parameters into consideration: blastocoele expansion, form of inner-cell mass (ICM) and trophectoderm (TE) cohesiveness.

4.1 Tripartite scoring of blastocysts

Gardner and Schoolcraft (1999) gave six numerical scores (1-6) to blastocysts regarding the degree of blastocoel expansion and status of hatching. The early blastocysts with the beginning of blastocoel formation are scored as 1 and hatched blastocysts as 6 (Figure 1).

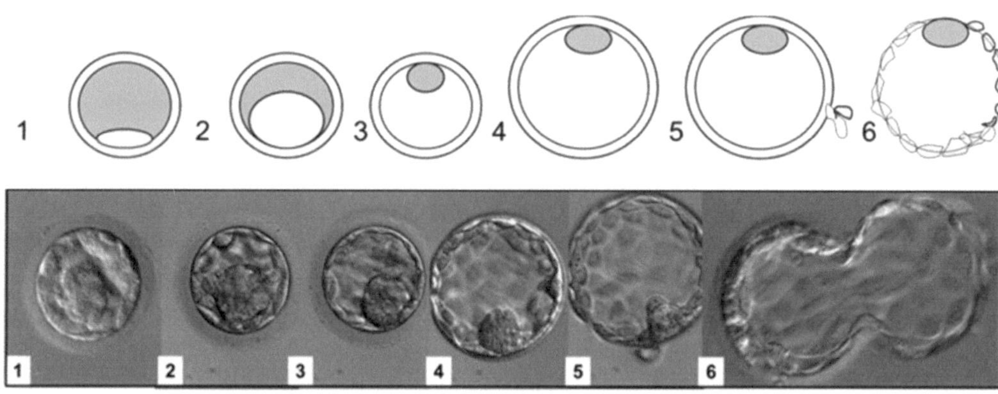

Fig. 1. Expansion and hatching status.
1 The blastocoel cavity represents less than half the volume of the embryo; **2** The blastocoel cavity is more than half the volume of the embryo; **3** Full blastocyst, cavity completely fills the embryo; **4** Expanded blastocyst, cavity is larger than the embryo with thinning of the shell; **5** Hatching out of the shell; **6** Hatched out of the shell. (Gardner & Schoolcraft, 1999).

ICM is only possible for assessment of full blastocysts graded 3-6. The ICM and TE were assessed each as A, B or C, where A is the score for optimal morphology and C for severe irregularities observed (Figure 2). By using this scheme, the transfer of blastocysts scored 3AA or greater results in a pregnancy rate of 60%.

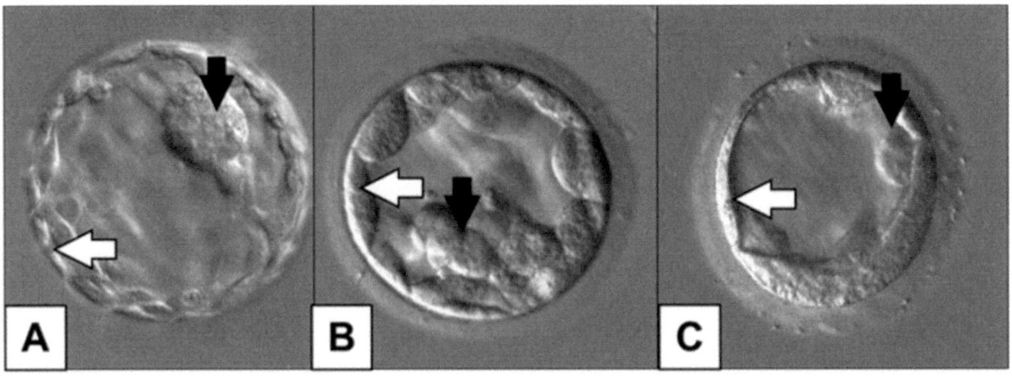

Fig. 2. Inner cell mass (black arrows) and trophectoderm (white arrows) scores.
Inner cell mass:**A** Many cells, tightly packed; **B** Several cells, loosely grouped; **C** Very few cells. Trophectoderm: **A** Many cells forming a cohesive layer; **B** Few cells forming a loose epithelium; **C** Very few large cells. (Gardner & Schoolcraft, 1999).

Gardner's system has been modified by Cornell's group (Veeck and Zaninović, 2009). The compact embryos with early cavitation and with blastocoels smaller than half the volume of the embryo was considered to be cavitating morulas and not blastocysts. Blastocysts were defined as having blastocoels filling greater than half the volume of the conceptus and should possess cells that suggest the formation of ICM. This means that Score 3 from Gardner's system is equal to Score 1 from Cornell's grading. Blastocysts with slightly thinner zona due to growing of the embryo are graded with Score 2. Score 3 is given to fully expanded blastocysts with thin zona. Scores 4 and 5 are equal to Gardner's Scores 5 and 6. Grade 6 was given to hatching or hatched blastocysts in which the zona has been opened due to blastomere biopsy or assisted hatching. Besides this, Cornell's system contains four alphabetical grades (A-D) for ICM and four for TE, where D is the score for degenerative ICM or TE.

By transferring one 1BD, an implantation rate of 59% was achieved, and replacement of one 3AA, 3AB or 3BA, resulted in implantation in 63% of cases. The difference was not significant and the authors concluded that any defined blastocyst on day 5 will lead to good pregnancy and implantation results. Lower success rates were obtained only after replacement of day-5 morulas (17%).

4.2 Grading of blastocysts

Too little attention has been given to individual grading parameters, and the main question in the selection process is which of the blastocyst structures is more important for achieving normal pregnancy. A tripartitive scoring system is therefore difficult to use in evaluating the implantation ability of various morphological types of blastocysts. It is not helpful in cycles in which the blastocysts for transfer have to be selected between suboptimal blastocysts.

From this reason, Kovačič et al. (2004) developed the simple blastocyst grading system. They took four morphological parameters into consideration: expansion of blastocoels, morphology of ICM, cohesiveness of TE and presence of excluded blastomeres or fragments from the formation of blastocysts (Figure 3). This system does not distinguish between different degrees of blastocoel expansion. The authors explained their decision with the fact that the blastocoel can fill and expands in a very short time. They described eight morphological types of day-5 embryos that are most frequently found in the cohort of vital embryos after prolonged cultivation in vitro. All eight types were ranked for their implantation abilities and live birth rates from B1 to B8 (live birth rates: 45.2%, 32.8%, 26.9%, 23%, 17.7%, 16.7%, 7.7%, 1.2%). ICM was found to be the most important factor for successful implantation.

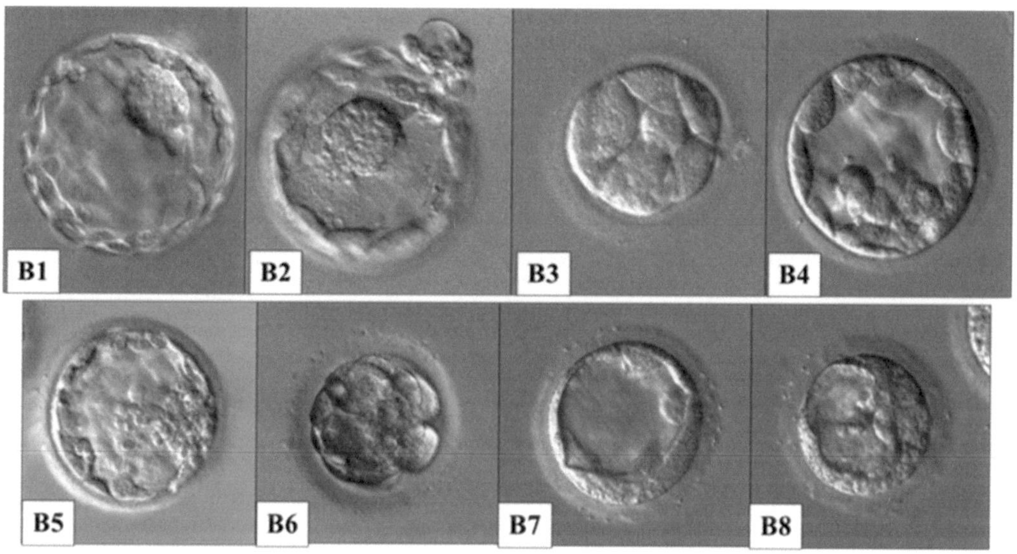

Fig. 3. Grading of blastocysts by Kovacic et al. (2004).
B1 Optimal blastocysts: full or expanded blastocysts with blastocoele filling the entire blastocyst, oval shaped and compact inner-cell mass (ICM) and multicellular cohesive trophectoderm (TE). **B2** Expanded blastocysts with normal ICM, but non-optimal (fragmented or necrotic) TE. **B3** Unexpanded blastocysts and compact morulae with beginning of cavitation. B**4** Expanded blastocysts with normal TE, but non-optimal (non-compact or fragmented) ICM. **B5** Expanded blastocysts with non-optimal ICM and TE. **B6** Slightly smaller blastocysts with up to 20% excluded blastomeres or fragments from the formation of blastocyst. **B7** Necrotic blastocysts without ICM and with large vacuole instead of blastocoel. **B8** Small blastocysts with less than 80% of embryonic mass transformed into compact morulae or blastocysts.

4.3 Other morphological characteristics with impact on implantation

Individual grading parameters were further studied by various groups.

Using morphometry of ICM, Richter et al. (2001) defined optimal blastocysts even more precisely. The authors discredited the previously described tripartitive scoring systems, stating that the observed differences using this system reflect differences in developmental timing rather than differences in actual quality. More attention in their own study was given to measuring of ICM size and shape. They found that the ICMs of implanting blastocysts were significantly larger than ICMs of non-implanting ones. A linear positive relationship between ICM size and implantation ability was revealed. Optimal ICM size was defined as measuring >4500 μm^2 and poor blastocysts with ICM size of <3800 μm^2 (implantation rates 45% vs. 32%). The ICM shape seems to play an important role in further embryo development as well, since blastocysts with optimal ICM sizes and oval shapes implanted in a higher proportion (60%) than the blastocysts with ICMs that were only optimally sized (29%) or shaped (32%).

Ebner et al. (2004) found a significant difference in blastocyst implantation rates when the location of herniation during hatching process is positioned in the ICM region or TE region (67% vs. 41%).

Between various morphological characteristics with possible influence on further embryo development, cytoplasmic strings that connect ICM with TE (Scott, 2000) and vacuoles in the ICM region were found to decrease implantation ability.

The proportion of cytoplasm excluded from the formation of blastocysts either as blastomeres or fragments is also in correlation with embryo ability to reach a morphologically optimal blastocyst (Ivec et al., 2011).

The effect of delay in development to blastocyst by one day was also analyzed by several groups. It can frequently occur that embryos reach blastocyst stage only on day 6. The reasons for this phenomenon are not exactly known. It was only hypothesized that cytoplasmic immaturity of oocytes, chromosomal abnormalities in blastomeres and suboptimal culture conditions could cause longer intermitotic periods and, consequently, slower embryo development. Our results (Ivec et al., 2011) showed that 84.4% of compact day-5 morulas are able to reach the blastocyst stage, but only 23.9% of them are morphologically optimal blastocysts.

Day-5 blastocysts usually result in better implantation rate than embryos that are transferred into the uterus as day-6 blastocysts (37.4% vs. 20.6% in Shapiro et al., 2001)(22.1% vs. 3.6% in Barrenetxea et al., 2005). However, the implantation rates can be improved when day-6 blastocysts are frozen and replaced during one of the next fresh cycles (Shapiro et al., 2008).

5. Blastocyst selection for transfer

Multiple pregnancies, the usual complications of an IVF program, present a serious perinatal risk for mother and child. The analyses of assisted reproductive technology outcomes from European and American registers reported that one half of children born after IVF/ICSI methods derived from multiple pregnancies (de Mouzon et al., 2010; Schieve et al., 1999).

Such a high rate of multiple pregnancies after IVF has been accepted in the past, since acceptable success rates have been achieved only after the transfer of three or four early cleavage stage embryos. By improving the culture conditions, developing culture media for prolonged cultivation of embryos in vitro and by introducing the blastocyst culture, reduction of the number of embryos for transfer was enabled (Vlaisavljević et al., 2008). Moreover, it has been proved in many studies that the transfer of only one blastocyst in a group of patients with the highest probability for conception can result in a similar pregnancy rate as the transfer of two blastocysts, but the proportion of multiple pregnancies is significantly reduced (Gerris et al., 2005). The analysis of outcomes of 904 IVF cycles from four randomized studies and 7404 cycles from six cohort studies showed a pregnancy rate of 33.9% after elective single embryo-transfers (eSET) and 35% after double embryo-transfers (DET), and a very high twins rate of 32.6% in the DET group (Gerris et al., 2005).

The success rate of eSET mainly depends on the ability of selection of the best embryo from all those available. The selection made among blastocysts is easier than selection of early cleavage stage embryos. Nevertheless, the morphology of blastocysts is very heterogeneous and a decision for single or double blastocyst transfer is sometimes very difficult, especially if only morphologically suboptimal blastocysts are available.

5.1 Transfer outcome in relation to blastocyst morphology

The analysis was made on 2779 blastocyst transfer cycles performed at the Maribor IVF Centre from 2001 to 2010 in a patient group with female ages of less than 36 and a maximum of one previous IVF attempt. Ovarian stimulation protocols with a combination of GnRH agonist/GnRH antagonist and recombinant FSH (Gonal-f®, Serono International SA, Geneva, Switzerland)/HMG (Menopur, Ferring Pharmaceuticals Inc., Saint-Prex, Switzerland) were used and described previously in detail (Vlaisavljević et al, 2008). The decision for short or prolonged embryo culture was made on the third day after oocyte insemination. The embryos were cultivated to day 5 if the cohort of day-3 embryos had more than two morphologically optimal embryos containing eight equally-sized blastomeres and less than 10% of cytoplasmic fragments in the periviteline space. Embryos were cultivated in sequential media (BlastAssist System, Medicult/Origio, Denmark) and were assessed daily by using the conventional grading system for early embryos and our blastocyst grading system (Kovačič et al., 2004). Single (SBT) or double blastocyst transfer (DBT) was selected with the agreement of patients. In 2008, the Health Insurance Institute of Slovenia strove to lower the number of multiple pregnancies. It widened the rights of patients by reimbursing them for two additional IVF cycles, allowing a total of six cycles to be reimbursed. But in women younger than 36, only one top-quality embryo in the first two IVF cycles should be transferred. According to this limitation, elective single blastocyst transfer was favoured from 2008 in this patient group.

The analysis shows similar delivery rates in groups of transfers of single optimal blastocyst, double optimal blastocysts or double optimal + non-optimal blastocysts (54.7% vs. 60.4% vs. 53.1%; P>0.05).

The twins rate was 51.9% in the group of double optimal blastocysts and only 10% less (41.5%) in double optimal + non-optimal blastocyst group.

Single non-optimal or double non-optimal blastocyst transfers resulted in equal delivery rates (32.6% vs. 34.7%), but they were significantly lower than the delivery rate obtained in the group of single optimal blastocyst transfers (54.7%)(p<0.05). Nevertheless, the twins rate in double non-optimal blastocyst transfer was still 28%.

A more detailed analysis of transfers of poor quality blastocysts graded B5 to B8 shows, again, very similar delivery rates after SBT and DBT (29.1% vs. 26.9%) and a twins rate of 21.7% in the DBT group.

	Single blastocyst transfer		Double blastocyst transfer		
Blastocyst quality	Optimal	Non-optimal	Optimal Optimal	Optimal Non-optimal	Non-optimal Non-optimal
No. of transfers	869	362	555	377	616
Clinical pregnancies	546 (62.8)	124 (34.3)	373 (67.2)	227 (60.2)	248 (40.3)
Deliveries	475 **(54.7)**	118 **(32.6)**	335 **(60.4)**	200 **(53.1)**	214 **(34.7)**
Singletons	469 (98.7)	115 (97.5)	157 (46.9)	115 (57.5)	154 (72)
Twins	6 **(1.3)**	3 **(2.5)**	174 **(51.9)**	83 **(41.5)**	60 **(28)**
Triplets	0	0	4 (1.2)	2 (1)	0

Values in parentheses are percentages.

Table 1. Delivery rates after single and double blastocyst transfers in a group of patients younger than 36 with one or fewer previous IVF treatments.

It is clear from previous reports (Henman et al., 2005; Lukassen et al., 2005; Vlaisavljević et al., 2008) that in women 36 years old and younger, where we expect a delivery rate per transfer of more than 30%, transferring two blastocysts will result in an unacceptably high percentage of multiple pregnancies. In some countries (like in Slovenia), the obligation for single embryo-transfer is not only related to patient age but also to embryo quality (for example: elected single embryo-transfer of top quality embryo). Some consider every blastocyst to be a top quality embryo, while others categorize them more precisely and decide for double transfer if blastocysts are not morphologically optimal.

Our blastocyst grading system (Kovačič et al., 2004) consists of 7 morphologically suboptimal blastocyst types, and for each, the expected live birth rate was calculated in a patient group younger than 40. All the categories of suboptimal blastocysts, graded from B4 to B8 had a live birth rate calculated at lower than 30%. According to the recommendation regarding the limitation of double embryo transfer in cycles with expected delivery rates of more than 30%, we can conclude that in cases with blastocysts graded B3 and higher, more than one blastocyst could be transferred. However, in our recent study (Table 2), the subpopulation of blastocyst transfers of very poor quality blastocysts was further analyzed. It was proven again that double blastocyst transfer does not improve delivery rate neither in cycles with optimal nor in cycles with very poor quality blastocysts.

One of the main reasons for doubts about the reasonability of single blastocyst transfer in the past was in the relatively low success of the blastocyst-freezing program. The pregnancy rate in European countries was around 15% per one thawing cycle. This was only half of the pregnancy rate achieved by fresh blastocysts (de Mouzon et al., 2010), but the modification of vitrification techniques in the last couple of years have much improved the survival and live birth rates (Mukaida et al., 2001; Hiraoka et al., 2004; Kuwayama et al., 2005).

	Single blastocyst transfer	Double blastocyst transfer
Blastocyst quality	B5 - B8	Both B5-B8
No. of transfers	172	308
Clinical pregnancies	57 (33.1)	99 (32.1)
Deliveries	50 **(29.1)**	83 **(26.9)**
Singletons	50 (100)	65 (78.3)
Twins	0 **(0)**	18 **(21.7)**
Triplets	0	0

Values in parentheses are percentages.

Table 2. Delivery and twins rate in a younger patient group after the transfer of one or two blastocysts of poor quality.

6. Blastocyst morphology after cryopreservation

Blastocyst is not the optimal stage for cryopreservation. It contains a large amount of liquid in the blastocoel, which must be eliminated before the embryo undergoes cooling. To achieve this, a high concentration of cryoprotectants must be used, despite that they can become toxic to an embryo after a longer exposure time. Vitrification is a two-step technique. In the first step, the blastocyst must be exposed to an equilibration medium, which causes partial dehydration and decreasing in the blastocyst volume and its re-expansion after a couple of minutes. The second step must be performed in one minute. After putting the blastocyst into the vitrification medium, its blastocoel quickly looses liquid. Blastocysts are therefore vitrified in a collapsed stage. When it is warmed, its embryonic mass fills only 50% of the volume within zona pelucida (Figure 4A). By

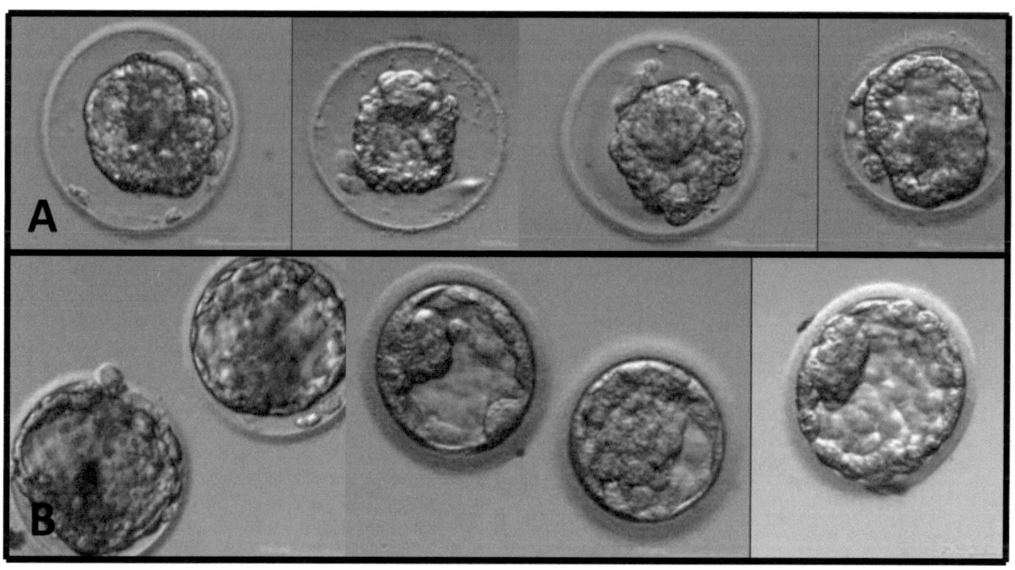

Fig. 4. Blastocysts that completely survived the vitrification/devitrification procedure. **A** Blastocysts in the collapsed stage immediately after devitrification. **B** Re-expanded blastocysts two hours later.

decreasing the concentration of cryoprotectants stepwise, the blastocyst should recover the volume of trophectoderm cells that they had before cryopreservation. The intracellular organelles must be redistributed forming polarized cells and a functional Na/K pump, responsible for filling the blastocoel with liquid. Two hours after warming, a blastocyst should partially or completely re-expand (Figure 4B) to the dimensions it had before vitrification. If the blastocyst survives, its ICM must be equally shaped and sized as before cryopreservation.

6.1 Impact of blastocyst expansion on survival after vitrification

Fresh blastocysts are heterogeneous in morphology and in the ability to survive vitrification. The aim of our study was to find out the implantation ability of various blastocyst types after vitrification, warming and embryo replacement (VER) and to estimate the prediction of live birth after VER.

Day-5 surplus blastocysts or compact morulae from IVF/ICSI cycles were scored before vitrification by using our grading system (Kovačič et al., 2004) (**Figure 3**). Surplus blastocysts were vitrified in Cryo Bio System Vitrification straws (France) by using Irvine Scientific (USA) Vitrification protocol and media. Blastocysts were frozen individually, thus, their quality (grade) was known when they were thawed.

Warmed blastocysts were replaced in natural cycles (n=327) or in cycles supported by estrogen/progesterone (n=103). In our retrospective study, we analyzed 430 devitrification cycles in which 750 blastocysts were devitrified and 642 (85.6%) embryos survived and were replaced.

Types of blastocysts before vitrification		**Expanded Blastocysts**	**Early blastocysts**	**Poor blastocysts**
Number of warmed blastocysts *(n)*		552	97	101
Morphology of warmed blastocysts				
a	100% intact, re-expanded *(n)*	224 **(40.6)**	63 **(64.9)**	38 **(37.6)**
b	<100% >50% intact, re-expanded *(n)*	200 (36.2)	21 (21.6)	32 (31.7)
c	<100% >50% intact, non-expanded *(n)*	40 (7.2)	7 (7.2)	17 (16.8)
d	Damaged *(n)*	88 (15.9)	6 (6.2)	14 (13.9)
Survival rate (a+b+c) *(%)*		**84.0**	**93.8**	**86.1**
Live births/warmed blastocysts *(%)*		82/552 (14.9)	14/97 (14.4)	8/101 (7.9)
Live births/transferred blastocysts *(%)*		82/464 **(17.7)**	14/91 **(15.4)**	8/87 **(9.2)**

Values in parenthesis are percentages.

Table 3. Survival and live birth rates after vitrification in variously expanded blastocyst groups.

All warmed blastocysts were assessed for morphology, first, immediately after warming and second, two hours later, before the transfer was performed. Warmed blastocysts were categorized into four groups (**A-D**), considering the proportion of intact cells and the ability of re-expansion. **A** were blastocysts with 100% intact cells and re-expansion within two hours after cryopreservation. **B** were blastocysts with less than 100% and more than 50% of intact cells with the ability to re-expand the blastocoel. **C** contained blastocysts that remained non-expanded even after two hours of incubation after thawing. **D** blastocysts degenerated or had less than 50% of intact cells.

Survival (more than 50% of intact cells), optimal survival (100% of intact cells and re-expansion), implantation (gestational sac with heart beats) and live birth rates were calculated for all three groups of warmed blastocysts for which the outcome after replacement was known (98.4% of all transferred blastocysts).

Blastocysts with optimal survival (a) contained all cells intact and were able to refill the blastocoel and expand after two hours of incubation. The rates of optimal survival differ significantly between expanded blastocysts (40.6%) and non-expanded blastocysts (64.9%) ($P<0.0001$). Among poor blastocysts, only 37.6% of them completely survived vitrification.

By regarding overall survival rates (at least 50% of intact cells), those embryos with no blastocoel or with the beginning of cavitation survived vitrification better than morphologically optimal blastocysts with expanded blastocoel and normal TE and ICM ($P<0.05$). The same has been reported by Van Landuyt et al. (2011). The survival rates in their study were higher for early blastocysts (86.7%) compared to full (78.7%) or expanded blastocysts (72.7%). Similar results were also obtained by Cho et al., 2002; Vandezwalmen et al., 2002; Mukaida et al., 2006; and Ebner et al., 2009. This is probably due to lower permeability of later blastocyst stages to the cryoprotectant (Cho et al., 2002; Vanderzwalmen et al., 2002).

6.2 Live birth rates after vitrification of variously expanded blastocysts

Meta analysis of studies comparing transfer outcomes of slowly frozen/thawed and vitrified/warmed embryos and blastocysts showed significantly better clinical results in the vitrification group (Loutradi et al., 2008). Vitrification is becoming an increasingly popular method of cryopreservation due to simplification of the procedure. It is evident that this method improved survival and implantation rates, especially in the blastocyst cryopreservation program. There are some technical details with great impact on blastocyst survival. First, expanded blastocysts are sometimes more difficult to equilibrate with cryoprotectant than other stage embryos, thus, exposure to equilibration solution should be modified from embryo to embryo depending on its expansion rate. However, all procedures are time limited due to possible toxic effects in cases of longer incubation of embryos in cryoprotectant. Secondly, faster rates of cooling and warming can be achieved by minimizing the volume of the cryoprotectant with which embryos are vitrified. Most published studies on blastocyst vitrification present survival rates that are higher than 85% (Mukaida and Takahashi, 2007). However, there are still big differences in implantation and pregnancy rates among published studies.

Mukaida and Takahashi (2007) achieved a pregnancy rate per warming of 48.4% and an implantation rate of 38.5% in 1500 warming cycles with 3500 warmed blastocysts by using the cryoloop technique. They much improved their results when artificial shrinkage was applied in expanded blastocysts before vitrification (60% pregnancy and 48% implantation rate).

Goto et al. (2011) demonstrated that there was a significant correlation between fresh blastocyst score and pregnancy outcome after vitrification, warming and transfer of blastocysts. The highest delivery rate was observed in the fully-expanded and hatching blastocyst group of transfers and the lowest success with early blastocysts (59.9% vs. 4.5%) in the young patient group. They reported the same success rate as is usually achieved with fresh optimal blastocysts. The blastocysts in this study were vitrified in open straws with a cooling rate of -23000°C/min.

In our study, we used closed vitrification straws, according to EU Directives concerning tissue and cell storage, in which the blastocysts were vitrified with a cooling rate of approximately -2000°C/min. Our delivery rates in the expanded blastocyst group deviate a lot from Goto's results (17.7%). We can't explain the difference in success rates with different cooling rates used in both studies, since some experiments have already demonstrated that the success rate of blastocyst vitrification in a closed or open system can be the same (Guns et al., 2008). The results from our study are completely comparable with results from the Belgian group (Van Landuyt et al., 2011) in which the vital clinical pregnancy rate per transferred full blastocyst was around 17.5% and per transferred early blastocyst was 10.6%.

In our and in Belgian studies, the blastocysts for vitrification were not rigorously preselected. Besides this, the difference from the Japanese studies is also in their waiting for blastocoels expansion or spontaneous hatching of blastocysts and in performing assisted collapsing before vitrification. All these details could be crucial for success, but their impact should be further investigated.

7. Conclusions

The calculated implantation ability of specific blastocyst type should help the clinicians in their decision regarding the number of fresh or frozen/thawed blastocysts for transfer and in predicting implantation and live birth after the transfer. Our results showed that single or double blastocyst transfer result in similar pregnancy rates in young patient groups, but the twin rate remains unacceptably high after the transfer of two blastocysts, especially if at least one of them is morphologically optimal. Double blastocyst transfer is therefore not advised in young patient groups.

Vitrification is a cryopreservation method for surplus blastocysts. It seems that non-expanded blastocysts are a more optimal stage for vitrification than expanded blastocysts, since the former survive vitrification at higher rates. Nevertheless, the implantation abilities of devitrified early blastocysts or expanded blastocysts were comparable, but significantly lower when compared to fresh blastocysts. It is not clear yet if the differences in success rates after the transfer of devitrified blastocysts between studies are the result of various preselection criteria for blastocysts suitable for vitrification or that there are details in vitrification techniques that are crucial for embryo survival and implantation. Further studies are required for analysis of the effect of open or closed vitrification systems, different cryopreservation media, assisted collapsing and times of exposing the embryos to vitrification solutions.

8. References

Abe, H. Otoi, T. Tachikawa, S. Yamashita, S. Satoh, T & Hoshi, H. (1999). Fine structure of bovine morulae and blastocysts in vivo and in vitro. *Anatomy and Embryology*, Vol.199(6), pp. 519-527

Balaban, B. Urman, B. Sertac, A. Alatas, C. Aksoy, S & Mercan, R. (2000). Blastocyst quality affects the success of blastocyst-stage embryo transfer. *Fertility and Sterility*, Vol.74, pp. 282-287

Barrenetxea, G. López de Larruzea, A. Ganzabal, T. Jiménez, R. Carbonero, K & Mandiola, M. (2005). Blastocyst culture after repeated failure of cleavage-stage embryo transfers: a comparison of day 5 and day 6 transfers. *Fertility and Sterility*, Vol.83(1), pp. 49-53

Braude, P. Bolton, V & Moore, S. (1988). Human gene expression first occurs between the four- and eight-cell stages of preimplantation development. *Nature*, Vol.332(6163), pp. 459-61

Cho, H.J. Son, W.Y. Yoon, S.H. Lee, S.W. & Lim, J.H. (2002). An improved protocol for dilution of cryoprotectants from vitrified human blastocysts. *Human Reproduction*, Vol.17(9), pp. 2419-2422

Conagham, J. Hardy, K. Handyside, A.H., Winston, R.M. & Leese, H.J. (1993). Selection criteria for human embryo transfer: a comparison of pyruvate uptake and morphology. *Journal of Assisted Reproduction and Genetic*, Vol.10, pp. 21-30

Croxatto, H.B. Ortiz, M.E. Díaz, S. Hess, R. Balmaceda, J. & Croxatto, H.D. (1978). Studies on the duration of egg transport by the human oviduct. II. Ovum location at various intervals following luteinizing hormone peak. *American Journal of Obstetrics and Gynecology*, Vol.132(6), pp. 629-634

Dardik, A. Doherty, A.S. & Schultz, R.M. (1993). Protein secretion by the mouse blastocyst: stimulatory effect on secretion into the blastocoel by transforming growth factor-alpha. *Molecular Reproduction and Development*, Vol.34(4), pp. 396-401

De Mouzon, J. Goossens, V. Bhattacharya, S. Castilla, J.A. Ferraretti, A.P. Korsak, V. Kupka, M. Nygren, K.G. Nyboe Andersen. A. & The European IVF-monitoring (EIM) Consortium. (2010). Assisted reproductive technology in Europe, 2006: results generated from European registers by ESHRE. *Human Reproduction*, Vol.25, pp. 1851-1862

Dokras, A. Sargent, I.L. & Barlow, D.H. (1993). Human blastocyst grading: an indicator of developmental potential. *Human Reproduction*, Vol.8, pp. 2119-2127

Ducibella, T. Albertini, D.F. Anderson, E. & Biggers, J.D. (1975). The preimplantation mammalian embryo: characterization of intercellular junctions and their appearance during development. *Developmental Biology*, Vol.45(2), pp. 231-250

Ebner, T. Gruber, I & Moser, M. (2004). Location of herniation predicts implantation behaviour of hatching blastocysts. *Journal of the Turkish-German Gynecological Association*, Vol.8, pp. 184-189

Ebner, T. Vanderzwalmen, P. Shebl, O. Urdl, W. Moser, M. Zech, NH & Tews, G. (2009). Morphology of vitrified/warmed day-5 embryos predicts rates of implantation, pregnancy and live birth. *Reproductive Biomedicine Online, Vol.*19(1), pp. 72-78

Gardner, D. Vella, P. Lane, M. Wagley, L. Schlenker, T & Schoolcraft, W. (1998). Culture and transfer of human blastocysts increases implantation rates and reduces the need for multiple embryo transfers. *Fertility and Sterility*, Vol.69, pp. 84-88

Gardner, D.K. & Lane, M. (1997). Culture and selection of viable human blastocysts: a feasible proposition for human IVF. *Human Reproduction Update,* Vol.3, pp. 367-382

Gardner, D.K. & Schoolcraft, WB. (1999). In vitro culture of human blastocysts. In: Jansen R, Mortimer D (eds) *Toward reproductive certainty: fertility and genetics beyond.* Parthenon Publishing, Carnforth, UK. pp. 378-388

Gardner, D.K. Lane, M. Stevens, J. & Schoolcraft, WB. (2001). Nonivasive assessment of human embryo nutrient consumption as a measure of developmental potential. *Fertility and Sterility,* Vol.76, pp. 1175-1180

Gardner, D.K. Lane, M. Stevens, J. Schlenker, T. & Schoolcraft, W.B. (2000). Blastocyst score affects implantation and pregnancy outcome: towards a single blastocyst transfer. *Fertility and Sterility,* Vol.73(6), pp. 1155-1158

Gardner, D.K. Lane, M.W. & Lane, M. (2000). EDTA stimulates cleavage stage bovine embryo development in culture but inhibits blastocyst development and differentiation. *Molecular Reproduction and Development,* Vol.57, pp. 256-261

Gardner, D.K. Pool, T.B. & Lane, M. (2000). Embryo nutrition and energy metabolism and its relationship to embryo growth, differentiation, and viability. *Seminars in Reproductive Medicine,* Vol.18(2), pp. 205-218

Garrod, D. Chidgey, M. & North, A. (1996). Desmosomes: differentiation, development, dynamics and disease. *Current Opinion in Cell Biology,* Vol.8(5), pp. 670-678

Gerris, J.M. (2005). Single embryo transfer and IVF/ICSI outcome: a balanced appraisal. *Human Reproduction Update,* Vol.11, pp. 105-121

Goto, S. Kadowaki, T. Tanaka, S. Hashimoto, H. Kokeguchi, S & Shiotani, M. (2011). Prediction of pregnancy rate by blastocyst morphological score and age, based on 1,488 single frozen-thawed blastocyst transfer cycles. *Fertility and Sterility,* Vol.95(3), pp. 948-952

Gualtieri, R. Santella, L & Dale, B. (1992). Tight junctions and cavitation in the human pre-embryo. *Molecular Reproduction and Development,* Vol.32(1), pp. 81-87

Guns, Y. Vandermonde, A. Vitrier, S. Sterckx, J. Devroey, P. Van den Abbeel, E. & Van Der Elst, J. (2008). Validation of media and devices for vitrification of human embryos: in search of an optimum. In: Abstracts of the 24th Annual Meeting of the ESHRE, Barcelona, Spain, O-134, pp. i55-i56

Henman, M. Catt, J.W. Wood, T. Bowman, M.C. de Boer, K.A. & Jansen, R.P. (2005). Elective transfer of single fresh blastocysts and later transfer of cryostored blastocysts reduces the twin pregnancy rate and can improve the in vitro fertilization live birth rate in younger women. *Fertility and Sterility,* Vol.84, pp. 1620-1627

Hiraoka, K. Hiraoka, K. Kinutani, M & Kinutani, K. (2004). Blastocoele collapse by micropipetting prior to vitrification gives excellent survival and pregnancy outcomes for human day 5 and 6 expanded blastocysts. *Human Reproduction,* Vol.19, pp. 2884-2888

Houghton, F.D. (2006). Energy metabolism of the inner cell mass and trophectoderm of the mouse blastocyst. *Differentiation,* Vol.74, pp. 11-18

Houghton, F.D. Hawkhead, JA. Humpherson, PG. Hogg, JE. Balen, AH. Rutherford, AJ & Leese, HJ. (2002). Non-invasive amino acid turnover predicts human embryo developmental capacity. *Human Reproduction,* Vol.17, pp. 999-1005

Ivec, M. Kovačič, B & Vlaisavljević, V. (2011). Prediction of human blastocyst development from morulae with delayed and/or uncomplete compaction. *Fertility and Sterility*, (In Press).

Kovacic, B. & Vlaisavljevic, V. (2008). Influence of atmospheric versus reduced oxygen concentration on development of human blastocysts in vitro: a prospective study on sibling oocytes. *Reproductive Biomedicine Online*, Vol.17, pp. 229-236

Kovačič, B. Sajko, M.C. & Vlaisavljević, V. (2010). A prospective, randomized trial on the effect of atmospheric versus reduced oxygen concentration on the outcome of intracytoplasmic sperm injection cycles. *Fertility and Sterility*, Vol.94, pp. 511-519

Kovacic, B. Vlaisavljevic, V. Reljic, M. & Cizek-Sajko, M. (2004). Developmental capacity of different morphological types of day 5 human morulae and blastocysts. *Reproduction Biomedicine Online*, Vol.8, pp. 687-694

Kuwayama, M. Vajta, G. Ieda, S & Kato, O. (2005). Comparison of open and closed methods for vitrification of human embryos and the elimination of potential contamination. *Reproductive Biomedicine Online*, Vol.11, pp. 608-614

Leese, H.J. Conaghan, J. Martin, KL & Hardy, K. (1993). Early human embryo metabolism. *Bioessays*, Vol.15, pp. 259-264

Lesny, P. Killick, S.R. Tetlow, R.L. Robinson, J. & Maguiness, S.D. (1998). Uterine junctional zone contractions during assisted reproduction cycles. *Human Reproduction Update*, Vol.4(4), pp. 440-445

Loutradi, K.E. Kolibianakis, E.M. Venetis, C.A. Papanikolaou, E.G. Pados, G. Bontis, I. & Tarlatzis, B.C. (2008). Cryopreservation of human embryos by vitrification or slow freezing: a systematic review and meta-analysis. *Fertility and Sterility*, Vol.90, pp. 186-193

Lukassen, H.G. Braat, D.D. Wetzels, A.M. Zeilhuis, G.A. Adang, E.M. Scheenjes, E. & Kremer, J.A. (2005). Two cycles with single embryo transfer versus one cycle with double embryo transfer: a randomized controlled trial. *Human Reproduction*, Vol.20, pp. 702-708

Mukaida, T & Takahashi, K. (2007). Vitrification of blastocysts using the Cryoloop technique. In Tucker MJ, Lieberman J (eds.) Vitrification in assisted reproduction, Informa Healthcare, London , pp. 219-238

Mukaida, T. Nakamura, S. Tomiyama, T. Wada, S. Kasai, M. & Takahashi, K. (2001). Successful birth after transfer of vitrified human blastocysts with use of a cryoloop containerless technique. *Fertility and Sterility*, Vol.76, pp. 618-620

Mukaida, T. Oka, C. Goto, T. & Takahashi, K. (2006). Artificial shrinkage of blastocoeles using either a micro-needle or a laser pulse prior to the cooling steps of vitrification improves survival rate and pregnancy outcome of vitrified human blastocysts. *Human Reproduction, Vol.*21(12), pp. 3246-3252

Richter, K.S. Harris, D.C. Daneshmand, S.T. & Shapiro, B.S. (2001). Quantitative grading of a human blastocyst: optimal inner-cell mass size and shape. *Fertility and Sterility*, Vol.76, pp. 1157-1167

Schieve, L.A. Peterson, H.B. Meikle, S.F. Jeng, G. Danel, I. Burnett, N.M. & Wilcox, L.S. (1999). Live-birth rates and multiple-birth risk using in vitro fertilization. *JAMA*, Vol.282, pp. 1832-1838

Scott, L.A. (2000). Oocyte and embryo polarity. *Seminars in Reproductive Medicine*, Vol.18, pp. 171-183

Shapiro, B.S. Daneshmand, S.T. Garner, F.C. Aguirre, M. & Ross, R. (2008). Contrasting patterns in in vitro fertilization pregnancy rates among fresh autologous, fresh oocyte donor, and cryopreserved cycles with the use of day 5 or day 6 blastocysts may reflect differences in embryo-endometrium synchrony. *Fertility and Sterility*, Vol.89(1), pp. 20-26

Shapiro, B.S. Richter, K.S. Harris, D.C & Daneshmand, S.T. (2001). A comparison of day 5 and day 6 blastocyst transfers. *Fertility and Sterility*, Vol.75, pp. 1126-1130

Shoukir, Y. Chardonnens, D. Campana, A. Bischof, P & Sakkas, D. (1998). The rate of development and time of transfer play different roles in influencing the viability of human blastocysts. *Human Reproduction*, Vol.13, pp. 676-681

Stojkovic, M. Kolle, S. Peinl, S. Stojkovic, P. Zakhartchenko, V. Thompson, JG. Wenigerkind, H. Reichenbach, H.D. Sinowatz, F. & Wolf, E. (2002). Effect of high concentrations of hyaluronan in culture medium on development and survival rates of fresh and frozen-thawed bovine embryos produced in vitro. *Reproduction*, Vol.124, pp. 141-153

Summers, M.C. & Biggers, J.D. (2003). Chemically defined media and the culture of mammalian preimplantation embryos: historical perspective and current issues. *Human Reproduction Update*, Vol.9, pp. 557-582

Van Landuyt, L. Stoop, D. Verheyen, G. Verpoest, W. Camus, M. Van de Velde, H. Devroey, P & Van den Abbeel, E. (2011). Outcome of closed blastocyst vitrification in relation to blastocyst quality: evaluation of 759 warming cycles in a single-embryo transfer policy. *Human Reproduction*, Vol.26, pp. 527-534

Vanderzwalmen, P. Bertin, G. Debauche, C.H. Standaert, V. van Roosendaal, E. Vandervorst, M. Bollen, N. Zech, H. Mukaida, T. Takahashi, K & Schoysman, R. (2002). Births after vitrification at morula and blastocyst stages: effect of artificial reduction of the blastocoelic cavity before vitrification. *Human Reproduction, Vol.*17(3), pp. 744-751

Veeck, L. & Zaninovic, N. (2009). Human blastocysts in vitro. In: Veeck L, Zaninovic N, eds. An Atlas of Human Blastocysts. Boca Raton, London, New York, Washington: Parthenon Publishing, pp. 99-137.

Veeck, L.L. (2003). Does the developmental stage at freeze impact on clinical results post-thaw? *Reproductive Biomedicine Online*, Vol.6(3), pp. 367-374

Vlaisavljevic, V. Dmitrovic, R. & Sajko, M.C. (2008). Should the practice of double blastocyst transfer be abandoned? A retrospective analysis. *Reproduction Biomedicine Online*, Vol.16, pp. 677-683

Watson, A.J. & Kidder, G.M. (1988). Immunofluorescence assessment of the timing of appearance and cellular distribution of Na/K-ATPase during mouse embryogenesis. *Developmental Biology*, Vol.126(1), pp. 80-90

Watson, AJ. (1992). The cell biology of blastocyst development. *Molecular Reproduction and Development*, Vol.33, pp. 492-504

Yoon, H.J. Yoon, S.H. Son, W.Y. Im, K.S. & Lim, J.H. (2001). High implantation and pregnancy rates with transfer of human hatching day 6 blastocysts. *Fertility and Sterility*, Vol.75, pp. 832-833

12

Pregnancy Rates Following Transfer of Cultured Versus Non Cultured Frozen Thawed Human Embryos

Bharat Joshi, Manish Banker, Pravin Patel, Preeti Shah and Deven Patel
Pulse Women's Hospital, Ahmedabad, Gujarat
India

1. Introduction

Frozen embryo transfers (FET) are increasingly becoming a routine part of *in*-Vitro Fertilization (IVF) programs at advanced assisted reproductive technology (ART) centers throughout the world. Comparatively FET yield lower pregnancy rates than fresh embryo transfers. Cryopreseravtion offers optimum utilization of embryos produced and is advantageous for the patients with the surplus embryos, ovarian hyper stimulation, radiotherapy or chemotherapy etc. It is of prime importance to dehydrate cells i.e. withdrawal of intracellular water. This is brought about by adding permeable and non permeable cryoprotective agents (CPA). These agents help to minimize the damage to the organelles within the cell and also help to maintain the osmolar changes taking place during the freezing and thawing process. Almost all the cryoprotectants exert some degree of toxic effect to the blastomeres in direct proportion to their concentration used and the time of exposure. The toxic effect can be reduced by step wise addition of cryoprotective agent during the freezing process. Freezing and thawing may damage the morphological characteristics of embryos and survival rate of blastomeres resulting into lower implantation rates. With the varying degrees of post-thaw survival (40% to 90%) and success rate (ranging from 7% to 40%) oocytes and embryos have been frozen in almost all developmental stages, e.g. oocyte (Chen,1986, Borini et al, 2004,2006), pronuclear (Barg et al.,1990, Van den Abbeel et al.,1997, Senn et al.,2000 and Al-Hasani et al.,2007), cleavage stage on day2 and day3 post OPU (Li et al.,2007, Mauri et al.,2001, Kuwayama et al.,2005, Van der Elst et al.,1997 and Rama Raju et al., 2005), morula stage (Tao et al.,2001) and blastocyst stage (Menezo,2004, Liebermann and Tucker,2006, Clifford et al.,2007).

2. Cryopreservation

Cooling exerts irreversible damage to the cytoplasmic lipid droplets and reversible damage to the microtubules. Further the damages are also shown in intracellular organelles, cytoskeleton and cell-to-cell contacts (Vincent and Jhonson, 1992; Massip et al.,1995; Dobrinsky,1996). Also, due to cooling and thawing process there is fracture damage to the zona pellucida leading to the varying survival of the frozen thawed embryos. As reviewed by Guiref et al,2002 and Abdel Hafez et al,2010 various factors affecting outcome are embryo cleavage stage, pre freeze appearance, hormone supplementation during the cycle, ovarian stimulation before Ovum Pick Up (OPU), outcome of fresh Embryo Transfer (ET) cycle, choice of cryoprotective agent, , freezing technique (Controlled rate slow vs Vitrification), type of carrier etc.

3. Slow freezing

Slow freezing is a process where embryos are equilibrated in 1-2 mol/l of permeable and non permeable cryoprotectants, cooled from room temperature to -7°C temperature in a controlled biological freezer, induce seeding at -7°C and than slowly cooled at 0.3 – 1.0°C/ minute up to -35°C, with a freefall up to -120°C. Embryos loaded in straws are plunged in to liquid Nitrogen for storage. Slow freezing causes damage to the embryos due to the intra cellular ice crystal formation but the toxic effect of low concentrations of cryoprotectants favours survival of embryos in slow freezing. This technique is expensive in its requirement of a programmable bio-freezer, liquid Nitrogen consumption, electricity, time of freezing etc. Still this is widely practiced freezing technique in many laboratories around the world.

4. Vitrification

Vitrification is the process of solidification of a solution at low temperatures without ice crystal formation, by extreme elevation in its viscosity using cooling rates of 15,000 to 30,000^{0}C/ min (Rama Raju et al, 2006). This phenomenon requires either rapid cooling rates (Rall,1987) or the use of high concentration of cryoprotectant solutions, which decrease ice crystal formation and increase viscosity at low temperatures until the molecules become immobilized and has the properties of solid (Fahy,1986). To achieve rapid cooling (2500°C/min), the exposure time of embryos to cryoprotectant solutions must be short due to the toxic effects of high cryoprotectant concentrations. However, if the exposure is too short, the penetration of the cryoprotectant will be inadequate and intracellular ice could form, even in the absence of extracellular ice (Otoi et al.,1998). The way to circumvent the noxious effects of cryoprotectants in the vitrification process could be through the use of high cryoprotectant concentrations for short periods of time (Vajta et al.,1998) or increasing the equilibration period by using lower cryoprotectant concentrations (Papis et al.,2000).

With the advances made in cryobiology by using combinations of freezing solution or/and thawing techniques there is an improvement in the pregnancy rates. This was extensively reviewed in a meta-analysis by Abdel Hafez et al, 2010 suggesting superiority of vitrification technology over slow freezing method in terms of significantly higher survival rate of embryos with an increased implantation and pregnancy rates. In terms of techniques employed for freezing, vitrification is gaining more and more support over slow freezing.

However, at our center vitrification has just been introduced and still in trial phase. Simultaneously we are putting in efforts to investigate factors which may enhance pregnancy rates using slow freezing with the aim to select embryos after freezing and thawing so as to get similar results as obtained by using fresh embryos.

5. Materials and methods

5.1 Embryo freezing and thawing at Pulse

With the aim to improve upon pregnancy rates (PR) and to get better selection of embryos from thawed embryos (culture vs non culture), a retrospective analysis of work done at Pulse Women's Hospital, Ahmedabad, India during 2006-2011 is presented here. Patients opting for ART procedure were stimulated using long or antagonist protocols. Ovulation was triggered when majority of the follicles attained 18-20mm diameter with human Chorionic Gonadotropin (hCG). Mature oocytes were inseminated within 4 hours of collection. Fertilization checks were carried out 16-20 hours post insemination. Not more than three embryos were transferred ~48 hours post egg collection. Surplus embryos were frozen in Embryo Freezing Media (Cook Medicals, Australia) using Cryologic programmable biofreezer (CL 8800) in mini straws (0.25 ml capacity). Seeding was induced at -7^{0}C followed by cooling with the rate -0.3^{0}C /minute up to -35^{0}C with a free fall to -120^{0}C. Thereafter the straws were stored in liquid Nitrogen. Embryos were thawed either on the ET day or a day prior to ET. Thawing was performed with stepwise removal of CPA using Embryo Thawing Media (Cook Medicals, Australia).

5.2 Results and discussion

Data created during 2006-2011 were analyzed using Chi-Square test. Out of total 1248 frozen thaw ET cycles, 275 pregnancies (PR-22.0%) were obtained, similar to the 28.8% pregnancy rates obtained by Ying-hui et al, 2002. Results were compared for parameters like patient's age, number of embryos transferred and the time interval between thawing and transfer.

5.3 Patient's age

Comparing the age of patient (Table:1), up to 30 years resulted in 25.4 % pregnancy rates which is significantly higher than the 18.6% rates obtained in patients with the age of >30 years ($p<0.01$).

Patient's AGE	No. of ET'S	PREGNANT	PREGNANCY RATE (%)
≤30	630	160	25.4
>30	618	115	18.6

Table 1. Pregnancy rates according to patient's age

5.4 Number of embryos transferred

FET of 3 embryos yielded 27.1% pregnancy rates, significantly higher to the 9.9% pregnancy rates (Table:2) obtained when upto 2 embryos were transferred ($p<0.0003$).

NO OF EMBRYOS	No. of ET	No. of pregnancy	PREGNANCY RATE (%)
≤ 2	365	36	9.9
3	883	239	27.1

Table 2. Pregnancy rates according to number of embryos transferred

5.5 Time interval between thawing and transfer

Data were further divided into two groups viz. group I in which embryos were thawed and cultured overnight before ET and group II in which embryos were thawed and transferred within two hours (Table: 3).

GROUP	MEAN AGE	No. of pregnancy/ ET	PREGNANCY	PREGNANCY RATE (%)
I (Overnight culture)	31.6 yrs.	1074	240	22.3
II (2 hours culture)	30.1yrs.	174	35	20.1

Table 3. Pregnancy rates according to time of ET

Embryos cultured overnight produced pregnancy rates of 22.3% while embryos transferred within 2 hours post thawing resulted in pregnancy rates of 20.1%, showing no significant difference between the two groups. Results are comparable with the pregnancy rates obtained by Karlstorm et al, 1997 (22%) and by Singh et al,2007 (16%).

Van der Elst et al,1997, Zeibe et al,1998 and Guiref et al,2002 proposed to evaluate resumption of mitosis by doing overnight culture and selection of thawed embryos before transfer. On this basis within group I i.e. the cultured group, embryos were assessed for further cleavage of the blastomeres. There was a significant difference ($p<0.0001$) when all non-cleaved embryos were transferred (7.1%) and when 1 to 3 cleaved embryos (31.9%) were transferred (Table:4). This is similar to the results obtained by Ying-hui et al,2002, where 35.2% pregnancy rate was achieved when at least one cleaved embryo was transferred against 10.2% when no cleaved embryo was transferred. Further pregnancy rates were significantly higher when two ($p=0.0004$) and three ($p=0.0005$) cleaved embryos were transferred compared to only one cleaved embryo. However, there was no significant difference between transfer of two and three cleaved embryos.

EMBRYOS CLEAVED	ET	PREGNANCY	PREGNANCY RATE (%)	p values
0	294	21	7.1[a]	
1	422	83	19.7[b]	<0.0001 a.b
2	258	93	36.1[c]	=0.0004 b,c
3	100	43	43[d]	=0.0005 b,d

Table 4. Comparison of pregnancy rate between numbers of cleaved embryos transferred

When 2 cleaved embryos after culture were transferred, 36.1% pregnancies were achieved and when all 3 cultured and cleaved embryos were transferred, 43.0% pregnancy rates were achieved, showing that these results are at par with those obtained in fresh embryo transfer cycle. This is much higher than the results obtained by Karlstorm et al,1997, where pregnancy rates was 23% when 2 cleaved embryos were transferred and 27% when 3 cleaved embryos were transferred.

Pregnancy rates have shown further increase when only the embryos which have cleaved to an eight cell stage during culture were transferred (Table:5) as compared to results shown in table 4.

EMBRYOS CLEAVED (only 8 cells)	ET	PREGNANCY	PREGNANCY RATE (%)	P values
0	294	21	7.1[a]	
1	302	67	22.2[b]	<0.0001 a,b
2	208	84	40.4[c]	<0.001 b,c
3	82	38	46.3[d]	<0.003 b,d

Table 5. Comparison of pregnancy rate when only 8-cell embryos were transferred

Highly significant difference ($p<0.0001$) in pregnancy rates was observed when all non-cleaved embryos were transferred compared to 1 to 3 cleaved 8-celled embryos. Pregnancy rates were significantly higher when two ($p<0.001$) and three ($p<0.003$) cleaved 8- celled embryos were transferred compared to only one cleaved 8- celled embryo. However, there was no significant difference between transfer of two and three cleaved 8-celled embryos.

6. Conclusion

Taking into account the results obtained in various categories it can be concluded that pregnancy rates can be improved through selection of better embryos and brought at par with that of fresh ET.

7. References

[1] Chen, C. (1986) Pregnancy after human oocyte cryopreservation. Lancet 1, 884-886.

[2] Borini, A., Bonu M.A., Coticchio. G., Bianchi, V., Cattoli, M and Flamigni, C. (2004) Pregnancies and births after oocyte cryopreservation. Fertility and sterility, 82, 601-605.

[3] Borini, A., Sciajno, R., Bianchi, V., Sereni, E, Flamigni, C. and Coticchio. G., (2006) Clinical outcome of oocyte cryopreservation after slow cooling with a protocol utilizing a high sucrose concentration. Human Reproduction, 21, 512-517.

[4] Barg, P.E., Barad, D.H. and Feichtinger, W. (1990). Ultrarapid freezing (URF) of mouse and human preembryos: a modified approach. J. In vitro Fertil. Embryo Transfer IVF 7, 355-357.

[5] Van den Abbeel, E., Camus, M., Van Waesberghe, L., et al., (1997) A randomized comparison of the cryopreservation of one-cell human embryos with a slow controlled-rate cooling procedure or a rapid cooling procedure by direct plunging into liquid nitrogen. Human Reproduction Vol.12, pp- 1554-1560.

[6] Senn, A., Vozzi, C., Chanson, A., et al. (2002) Prospective randomized study of two cryopreservation policies avoiding embryo selection: the pronucleate stage leads to a higher cumulative delivery rate than the early cleavage stage. Ferti. Steril. 74, 946-952.

[7] Al-Hasani, S., Ozmen, B., Koutlaki, N., et al (2007) Three years of routine vitrification of human zygotes: is it still fair to advocate slow-rate freezing? Reproductive BioMedicine Online 14, 288-293.

[8] Li, Y., Chen, Z.J., Yang, H.J, et al, (2007) Comparison of vitrification and slow freezing of human day 3 cleavage stage embryos: post vitrification development and pregnancy outcomes. Zhonghua Fu Chan Ke Za Zhi, 42, 753-755.

[9] Mauri, A.L., Petersen, C.G., Baruffi, R.L., et al., (2001) Comparison of the cryopreservation of human embryos obtained after intracytoplasmic sperm injection with a slow cooling or an ultrarapid cooling procedure. J. Assist. Reprod. Genet. 18, 257-261.

[10] Kuwayama, M., Vajta, G., Ieda, S., Kato, O., (2005) Comparison of open and closed methods for vitrification of human embryos and the elimination of potential contamination. Reproductive BioMedicine Online. Vol 11, pp-608-614.

[11] Van der Elst, J., Van den Abbeel, E., Vitrier, S., Camus, M., Devroey P. and Van Steirteghem, A.C. (1997) Selective transfer of cryopreserved human embryos with further cleavage after thawing increases delivery and implantation rates. Human Reproduction. Vo. 12, pp-1513-1521.

[12] Rama Raju, G.A., Haranth, G.B., Krishana, K.M., Jaya Prakash, G. and Madan, K. (2005) Vitrification of human 8-cell embryos, a modified protocol for better pregnancy rates. Reproductive BioMedicine Online, Vol 11, 434-437.

[13] Tao. J., Tamis, R., Fink, K., (2001) Pregnancies achieved after transferring frozen morula/ compact stage embryos. Fertility and Sterility, 75, 629-631.

[14] Menezo, Y., (2004) Cryopreservation of IVF embryos: which stage? Eur. J. Obstet. Gynecol. Reprod. Biol. 113, (Suppl. 1) S28-S32.

[15] Liebermann, J., and Tucker, M.J., (2006) Comparison of vitrification and conventional cryopreservation of day 5 and day 6 blastocysts during clinical application. Fertility and Sterility, 86, pp- 20-26.

[16] Clifford, A.L., Jilbert, P.M., Gentry, W.L., et al., (2007) Better ongoing pregnancy rates from frozen embryo transfers when vitrified blastocysts are used. Fertility and Sterility. 88 (Suppl. 1), S349-S350.

[17] Vincent, C. and Jhonson, J.H. (1992) Cooling cryoprotectants and the cytoskeleton of the mammalian oocyte. Oxford Review in Reproductive Biology, 14, 73-100.

[18] Massip, A., Mermillod, P., Dinnyes, A. (1995) Morphology and biochemistry of in-vitro produced bovine embryos: implications for their cryopreservation. Human Reproduction, 10, 3004-3011.

[19] Dobrinsky, J.R. (1996) Cellular approach to cryopreservation of embryos. Theriogenology, 45, 17-26.

[20] Guiref, F., Bidault, R., Cadoret, V., Couet, M., Lansac, J and Royere D. (2002) Parameters guiding selection of best embryos for transfer after cryopreservation: a reappraisal. Human Reproduction Vol.17, No.5 PP. 1321-1326.

[21] Abdel Hafez, F.F., Desai, N, Abou-setta, A.M. Falcone T and Goldfarb J. (2010) Slow freezing, vitrification and ultra-rapid freezing of human embryos: a systematic review and meta analysis.

[22] Rama Raju G A, Murali Krishna K, Prakash G J and Madan K. 2006. Vitrification: An emerging Technique for Cryopreservation in Assisted Reproduction Programmes. Embryo Talk Vol 1.4 : 210- 227.

[23] Rall W F. 1987. Factors affecting the survival of mouse embryos cryopreserved by vitrification. Cryobiology 24, 387-402.

[24] Fahy G M. 1986. vitrification: a new approach to organ cryopreservation. In:Meryman HT (ed.), Transplantation: approaches to graft rejection, Alan R Liss, New york, PP: 305-355.

[25] Otoi T, Yamamoto K, Koyama N, Tachikawa S, Suzuki T. 1998, Cryopreservation of mature bovine oocytes by vitrification in straws. Cryobiology. Aug;37 (1):77-85.

[26] Vajta G, Holm P, Kuwayama M, Booth P J, Jacobsen H, Greve T, Callesen H. 1998. Open pulled straw vitrification: a new way to reduce cryoinjuries of bovine ova and embryos. Mol Reprod Dev. 51: 53-58.

[27] Papis K, Shimizu M, Izaike Y. 2000. Factors affecting the survivability of bovine oocytes vitrified in droplets. Theriogenology. Sep 15;54(5):651-8.

[28] Ying-hui, Y.E., Fan, J.I.N., Chen-ming, X.U.,Lan-feng, X.I.N.G, (2002) Factors influencing the outcome of embryo freezing and thawing program. Journal of Zhejiang University Science V.3.pp-493-496

[29] Karlstorm, P.O., Bergh, T., Forsberg, A.S. Sandkvist, U., Wikland, M. (1997) Prognostic factors for the success rate of embryo freezing. Human Reproduction. Vol 12, pp-1263-1266.
[30] Singh, P.M., Vrotson, K., Balen, A.H., (2007) Frozen embryo replacement cycle: An analysis of factors influencing the outcome. J. Obstet Gynecol India. Vol 57, pp-240-244.
[31] Zeibe, S., Bech, B., Petersen, K., et al., (1998) Resumption of mitosis during post-thaw culture: a key parameter in selecting the right embryos for transfer. Human Reproduction. Vol 13, pp-178-181.

13

Intercourse and ART Success Rates

Abbas Aflatoonian[1], Sedigheh Ghandi[2] and Nasim Tabibnejad[1]
[1]*Department of Obstetrics and Gynecology, Research and Clinical Center for Infertility Shahid Sadoughi University of Medical Sciences, Yazd*
[2]*Department of Obstetrics and Gynecology Sabzevar University of Medical Sciences, Sabzevar Iran*

1. Introduction

Embryo implantation is critically dependent on a supportive uterine environment. Uterine receptivity is the culmination of a cellular and molecular transformation mediated locally by paracrine signals under the governance of ovarian steroid hormones, with cells and cytokines of the immune system playing integral roles in this process (1,2). The implantation rates and subsequent pregnancy rates in In Vitro Fertilization (IVF) programs are lower than the normal fertile population. During IVF treatment regimens, intercourse is not allowed and artificial insemination is excluded. There is a substantial body of evidence supporting the need for exposure of the female reproductive tract to semen / seminal plasma around the time of embryo implantation in order to maximize reproductive efficiency (3). The aim of this chapter is to examine the available evidences suggesting why intercourse is beneficial or harmful to assisted reproductive techniques outcome.

In the reproductive process, seminal plasma is viewed primarily as a transport medium for spermatozoa traversing the female cervix and uterus after coitus (4, 5). However, studies in animal species show that seminal plasma also delivers to the female an array of signaling molecules that interact with epithelial cells lining the female reproductive tract. This interaction triggers local cellular and molecular changes that resemble an inflammatory response (6). In mouse and pig experiments, seminal fluid activates expression of several pro-inflammatory cytokines and chemokines in uterine epithelial cells (7-9). In turn, these factors amplify the actions of seminal fluid chemotactic agents resulting in vascular changes and recruitment and activation of macrophages, granulocytes and dendritic cells. These cells accumulate in the uterine endometrial tissue subjacent to the epithelial surface, and migrate between epithelial cells into the luminal cavity (9-11). The infiltrating leukocytes are implicated in clearance of seminal debris from the female tissues and potentially selection of fertilizing sperm (12,13). The infiltrating leukocytes may also influence the female immune response to seminal antigens and evoke tissue remodelling changes to condition the endometrial environment in preparation for pregnancy (3,6).

In mice and pigs, the epithelial cells of the uterine endometrium are the primary site of seminal fluid interaction and, the induced key cytokines are GM-CSF and IL-6, as well as the chemokines KC (mouse IL-8 homologue) and MCP-1 (7-9). Experiments with male mice by vasectomy or surgical removal of the seminal vesicle gland show that the active signaling moieties (signaling molecules) are contained within the seminal plasma fraction of the ejaculate and are derived from the seminal vesicle (8). Cytokines of the transforming growth factor-β (TGF-B) family are identified as the major active factors in mouse seminal plasma (14). Seminal TGF-B is synthesized in the latent form in the seminal vesicle gland and is activated in the female tract upon deposition at mating (14).

However, how seminal fluid activates inflammatory cytokine synthesis or leukocyte infiltration in any compartment of the human female tract is unclear. Two previous *in vivo* studies in women have shown neutrophil exocytosis in the cervical tissues following either sexual intercourse or artificial insemination and they reported that sperm, but not seminal plasma, is required to elicit this "leukocytic reaction" (15,16). There are preliminary indications that signaling activity is also associated with the cell-free, plasma fraction of semen. *In vitro* studies demonstrate that human female reproductive tract cells can respond to seminal plasma, with increased IL-8 and secretory leukocyte protease inhibitor (SLPI) secretion from cervical explants (17). Endometrial epithelial cells are reported to show elevated synthesis of IL-1β, IL-6 and leukaemia inhibitory factor (LIF) after culture with seminal plasma (18). Seminal fluid might also target infiltrating leukocytes directly, since IL-10 production in human monocyte U937 cells can be induced in response to seminal fluid constituents (17).Transmission of seminal factors in the female reproductive tract organizes molecular and cellular changes in the endometrium to facilitate embryo development and implantation.

2. Clinical studies

The available literature on the potential benefit of intercourse in patients undergoing assisted reproduction techniques is not extensive. To date; only two studies have examined the effect of intercourse around the time of embryo transfer on ART cycles (19, 20), while several studies have looked at the effect of artificial insemination with whole semen or seminal plasma (21-23). In a multicenter randomized study, patients undergoing fresh (400 cycles) and thawed (200 cycles) embryo transfer were randomized either to abstain or to engage in vaginal intercourse around the time of embryo transfer. There were no significant difference in pregnancy rates between the intercourse and abstinence groups but viability of transferred embryos at 6 - 8 weeks was significantly higher in the exposed semen group than abstained group. The authors' result indicates that exposure to semen around the time of embryo transfer increases the likelihood of successful early embryo implantation and development (19). In another study, 390 women were randomly divided into intercourse and abstinence groups during embryo transfer period and results indicated that intercourse did not significantly increase the pregnancy and implantation rates in ART cycles (20). Clinical pregnancy rates were not significantly different in two groups. In a prospective trial, Bellinge demonstrated an improved implantation rate with high vaginal deposition of a portion of their partners' semen samples compared with controls (21). However, in a subsequent prospective trial, Fishel found no significant effect of the use of high vaginal insemination at the time of oocyte recovery in patients undergoing IVF (22). Neither of these two reports utilized true randomization methods to assign treatment - control protocols. The final randomized control trial allocated patients to high vaginal insemination with either their partners' seminal plasma or a saline placebo at the time of oocyte retrieval (23). This study of 168 patients reported a 45% relative increase in implantation rates in the seminal plasma exposed group, but it did not reach statistical significance. In one retrospective study, postoperative intrauterine and intracervical insemination was performed in gamete intrafallopian transfer (GIFT) program and the result showed that clinical pregnancy rates were higher in patients with additional postoperative insemination (24). In one randomized, double blind study, the absence or presence of seminal fluid in patients undergoing ovulation induction with intrauterine insemination was investigated. Intercourse was restricted. A comparison of clinical pregnancy rates between two groups showed no significant difference. Further in non-participants with unregulated intercourse, the pregnancy rates were not significantly different (25). Coulam and Stern suggested that higher implantation rates were obtained in a group of women experiencing infertility and/or recurrent spontaneous abortion who received vaginal capsules of seminal plasma versus placebo, however this difference was not significant (26). The same group reported that in women experiencing a history of recurrent spontaneous abortion, seminal plasma enhanced the probability of live birth by 21% (27). Therefore the vast majority of evidence suggests that exposure of the female reproductive tract to sperm/seminal plasma through either artificial insemination or intercourse does not have negative impact on outcome.

3. Discussion

Theoretically, intercourse can impair implantation by these mechanisms:

i. the introduction of infection,
ii. initiation of uterine contractions (at orgasm),
iii. pressure created by penile contact with the cervix may dislodge the embryos, furthermore intercourse may produce painful rupture of ovarian follicles.

Intercourse has been linked with ascending uterine infection during late pregnancy (28), and subclinical infection of the upper reproductive tract is associated with poor IVF embryo transfer outcome (29). During an IVF cycle the uterine cavity is vulnerable to intercourse related infection since the cervical mucus barrier that prevents ascending infection is disrupted by passage of the embryo transfer catheter. On the other hand, Sharkey et al investigated seminal plasma induction of inflammatory cytokines and chemokines gene regulation in human cervical vaginal epithelial cells in vitro. These experiments show that seminal plasma can elicit expression of a range of inflammatory cytokines and chemokines in reproductive epithelia, and implicate the ectocervix as the primary site of responsiveness. Seminal factor regulation of inflammatory cytokines in the cervical epithelium is implicated in controlling the immune response to seminal antigens. This inflammatory cytokines also is responsible for defense against infectious agents introduced at intercourse (30). Intercourse increases uterine myometrial activity during female orgasm (31) and these contractions may interfere implantation of early embryo since high levels of spontaneous uterine activity are associated with poor IVF outcome (32, 33). On the positive side, intercourse may act to assist implantation. Seminal plasma induction of the pro - inflammatory and chemotactic cytokines supports the interpretation because one function of seminal fluid is to activate an inflammatory cascade after deposition in the human female reproductive tract at intercourse, analogous to the consequences of mating in mice (6) and in pigs (8). Since each of these factors also regulates leukocyte recruitment and activation in humans, it is likely that elevated production of the pro - inflammatory and chemotactic cytokines in the cervix elicits changes in local leukocytes, which manifest as the post - coital leukocytic reaction in women (15, 16). Epithelial cell regulation of this response is consistent with the notion that epithelial cytokines control accumulation and functional behavior of local dendritic cell, macrophage and granulocyte populations in other epithelia (34). However, since the effects of seminal fluid on leukocytes have not examined, the possibility of direct seminal fluid signaling in these cells contributing to the response, cannot be excluded. Active synthesis of a wider range of cytokines in the cervix after intercourse would facilitate optimal competence in protecting the higher reproductive tract from pathogen invasion and in reinforcing the defensive barrier function of this epithelial surface (35).

Induction of GM-CSF and IL-6 in the cervical tissues would influence the activation status of local antigen-presenting cells, programming phenotypes that impact the ensuing response to antigens processed by those cells (36-39). The significance of these two cytokines being preferentially expressed in the ectocervix is consistent with this tissue being the primary site for female 'sampling' of paternal antigens. Their presence together with the action of the immune-deviating agents TGFβ and prostaglandin E_2 (PGE_2) in seminal fluid would be expected to ensure that the outcome of any antigen-specific immune response did not adversely affect female tolerance of any future exposure to semen. Similarly, uptaking and processing of male antigens in semen may provide an opportunity for priming the maternal immune response in preparation for an ensuing pregnancy fathered by the same male, since the conceptus shares many of the same paternal antigens (13, 39). IL-6, together with LIF and IL-1β, can also be induced in uterine endometrial cells by seminal factors *in vitro* (18), where it appears to be a key determinant of uterine receptivity at embryo implantation (40,41). This suggests that the action of seminal fluid in regulating the quality of female tract immune responses may extend higher into the female tract, after transport of active seminal constituents by uterine peristaltic contractions which transport macromolecular material as high as the fallopian tube (42). Whether GM-CSF, IL-8 and IL-6 can also be induced in endometrial cells or not needs to be examined.

4. Conclusion and recommendations

A large of randomized control trials suggest that intercourse around the time of embryo transfer improve IVF implantation rates and increase pregnancy rates in ART cycle, but some studies thought that intercourse did not significantly increase pregnancy rate. While this mechanism of intercourse improving pregnancy rate is not fully understood, it seems that semen/seminal plasma could induce immune reactions in female reproductive tract that augments embryo development and endometrial receptivity. On the negative side, hyperstimulated ovaries are vulnerable to rupture during intercourse. Therefore, we suggest that intercourse around the time of embryo transfer should be encouraged, except in the small subgroup of women with large hyperstimulated ovaries.

5. References

[1] Rogers PAW, Murphy CR. Uterine receptivity for implantation: human studies. In: Yoshinaga K , editors . Blastocyst implantation. Norwell , MA: Serono Symposia Press. 1989; 231 - 280

[2] Finn CA, Martin L. The control of implantation. J Reprod Fertil. 1974; 39(1): 195-206.

[3] Robertson SA, Mau VJ, Hudson SA, et al. Cytokine-leukocyte networks and the establishment of pregnancy. Am J Reprod Immunol 1997;37:438-442.

[4] Mann T. The Biochemistry of Semen and the Male Reproductive Tract. John Wiley and Sons, Inc., New York; 1964

[5] Aumuller G, Riva A. Morphology and functions of the human seminal vesicle. Andrologia 1992;24:183-196.
[6] Robertson SA. Seminal plasma and male factor signalling in the female reproductive tract. Cell Tissue Res 2005;322:43-52.
[7] Robertson SA, Mayrhofer G, Seamark RF. Uterine epithelial cells synthesize granulocyte-macrophage colony-stimulating factor and interleukin-6 in pregnant and nonpregnant mice. Biol Reprod 1992;46:1069-1079.
[8] Robertson SA, Mau VJ, Tremellen KP, et al. Role of high molecular weight seminal vesicle proteins in eliciting the uterine inflammatory response to semen in mice. J Reprod Fertil 1996;107:265-277.
[9] O'Leary S, Jasper MJ, Warnes GM, et al. Seminal plasma regulates endometrial cytokine expression, leukocyte recruitment and embryo development in the pig. Reproduction 2004;128:237-247.
[10] Phillips DM, Mahler S. Migration of leukocytes and phagocytosis in rabbit vagina. J Cell Biol 1975;67:334a.
[11] McMaster MT, Newton RC, Dey SK, et al. Activation and distribution of inflammatory cells in the mouse uterus during the preimplantation period. J Immunol 1992;148:1699-1705.
[12] Mattner PE. Phagocytosis of spermatozoa by leucocytes in bovine cervical mucus in vitro. J Reprod Fertil 1969;20:133-134.
[13] Roldan ER, Gomendio M, Vitullo AD. The evolution of eutherian spermatozoa underlying selective forces: female selection sperm competition. Biol Rev Camb Philos Soc 1992;67:551-593.
[14] Tremellen KP, Seamark RF, Robertson SA. Seminal transforming growth factor beta1 stimulates granulocyte-macrophage colony-stimulating factor production and inflammatory cell recruitment in the murine uterus. Biol Reprod 1998;58:1217-1225.
[15] Pandya IJ, Cohen J. The leukocytic reaction of the human uterine cervix to spermatozoa. Fertil Steril 1985;43:417-421.
[16] Thompson LA, Barratt CL, Bolton AE, et al. The leukocytic reaction of the human uterine cervix. Am J Reprod Immunol 1992;28:85-89.
[17] Denison FC, Grant VE, Calder AA, et al. Seminal plasma components stimulate interleukin-8 and interleukin-10 release. Mol Hum Reprod 1999;5:220-226.
[18] Gutsche S, von Wolff M, Strowitzki T, et al. Seminal plasma induces mRNA expression of IL-1beta, IL-6 and LIF in endometrial epithelial cells in vitro. Mol Hum Reprod 2003;9:785-791.
[19] Tremellen KP, Valbuena D, Landeras J, Ballesteros A, Martinez J, Mendoza S,et all. The effect of inter course on pregnancy rates during assisted human reproduction. Hum Reprod.2000;15(12):2653-2658.
[20] Aflatoonian A., Ghandi S., Tabibnejad N. The effect of entercourse around Embryo Transfer on Pregnancy Rate in Assisted Reproductive Technology Cycles. IJFS 2009;2: 169-172
[21] Bellinge BS, Copeland CM , Thomas TD, et al. The influence of patient insemination on the implantation rate in an in vitro fertilization and embryo transfer program. Fertil Steril 1986; 46: 252 - 6.
[22] Fishel S, Webster J, Jackson P, Faratian B. Evaluating of high vaginal insemination at oocyte recovery in patients undergoing *in vitro* fertilization. Fertil Steril. 1989;51:135-138.
[23] Von Wolff M, Rosner S, Thone C, et al. Intravaginal and intracervical application of seminal plasma in in vitro fertilization or intracytoplasmic sperm injection treatment

cycles - a double blind , placebo - controlled , randomized pilot study . Fertil Steril 2009 ; 91:167 - 72
[24] Tucker MJ, Wong CJ, Chan YM, Leong MK, Leong CK. Post-operative artificial insemination -does it improve GIFT outcome? Hum Reprod. 1990;5(2):189-192.
[25] Qasim SM, Trias A, Karacan M, Shelden R, Kemmann E. Does the absence or presence of seminal fluid matter in patients undergoing ovulation induction with intrauterine insemination? Hum Reprod. 1996; 11(5):1008-1010.
[26] Coulam C.B and Stern, J.J. Effect of seminal plasma on implantation rates. Early pregnancy: Biol. Med, 1995;1: 33 - 36.
[27] Stern, J.J, Coulam, C.B, Wagenknecht, D.R, Peters AJ, et al. Seminal plasma treatment of recurrent spontaneous abortion. Am J Reprod Immunol, 1992;27,50.
[28] Naeye RL. Coitus and associated amniotic-fluid infection. N Engl J Med. 1979;29;301(22):1198-200.
[29] Fanchin R, Harmas A, Benaoudia F. Microbial flora of the cervix assessed at the time of embryo transfer adversely affects *in vitro* fertilization outcome. Fertil Steril. 1998;70(5):866-870.
[30] Sharkey DJ, Macpherson Am, Tremellen KP, Robertson SA. Seminal plasma differentially regulates inflammatory cytokine gene expression in human cervical and vaginal epithelial cells. Mol Hum Reprod. 2007 Jul;13(7):491-501.
[31] Fox CA, Wolff HS, Baker JA. Measurement of intra-vaginal and intra-uterine pressures during human coitus by rodio-telemetery. J Reprod Fertill. 1970;22(2)243-251.
[32] Fanchin R , Righini C , Olivennes F . Uterine contractions at the time of embryo transfer alter pregnancy rates after in vitro fertilization . Hum Reprod . 1998 ; 13(7):1968 - 1974
[33] Fanchin R , Righini C , Ayoubi JM, Olivennes F , de Ziegler D . Uterine contractions at the time of embryo transfer : a hindrance to implantration ? Contracept Fertil Sex . 1998 jul - Aug : 26(7 - 8): 498 - 505
[34] Barker JN, Mitra RS, Griffiths CE, et al. Keratinocytes as initiators of inflammation. Lancet 1991;337:211-214
[35] Quayle AJ. The innate and early immune response to pathogen challenge in the female genital tract and the pivotal role of epithelial cells. J Reprod Immunol 2002;57:61-79.
[36] Sallusto F, Lanzavecchia A. Efficient presentation of soluble antigen by cultured human dendritic cells is maintained by granulocyte/macrophage colony- stimulating factor plus interleukin 4 and downregulated by tumor necrosis factor alpha. J Exp Med 1994;179:1109-1118.
[37] Burnham K, Robb L, Scott CL, et al. Effect of granulocyte-macrophage colony-stimulating factor on the generation of epidermal Langerhans cells. J Interferon Cytokine Res 2000;20:1071-1076.
[38] Diehl S, Rincon M. The two faces of IL-6 on Th1/Th2 differentiation. Mol Immunol 2002;39:531-536.
[39] Thompson LA, Barratt CL, Bolton AE, et al. The leukocytic reaction of the human uterine cervix. Am J Reprod Immunol 1992;28:85-89.
[40] Lim KJ, Odukoya OA, Ajjan RA, et al. The role of T-helper cytokines in human reproduction. Fertil Steril 2000;73:136-142.
[41] Jasper MJ, Tremellen KP, Robertson SA.Reduced expression of IL-6 and IL-1alpha mRNAs in secretory phase endometrium of women with recurrent miscarriage. J Reprod Immunol 2007;73:74-84.
[42] Kunz G, Leyendecker G. Uterine peristaltic activity during the menstrual cycle: characterization regulation function dysfunction. Reprod Biomed Online 2002;4 Suppl 3:5-9.

Part 5

Embryo Implantation and Cryopreservation

14

Implantation of the Human Embryo

Russell A. Foulk
University of Nevada, School of Medicine
USA

1. Introduction

Implantation is the final frontier to embryogenesis and successful pregnancy. Over the past three decades, there have been tremendous advances in the understanding of human embryo development. Since the advent of *In Vitro Fertilization,* the embryo has been readily available to study outside the body. Indeed, the study has led to much advancement in embryonic stem cell derivation. Unfortunately, it is not so easy to evaluate the steps of implantation since the uterus cannot be accessed by most research tools. This has limited our understanding of early implantation. Both the physiological and pathological mechanisms of implantation occur largely unseen. The heterogeneity of these processes between species also limits our ability to develop appropriate animal models to study. In humans, there is a precise coordinated timeline in which pregnancy can occur in the uterus, the so called "window of implantation". However, in many cases implantation does not occur despite optimal timing and embryo quality. It is very frustrating to both a patient and her clinician to transfer a beautiful embryo into a prepared uterus only to have it fail to implant. This chapter will review the mechanisms of human embryo implantation and discuss some reasons why it fails to occur.

2. Phases of human embryo implantation

The human embryo enters the uterine cavity approximately 4 to 5 days post fertilization. After passing down the fallopian tube or an embryo transfer catheter, the embryo is moved within the uterine lumen by rhythmic myometrial contractions until it can physically attach itself to the endometrial epithelium. It hatches from the zona pellucida within 1 to 2 days after entering the cavity thereby exposing the trophoblastic cells of the trophectoderm to the uterine epithelium. Implantation occurs 6 or 7 days after fertilization. During implantation and placentation, a human embryo must attach itself to the uterus under conditions of shear stress. The embryo is rolling about within a mucus rich environment between the opposing surfaces of the endometrial walls of the uterus. This interactive process is a complex series of events that can be divided into three distinct steps: apposition, attachment and invasion (Norwitz et al., 2001).

2.1 Apposition

Once the human blastocyst hatches from the zona pellucida, the free-floating sphere of cells must orient itself as it approaches the endometrial surface and form an initial adhesion (apposition) before it can firmly attach and begin the process of invasion. The apposition step is a transient and dynamic process whereby the embryo "tethers" itself to the endometrial surface. Uterine contractions and mucin secretion within the uterine cavity propel the blastocyst around the cavity. Despite these fluid dynamics which creates shear stress, the embryo is able to approach the wall, roll around to right itself so that the trophectoderm overlying the inner cell mass apposes to the endometrial surface. During this apposition phase, there is a dialogue between the floating blastocyst and endometrium using soluble mediators such as cytokines and chemokines acting in a bidirectional fashion to guide the blastocyst onto a 3-dimensional "docking" structure. The hormone-regulated pinopodes at the endometrial surface have been shown to mark the timing and appearance of optimal endometrial receptivity (Bentin-Ley et al., 2000).

Chemokines such as IL-8, RANTES, or MCP-1 are secreted locally by both the endometrium and blastocyst during the implantation window during the apposition phase. The L-selectin system, in particular, has been shown to be critically important during the blastocyst apposition phase (Genbacev et al., 2003). Selectins are lectin-like glycoproteins that include E-, L- and P-selectin, all of which were originally thought to be expressed exclusively by hemangioblast descendents. E-selectin is expressed on activated endothelial cells, P-selectin is expressed on the surfaces of activated platelets and endothelial cells and L-selectin is expressed on lymphocytes. Initial interest in the selectin system came because the implantation process bears some similarity to leukocyte transmigration across the blood vessel wall. Similar to a rolling blastocyst, the selectin adhesion systems allow leukocytes to tether and roll on the endothelial surface before invading into the interstitium. Leukocytes use specialized mechanisms, which involve the L-selectin adhesion system, to extravasate from flowing blood, under shear stress, into the endothelial wall. These specialized mechanisms in the vasculature enable cell adhesion to occur under shear flow. Interactions between leukocytes and endothelium are mediated by carbohydrate-binding proteins (selectins) that recognize specific oligosaccharide structures as their ligands. These interactions allow leukocytes to slow their passage on the endothelial surface (Alon & Feigelson, 2002). This step is followed by integrin activation which enable leukocytes to form a firm adhesion with the vascular endothelial surface and, subsequently, to transmigrate into tissues (Alon & Feigelson, 2002 and McEver, 2002). Selectins on the cell surface initiate tethering to their complementary ligands on specialized endothelial cells along the vascular wall until they become firmly attached (McEver, 2002). These lectin-like molecules recognize specific oligosaccharide structures carried on some glycoproteins including PSGL-1, CD34, GlyCAM-1, MAdCAM-1, podocalyxin and endoglycan. They are made up of at least 30% carbohydrates and bind to mucin oligosaccharide ligands on the endothelium. These types of interactions have rapid and reversible properties such that traveling leukocytes slow down, tether, release and roll on the epithelial cell surface until finally attaching at the site of extravasation. Once arrested, integrin activation triggers stable adhesion (shear-resistant) and subsequent transmigration through the vascular endothelium.

At morphological level, there are parallels between leukocyte extravasation from the vasculature and attachment of embryo to the uterine wall since both types of adhesion occur under shear flow and are followed by integrin activation. Genbacev et al. (2003) have shown that the L-selectin adhesion system plays a crucial role during an initial step of blastocyst implantation. Hatched blastocyst expresses L-selectin and uses this molecule to mediate its attachment to the luminal epithelial surface via its carbohydrate ligands, MECA-79 and related epitopes. Two different in vitro models illustrating L-selectin mediating adhesion were used to confirm the in-situ observations. In the first model, beads coated with synthetic L-selectin carbohydrate ligands were overlaid on placental chorionic villous explants under shear stress. It was shown the beads bound to cell column cytotrophoblasts (CTBs) on the explants and the binding was blocked by antibody to L-selectin. Additional immunolocalization experiment confirmed that the CTBs did express L-selectin. In the second model, isolated CTBs were overlaid on endometrial tissue sections under shear stress. It was shown that CTBs bound to epithelial surface of the endometrium tissues that were obtained during the luteal phase and did not bind to those that were obtained during the follicular phase. Again, the binding was blocked by anti-L-selectin antibody. Concurring with these observations, immunolocalization study of endometrial tissue demonstrated that the L-selectin carbohydrate ligand MECA-79 was upregulated from the day of ovulation to a peak 6 days post ovulation at the middle of the implantation window. It was negative throughout the follicular phase and remained negative if ovulation did not occur. Carson et al (2006) have shown that MUC-1, a transmembrane mucin glycoprotein expressed at the apical surface of the uterine epithelia, likely serves as a scaffold for these L- selectin carbohydrate ligands. Together, these studies suggests that the human embryo uses a mechanism well studied in leukocytes to mediate rolling and tethering onto the endometrial wall prior to firm adhesion when integrins begin their crucial role.

2.2 Embryo attachment

Shortly after the apposition step, integrin-dependent adhesion and attachment occurs. This receptor mediated event allows the blastocyst to attach firmly to the uterine wall and trophoblasts transmigrate across the luminal epithelium, burying the embryo beneath the uterine wall. Integrins are a family of cell adhesion molecules present on the plasma membrane as heterodimeric α and β glycoprotein subunits. These cell surface receptors on both the trophoblasts and the endometrium are involved at multiple functional levels during implantation. The trophoblast integrins have been shown to mediate cell-cell and cell-matrix interaction in trophoblast attachment, migration, differentiation and apoptosis. On the endometrial surface, most of the integrins serve housekeeping roles, but there are three heterodimers whose expression marks the boundaries of the implantation window (Lessey, 2002). The endometrial integrin $\alpha1\beta1$ is expressed during the full span of the implantation window from ovulation to the late luteal phase. The expression of $\alpha4\beta1$ begins with ovulation, but ceases as the window closes on cycle day 24. The endometrial integrin $\alpha v\beta3$ appears on the apical surface of the endometrial epithelium on cycle day 19 to 20, the opening of the implantation window and diminishes quickly through the next week. Its ligand, osteopontin is found concurrent with $\alpha v\beta3$ and might play a role in endometrial or embryo signaling, facilitating embryo attachment to the apical surface prior to invasion.

Absence of $\alpha v\beta3$ expression during the window of implantation has been reported with luteal phase deficiency and in some women with endometriosis, unexplained infertility and hydrosalpinges. This loss of normal integrin expression is thought to lead to implantation failure. Integrin knockout studies found that $\beta1$ null mice embryos develop normally to the blastocyst stage but fail to implant (Stephens et al., 1995). The human embryo regulates these integrins in the human endometrium at the protein level in the apposition phase (Simon et al., 1997). Therefore, after the human blastocyst tethers to and breaks through the glycocalix barrier, it then induces by paracrine crosstalk a favorable epithelial integrin pattern for its firm attachment.

2.3 Trophoblast Invasion

The final phase of implantation is invasion which permits the creation of the hemochorial placenta. The term invasiveness implies the ability of cells to cross anatomic barriers. The first barrier is the layer of endometrial epithelial cells upon which the trophoblasts are attached. Immediately beneath the epithelial layer of cells is a specialized type of matrix called the basement membrane, a thin continuous layer composed mainly of type IV collagen. The basement membrane functions as an anchor for surface epithelium and a separating layer by ensheathing blood vessels, muscle cells and nervous tissue. Beyond the basement membrane lies a highly variable matrix, called the interstitial stroma which contains other tissue cells, vessels and lymphatic channels. Since the blastocyst is too large to squeeze through the epithelial layer, the attached trophoblasts use paracrine activity to induce an apoptotic reaction in the underlying endometrial epithelial cells (Galan et al., 2000).

To achieve successful invasion, trophoblasts then differentiate in a tightly regulated manner producing anchoring cytotrophoblasts and highly secretory synciotrophoblasts that degrades the extracellular matrix with several proteases. The expression of matrix metalloprotease - 9 coincides with the peak invasive potential of trophoblasts. By the 10th day after fertilization, the blastocyst is completely embedded in the stromal tissue of the endometrium with the epithelium regrown over to cover the site of implantation. Eventually, the cytotrophoblasts invade the entire endometrium, the uterine vasculature and into the inner third of the myometrium. The access to the uterine vessels creates the lacunar networks comprising the uteroplacental circulation which places the placental trophoblasts in direct contact with maternal blood. The placenta then serves its vital role as the transfer organ between mother and fetus for nutrients, gas and waste products, hormones and growth factors, among others.

Improper invasion can lead to compromised placental development and complications of pregnancy. Where there is excessive invasion, a placenta may attach onto the myometrium (accreta), into the myometrium (increta) and completely through the myometrium (percreta). Each of these is associated with higher risks of hemorrhage, operative delivery and hysterectomy. If invasion is too shallow, it may lead to intrauterine growth restriction and/or preeclampsia (Zhou et al., 1997).

3. Optimizing embryonic implantation

For couples who suffer from infertility, assisted reproductive techniques have proven to be the most effective in overcoming the majority of barriers. The effectiveness of in vitro fertilization (IVF) is achieved by the ability to bypass certain barriers such as low sperm counts or tubal dysfunction and to choose the most competent embryo to be placed in the uterine cavity at the best time. The factors that limit IVF success can be generally be distilled down to the health of the embryo versus the health of the endometrium, or in essence an evaluation of the seed versus the soil.

3.1 Embryo (seed)

In the past decade, there have been tremendous strides into the study of embryonic competence, or the assessment of what constitutes the embryo with the highest potential to implant and create a baby. Historically, the most common means of assessment is based on morphological observation of an embryo's development in optimal culture conditions. Although this has steadily improved the ability to select the embryos with the highest reproductive potential, thereby increasing pregnancy rates while decreasing multiple gestations, the vast majority of embryos fail to implant. These failures and frustrations have led to the expansion of tools and means to better evaluate the embryo. Metabolomics and proteomics are fields of study into the culture conditions of the embryos looking for soluble markers of improved embryo health. Unfortunately, assessment by morphology and/or culture conditions are not enough since aneuploidy contributes to the majority of unhealthy embryos. Genomics has much promise since chromosomal abnormalities represent a substantial prevalence of reproductive waste (Hassold, 2007). Clinically, this is demonstrated by a woman's age with reduced fecundity, greater miscarriage rates and higher numbers of births with aneuploidy. Indeed, in clinical practice, the age of the oocyte is the single most important variable influencing the outcome of assisted reproduction.

This has led to preimplantation genetic diagnosis (PGD) or assessment to determine the chromosomal constitution before embryo transfer. Initially, polar body biopsy and blastomere biopsies from day 3 embryos were assessed with fluorescent-in-situ hybridization (FISH) for evaluation of a select number of chromosomes. A full discussion of PGD assessment is outside the scope of this chapter but briefly, because of the limitations of FISH, the assay techniques and timing of biopsy have continued to evolve into the development of comprehensive chromosomal screening platforms (Schoolcraft et al., 2011). Several advancements have improved the ability to correctly determine the reproductive potential of a single blastocyst. Combining the technique of trophectoderm biopsy, vitrification and 23 chromosome assessment by single-nucleotide polymorphism (SNP)-based microarray screening has shown promising data at markedly improving the implantation rate to over 60% and reducing the miscarriage rate. This represents an improvement in implantation rates simply by selecting the most reproductively competent seed. However, it is sobering to note that an implantation rate as high as 60% still means that 40% of the most highly selected embryos with a normal chromosome complement still fail to implant. Hence, the health of the seed is not the only component. Undoubtedly, further answers will come from the endometrial side of the equation.

3.2 Endometrium (soil)

Prior to implantation the endometrium undergoes extensive hormonal preparation to produce an epithelium capable of implantation. The development of the receptive endometrium is dependent on estrogen inducing rapid proliferation of the tissue followed by progesterone inducing a secretory pattern. The importance of these steroids cannot be understated as pregnancy cannot occur without them. Their effect is to organize the endometrium or "soil" appropriately so that local cytokines and chemokines can direct the activities in implantation. If the soil is ill prepared by improper hormonal signaling, the following events are much less likely to occur. When optimally primed, the endometrium becomes the most receptive. During the menstrual cycle between cycle days 20-24, or 6 – 10 days post ovulation, the endometrium becomes receptive to implantation during a well defined span of time, the so called "window of implantation". Outside this window, the endometrium is refractory to implantation. It is as if there are resistant factors that inhibit implantation. In fact, an embryo has a better chance of implanting in a fallopian tube or on the peritoneal surface then it does on the unreceptive endometrium. The acquisition of receptivity is a regulated process. Certain disorders that can lead to infertility may be either the absence of receptive molecules or the presence of resistant molecules that inhibit implantation. It has been suggested that MUC1 may act as an anti-adhesion molecule during embryo attachment in the mouse (Surveyor et al., 1995). One theory proposed is that MUC1 acts like bare branches on a Christmas tree that are resistant until adorned with ornaments that serve as ligands to embryonic receptors (see fig. 1). Since MUC1 acts as a scaffold to ligands of L-selectin, it is possible that a disruption of this glycoprotein complex may lead to failed implantation.

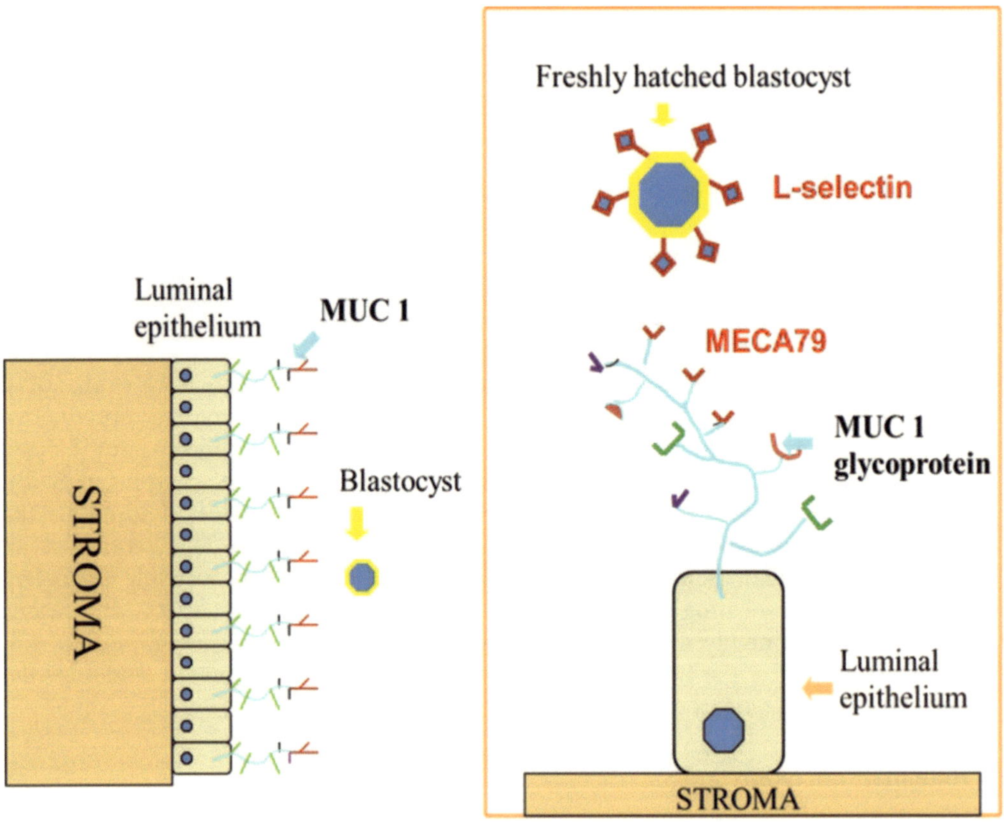

Fig. 1. Model of initial apposition of hatched blastocyst to uterine luminal epithelium

Unlike soil which takes a relatively passive role to the active functions of a seed, the endometrium must engage equally to become receptive and permit the peaceful invasion of a foreign group of cells. The critical component creating this receptivity is the dialogue that occurs between the endometrium and the attaching blastocyst. The endometrium prepares its "landing zones" at the same time a hatching blastocyst prepares it's "tethering tentacles" as it moves about the lumen. As the two appose one another the receptive endometrium actively participates in the implantation process through paracrine bidirectional cross-talk. Using the analogy above, the approaching embryo instructs the tree branches (i.e. endometrium) to self decorate with appropriate ornaments or ligands for tethering by the L-selectin molecules expressed on the exposed trophectoderm. One could hypothesize that infertile patients who suffer from repeated implantation failure would either lack or have diminished ligands on their endometrium during the window of implantation.

4. Study into the failure of implantation

Given the many and varied causes of infertility and early pregnancy loss, we hypothesized that defects in the selectin adhesion system could account for a portion of unexplained reproductive failures. In practice, there are subgroups of women undergoing in vitro fertilization who repeatedly fail to implant despite the transfer of top quality embryos. Our goal was to assess whether the absence of the L-selectin ligand MECA-79 on the endometrium occurs more frequently in patients with repeated implantation failure (RIF), and if the lack of the endometrial L-selectin ligand correlates with unsuccessful implantation.

4.1 Study design

We compared the presence of endometrial L-selectin ligand in a fertile population to a subgroup of patients with a history of repeated implantation failures. The subjects underwent endometrial biopsies during the mid luteal phase (e.g. implantation window) of an ovulation induction cycle. Those patients with implantation failure continued their pursuits of pregnancy through further treatments. The outcome of each patient was followed and tabulated according to whether they did or did not have the L-selectin ligand recognized by immunostaining with the antibody MECA-79.

4.2 Patient selection

Control subjects were healthy young women with proven fertility who were serving as anonymous ovum donors. Twenty RIF patients were recruited at the Nevada Center for Reproductive Medicine. Approval for this research was obtained from the Renown Medical Center Institutional Review Board of the Committee for Human Rights in Research. Patients were recruited if they had at least two unsuccessful in-vitro fertilization cycles due to implantation failure. The diagnosis of implantation failure was made if no implantation occurred despite the transfer of top-quality embryos into a normal appearing endometrial cavity. The embryo morphology was scored according to criteria by Veeck (Veeck, 1999). Only patients who had 6-8 cell stage embryos, grade 1 and 2 transferred were included. The uterine cavity was assessed pre-cycle by sonohysterography and in cycle by transvaginal sonographic evaluation of the endometrial thickness and appearance. Only patients with an endometrial thickness greater than 7 mm and a trilaminar appearance were included.

4.3 Endometrial biopsy

Informed consent was obtained from all patients using an IRB protocol that was approved by the Renown Medical Center Committee on Human Research. The phase of menstrual cycle was confirmed by either a controlled stimulation cycle or a natural cycle monitoring. The stimulation comprised 14 days of estradiol (estrace 2 mg orally bid), followed by micronized progesterone (prometrium 200 mg orally bid) plus estradiol (estrace 2 mg orally qd). In the natural cycles ovulation was confirmed by both a late follicular ultrasound and LH monitoring. An endometrial biopsy was obtained on day 6 of progesterone or the 7th day post LH surge by advancing a Unimar pipelle to the fundus, creating negative pressure and pulling the catheter out in a spiral fashion. The tissue was immediately fixed in 3% paraformaldehyde for 24 hrs. It was rinsed three times in PBS, infiltrated with 5 to 15% sucrose followed by OCT compound and frozen in liquid nitrogen. The tissue was sectioned (5 μm) using a cryomicrotome (Leica Microsystems, Bannockvurn, IL) for immunolocalization.

4.4 Endometrial dating

The morphology of the endometrial biopsies was scored according the dating criteria of Noyes by an experienced histologist (Noyes, 1950). The histologist was blinded to the patient history, including the cycle day of endometrial biopsy.

4.5 Immunohistochemistry

Rat monoclonal antibodies that recognize L-selectin ligand, MECA-79, were from BD Biosciences, San Jose, CA. The MECA-79 antibody recognizes a high-affinity L-selectin ligand carbohydrate epitope containing $SO3 \rightarrow 6GlcNAc$ (Yeh, 2001). The primary antibody was added at a concentration of 5 μg/μl. After the specimens were incubated at 4 °C overnight, they were washed three times in PBS and incubated with goat FITC-conjugated anti-rat IgM (Jackson ImmunoResearch Laboratories). As controls, an irrelevant rat IgM antibody (anti-KLH, eBioscience) or PBS was substituted for primary antibody. Staining was evaluated by using a Zeiss Axiophot fluorescence microscope.

4.6 Results

First we tested the expression of MECA-79 in the endometrial biopsies from control group that consisted of 20 healthy women who were proven to be fertile. All biopsy specimens had morphological characteristics of mid-luteal phase endometrium. The immunostaining with MECA-79 antibody revealed that this L-selectin ligand was present in all samples from the control group and that positive immunostaining was associated with the surface of the luminal and glandular epithelium.

Interestingly, one control patient who initially stained negative for MECA-79 was found to be out of phase during a natural cycle. Later we discovered she had not ovulated. She was placed on a controlled stimulation cycle and subsequently stained positive at the mid-luteal phase. The group of RIF patients was very heterogeneous. The immunostaining with MECA-79 was positive in 15 out of 20 specimens (i.e., in 75% of examined biopsies - see Figure 2). Of these 15 positive specimens, four exhibited weak or patchy staining and eleven were normal. All five MECA-79 negative samples were associated with severe uterine anomalies, including congenital anomalies (i.e. unicornuate uterus), asherman's syndrome, adenomyosis and multiple myomectomies. None of these patients became pregnant after an average of five separate attempts of embryo transfer (see Table 1). Out of 15 patients with MECA-79 positive biopsies, ten became pregnant and 5 quit treatments after an average of one more transfer following the biopsy.

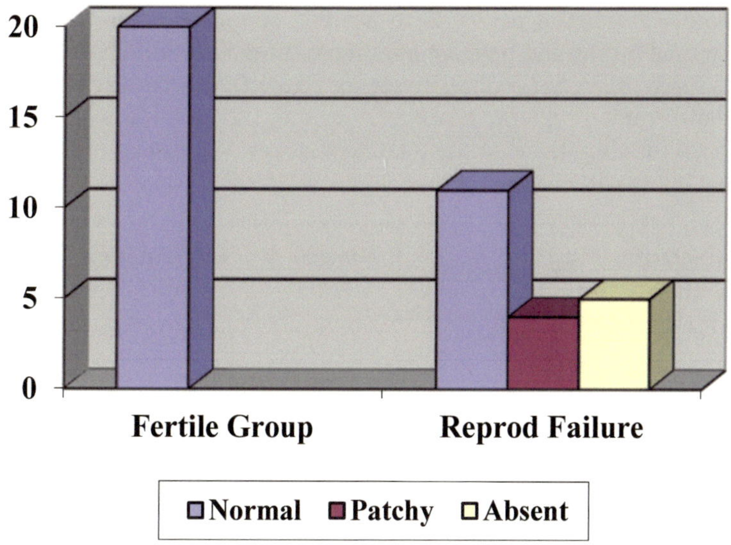

Fig. 2. Presence of L-selectin ligand MECA-79 immunostaining among patients

Of those that continued, the majority became pregnant over an average of two more transfers (see Table 2). Those patients that were positive for the ligand, but did not conceive stopped their treatments an average of 1.5 cycles sooner than those that did get pregnant (2.8 vs. 4.3 cycles respectively). There were no complications with the pregnancies to date.

L-Selectin Ligand (N)	Age (SD)	Uterine History	IVF History (no. of cycles)	Implantation Rate (pregnancies / no. embryos)
Absent (5)	39.0 (1.67)	Unicornuate (2) Asherman's syndrome Adenomyosis Many myomectomies	25/5 (5)	0/72
Patchy (4)	34.7 (4.43)	Normal (1) Hydrosalpingectomy(2) Postpartum curettage	17/4 (4.25)	3/47 (15.7%)
Normal (11)	40.1 (6.73)	Normal (6) Myomectomy (2) Mural myomas (2) Uterine septoplasty	40/11 (3.6)	11/76 (14.5%)

Table 1. Summary of Patients with Repeated Implantation Failure

The results of this pilot study have some important implications. First, the lack of expression of L-selectin ligand MECA-79 in the mid-luteal endometrial biopsy specimen in this group of patients was indicative of a very low or no chance of pregnancy. The predictive value is 100% with a sensitivity of 50% and specificity of 100% (see Table 3). Undoubtedly, the sensitivity would improve if the patients that quit treatments had persisted and become pregnant. Second, patients with a positive MECA-79, that had failed two good prognosis cycles, had about 32% chance per cycle to achieve pregnancy subsequently. Third, in 8 patients with normal uterus and positive immunostaining with MECA-79 the probability of pregnancy was higher than 85% cumulatively, or 53.8% (7/13) per cycle. The implantation rate of those that became pregnant, however, was only 12% overall which is less than one third the rate seen for all patients at the treatment center. Regardless of the presence of the L-selectin ligand, these patients clearly represent a sub-fertile group.

Patients	L-selectin ligand	Implantation	Normal Uterus	Implantation Rate (%)	Mean Number of Cycles
5	Absent	None	0/5	0/72 embryos	5
10	Present	10	7/10	14/116 (12.1%) --after endometrial biopsy 14/57(25%)	4.3
5	Present	None	1/5	0/37	2.8

Table 2. L-selectin ligand and outcome in RIF patients

L-Selectin Ligand	Not Pregnant	Pregnant	Positive Predictive Value	Negative Predictive Value	# subsequent cycles	Pregnancy per cycle (%)
Absent	5	0	100%		15	0/15
Present	5	30		86%	31	10/31 (32.2)

Table 3. Predictive value of L-selectin ligand absence to the lack of a subsequent pregnancy (screening test performed after at least two failed cycles)

4.7 Discussion

The apical surface of the endometrium contains key elements for the initiation of molecular interactions to capture the human blastocyst. The endometrium becomes hormonally primed through the menstrual cycle to create a period of optimal receptivity to successful embryonic implantation. This "window of implantation" occurs between days 20 to 24. Outside this window, the endometrium is resistant to embryo attachment (Navot, 1991). Lai, et. al described the expression of L-selectin ligand throughout the natural menstrual cycle (Lai, 2005) and controlled ovarian stimulation cycle (Lai, 2006). Its expression increased from the periovulatory interval to the mid-secretory phase. Peak immunostaining for L-selectin ligand was seen at the early to midsecretory interval on the luminal surface which coincides with the window of implantation. Interestly, a reduction in expression was seen in subjects who received ovulation induction medication. Vlahos, et. al found that progesterone supplementation enhances L-selectin ligand expression in the luteal phase following controlled ovarian stimulation (Vlahos, 2006). Preliminary work by Khan et al (Khan, 2005) found that N-acetylglucosamine-6-O-sulfotransferase (GlcNAc-6-OST), the gene responsible for high affinity L-selectin ligand epitope production, is regulated by estrogen and progesterone. Estrogen up regulates the gene, while progesterone amplifies this action. Progesterone alone however will suppress GlcNAc -6-OST expression, presumably rendering the endometrium non-receptive.

In our study group, those patients who lacked the ligand all had high risk histories for uterine defects. Iatrogenic causes include curettage and myomectomy while natural states like a congenital anomaly can also give rise to endometrial defects. Clearly, not all patients with such histories fail to achieve pregnancy, but perhaps the L-selectin ligand MECA-79 may act as a marker for the extent of injury or anomaly prior to attempts at pregnancy in high risk groups.

There could be other disease states that affect the expression of L-selectin ligand. Lessey et al described aberrant integrin expression in the endometrium of women with endometriosis (Lessey, 1994). Similarly, Kao et al found the gene, GlcNAc -6-OST, is down-regulated in patients with endometriosis (Kao, 2003). Mak et al found androgens suppress the gene expression which may play a role in poorer reproductive outcomes among patients with polycystic ovarian syndrome (Mak, 2005).

Shamonki et al correlated L-selectin ligand expression with the pregnancy rate in subsequent donor egg cycles (Shamonki, 2006). They demonstrated significantly higher immunohistochemical reactivity for the L-selectin ligand at the apex of endometrial surface epithelium obtained during mock cycle from donor egg recipients who subsequently conceived compared to those who did not. They scored the intensity of staining and correlated it to pregnancy rate, rather than the presence or absence as we have done. The study further supports our finding that L-selectin plays a role in implantation not only by its presence but also by its degree.

We demonstrated that the absence of L-selectin ligand in patients with multiple failed implantation cycles will continue to fail further attempts at implantation. Those who have failed but test positive for the L-selectin ligand, have a very good prognosis on subsequent trials of implantation despite having other unknown contributors to their subfertility.

5. Conclusion

Implantation of the human embryo is complex interaction between the endometrium and the mobile blastocyst. It must occur within a relatively narrow time frame under conditions of a primed receptive surface epithelium and a morphologically changing trophectoderm. Mechanically, the movement of the blastocyst must be arrested in order for attachment and then invasion can occur. The L-selectin ligand adhesion system is becoming more convincingly believed to play a major role in mediating initial embryonic apposition. By loose tethering, the blastocyst is able to attach despite the shear forces within the uterine lumen and orient itself for stable attachment. Once anchored, a cascade of events unfolds allowing the embryo to burrow into the endometrial wall and establish a hemochorial placenta.

Dysfunction in either the blastocyst or the endometrium can limit the implantation efficiency. Many studies into embryo reproductive competence have demonstrated that improved selection of the embryo can drastically improve the implantation rate. While the endometrial side of the equation is more challenging to study, we are uncovering areas where proper preparation and determination of a receptive endometrium is improving outcomes. At each phase along the implantation process, certain disease states have been shown to disrupt the delicate dialogue required for implantation. Regarding the apposition step, the L-selectin ligand may be used as a marker for implantation efficiency. Clinically, in high risk groups, one could biopsy a patient and potentially prevent many futile attempts of costly treatments if the ligand is absent. This would provide the patient with important information as to why she is unable to become pregnant and open options such as gestational surrogacy to help her to become a mother. Beyond apposition, defects that disrupt integrin expression have been shown in disease states such as endometriosis and hydrosalpinges. Treatment of these defects have improved outcomes. Finally, the invasion of cytotrophoblasts to the proper depth of the uterus is critical in determining the outcome of pregnancy. Excessive invasion leads to placenta accreta, while inadequate invasion has been implicated in the pathophysiology of preeclampsia, the leading cause of maternal death in the industrialized world.

Normal implantation is crucial for successful pregnancy. For the infertile couple and their treating physician, a better understanding of the processes of implantation will enable better diagnosis and treatments to overcome the reasons why they cannot have a healthy child. Together, by selecting of the healthiest embryo and establishing the most receptive endometrium we can increase implantation efficiency. Future research into markers of endometrial receptivity will allow clinicians to define the optimal environment in which to transfer the best embryos, thereby improving pregnancy rates and decreasing complications such as multiple pregnancies, miscarriages and ultimately conditions that compromise the healthy intrauterine development of baby.

6. References

Alon R., Feigelson S. (2002). From Rolling to Arrest on Blood Vessels: leukocyte tap dancing on endothelial integrin ligands and chemokines at sub-second contacts. *Semin Immunol,* Vol. 14, pp 93-104

Bentin-Ley U., Sjogren A., Nilsson L., Hamberger L., Larsen J.F., Horn T. (2000). Relevance of endometrial pinopodes for human blastocyst implantation. *Hum Reprod Suppl.,* Vol. 6, pp. 67-73

Carson D.D., Julian J., Lessey B., Prakobphol A., Fisher S. (2006). MUC1 is a Scaffold for Selectin Ligands in the Human Uterus. *Frontiers in Bioscience,* Vol. 11, pp. 2903-2909

Galan A., Herrer R., Remohi J., Pellicer A., Simon C. (2000). Embryonic regulation of endometrial epithelial apoptosis during human implantation. *Hum Reprod.,* Vol. 15(suppl. 6), pp. 74-80

Genbacev O., Prakobphol A., Foulk R., Krtolica A., Ilic D., Singer M., Yang Z.Q., Kiessling L., Rosen S., Fisher S. (2003). Trophoblast L-Selectin-Mediated Adhesion at the Maternal-Fetal Interface. *Science,* Vol.299, pp. 405-408

Hassold T., Hall H., Hunt P. (2007). The origin of human aneuploidy: where we have been, where we are going. *Hum Mol Genet,* Vol. 16, pp. R203-208

Kao L.C., Germeyer A., Tulac S. (2003). Expression profiling of endometrium from women with endometriosis reveals candidate genes for disease-based implantation failure and infertility. *Endocrinology,* Vol. 144, pp. 2870-2881

Khan S., Pisarska D., Kao L.C. (2005). Hormonal Regulation of N-acetylglucosamine-6-O-sulfotransferase (GlcNAc-6-OST), Expression in a Human Endometrial Cell Model. *Abs presented at conjoint meeting ASRM/CFAS* Sept.2005, Vol. 85:suppl 1:S434

Lai T.H., Shih I.M., Vlahos N., Ho C.L., Wallach E., Zhao Y. (2005). Differential Expression of L-selectin ligand in the Endometrum During the Menstrual Cycle. *Fertil Steril*, Vol. 83, pp. 1297-1302

Lai T.H., Zhao Y., Shih I.M., Ho C.L., Bankowski B., Vlahos N. (2006). Expression of L-selectin ligands in human endometrium during the implantation window after controlled ovarian stimulation for oocyte donation. *Fertil Steril* Vol. 85(3), pp. 761-763

Lessey B., Castlebaum A., Sawin S. (1994). Aberrant integrin expression in the endometrium of women with endometriosis. *J Clin Endocrinol Metab*, Vol. 79, pp. 643-649.

Lessey B.A. (2002). Adhesion molecules and implantation. *J Reprod Immunol* Vol. 55, pp. 101-112

Mak W., Khan S., Pisarska D. (2005). Androgen Suppression of a target human implantation gene N-acetylglucosamine-6-O-sulfotransferase (GlcNAc-6-OST) in a human endometrial cell model. *Abs presented at conjoint meeting ASRM/CFAS* Sept.2005, Vol 85:suppl 1:S10

McEver R.P. (2002). Selectins: lectins that initiate cell adhesion under flow. *Curr Opin Cell Biol*, Vol. 14, pp. 581

Navot D., Scott R.T., Droesch K. (1991). The Window of Embryo Transfer and the Efficiency of Human Conception in vitro. *Fertil Steril*, Vol. 55, pp.114-118

Norwitz E., Schust D., Fisher S. (2001). Implantation and the survival of early pregnancy. *NEJM*, Vol. 342,19, pp 1400-1408

Noyes W., Hertig A.I., Rock J. (1950). Dating the endometrial biopsy. *Fertil Steril* Vol. 1, pp. 3-25.

Prakobphol A., Thomsson K., Hansson G., Rosen S., Singer M., Phillips N., Medzihradszky K., Burlingame A., Leffler H., Fisher S. (1998). Human low-molecular-weight salivary mucin expresses the sialyl lewis - X determinant and has L-selectin ligand activity. *Biochemistry* Vol. 37, pp. 4916–4927

Prakobphol A., Boren T., Ma W., Zhixiang P., Fisher S. (2005). Highly glycosylated human salivary molecules present oligosaccharides that mediate adhesion of leukocytes and Helicobacter pylori. *Biochemistry* Vol. 44, pp. 2216–2224

Rosen S. (2004). Ligands for L-selectin: homing, inflammation, and beyond. *Annul. Rev. Immunol*. Vol. 22, pp. 129–156

Schoolcraft W., Treff N., Stevens J., Ferry K., Katz-Jaffe M., Scott R. (2011). Live birth outcome with trophectoderm biopsy, blastocyst vitrification, and single-nucleotide polymorphism micro-array-based comprehensive chromosomal screening in infertile patients. *Fertil Steril*, Vol96(3), pp. 638-642

Shamonki M.I., Kligman I., Shamonki J.M. (2006). Immunohistochemical expression of endometrial L-selectin ligand is higher in donor egg recipients with embryonic implantation. *Fertil Steril* Vol.86(5), pp. 1365-1375

Simon C., Gimeno M.J., Mercader A., O'Connor J.E., Remohi J., Polan M.L., Pellicer A. (1997). Embryonic regulation of integrins beta 3, alpha 4, and alpha 1 in human endometrial epithelial cells in vitro. *J Clin Endocrinol Metab*, Vol. 82, pp. 2607-2616

Stephens L.E., Sutherland A.E., Klimanskaya I.V., Andreiux A., Meneses J., Pedersen R.A., Damsky C.H. (1995). Deletion of beta 1 integrins in mice results in inner cell mass failure and peri-implantation lethality. *Genes Dev,* Vol. 9, pp. 1883-1895

Surveyor G.A., Gendler S., Pemberton L., Das S., Chakraborty I., Pimental R. (1995). Expression and steroid hormonal control of muc-1 in the mouse uterus. *Endocrinology,* Vol. 136, pp. 3639-3647

Veeck L.L. (1999). *An atlas of human gametes and conceptuses.* New York, Parthenon, pp. 46-51

Vlahos N.F., Lipari C.W., Bankowski B. (2006). Effect of luteal-phase support on endometrial L-selectin ligand expression after recombinant follicle-stimulating hormone and ganirelix acetate for in Vitro Fertilization. *Clin Endocrine Met,* Vol. 91(10), pp. 4043-4049

Yeh, J.C., Hiraoka N. (2001). Novel Sulfated Lymphocyte Homing Receptors and Their Control by a Corel Extension Beta 1,3-N,acetylglucosaminyltransferase. *Cell* Vol.105, pp. 957-969

Zhou Y., Damsky C., Fisher S. (1997). Preeclampsia is associated with failure of human cytotrophoblasts to mimic a vascular adhesion phenotype: one cause of defective endovascular invasion in this syndrome? *J Clin Invest.* Vol.99, pp. 2152-2164

15

Biomarkers Related to Endometrial Receptivity and Implantation

Mark P. Trolice[1] and George Amyradakis[2]
[1]Associate Professor, Department of Obstetrics & Gynecology, University of Central Florida School of Medicine, Orlando, FL
Director, Fertility Center of Assisted Reproduction & Endocrinology, Winter Park, FL
[2]Resident Physician, Winnie Palmer Hospital for Women & Babies, Orlando, FL
USA

1. Introduction

Implantation is a process requiring the delicate interaction between the embryo and a receptive endometrium. This intricate interaction requires a harmonized dialogue between embryonic and maternal tissues. [Aghajanova et al., 2008; Simon et al., 2000] The three stages of implantation are: apposition, adhesion, and invasion. Apposition describes trophoblast cells adhering to the receptive endometrial wall. Adhesion to the basal lamina and stromal extracellular matrix occurs in the presence of specific hormones, cytokines, and adhesion molecules. Once the blastocyst is anchored to the endometrial wall, it will become enclosed by an outer layer of syncytiotrophoblast, and an inner layer of cytotrophoblast. As the syncytiotrophoblast erodes the endometrium, the blastocyst will burrow into it and implantation will occur. [Ganong, 2005] During the last few years, research pursues enhancing both the quality of the embryo as well as understanding the highly dynamic tissue of the endometrial wall. Despite morphological and chromosomal criteria to improve the quality of transferred embryos, implantation rates remain at 25-35%. [Boomsma &Macklon, 2006]

The priming of the endometrium to optimize the window of implantation phase has been a subject of interest for decades, and much work has gone into understanding the preparation and capability of the endometrial wall to create a hospitable environment for the interaction with the blastocyst. While an embryo factor accounts for one third one implantation failure, lack of uterine receptivity explains approximately two thirds of implantation failures. [Achache, 2006; Ledee-Bataille et al., 2002] The actions of numerous cytokines, hormones, immunoglobulins, and other factors, are all orchestrated into preparing the endometrium for implantation. The morphological changes towards a receptive endometrium have been described as early as 1950 by Noyes, Hertig, and Rock [Strowitzki, 2006] and occur under the control of the sexual steroid hormones estrogen, and progesterone; with estrogen being the determinant hormone in the proliferative phase and progesterone being the determinant hormone in the secretory phase

During the luteal implantation phase; corresponding to cycle days 20-24, or seven to nine days after ovulation, the endometrium is receptive to the oncoming blastocyst. [Goiran &

Mignot, 1999] Essential expression of proteins, cytokines, and peptides can be detected at this time and serve as biomarkers for maximal endometrial receptivity. [Singh & Aplin, 2009; Lessey et al., 2002] The detection and investigation of biochemical markers during the implantation phase is an area of research receiving much interest and may serve to establish future treatments to help maximize the effectiveness of assisted reproductive techniques (ART) in the near future. According to Zhu, biomarkers are those that are present in the endometrium during the implantation phase, close to the implantation site, and disappear thereafter. [Cavagna & Mantese, 2003] This chapter will discuss biomarkers and their role in the attachment and invasion process during the implantation phase.

2. Biomarkers

HLA-G

Human leukocyte antigen G (HLA-G) is a major histocompatability complex (MHC) class Ib gene thought to play an essential role in implantation by modulating cytokine secretion to maintain local immunotolerance and modulate cytokine secretion to control trophopblastic cell invasion. [Roussev & Coulam, 2007] At first, HLA-G was proposed as a protector against natural killer (NK)-cell-mediated cytolysis of target cells and to prevent allorecognition by maternal cytotoxic lymphocytes. Recently, it has been shown tha these proteins regulate immune cells including T cells, NK cells, and antigen-presenting cells. [Fournel, 2000] Due to its essential role in the implantation process, recent attention has been focused on HLA-G and its diagnostic and therapeutic clinical applications. This has included the evaluation of couples with recurrent miscarriages and the mutation of the HLA-G gene. Serum sHLA-G levels during pregnancy may in the future become a diagnostic tool for evaluation of successful implantation but has yet to be established. [Roussev & Coulam, 2007]

Pinopodes

Pinopodes are organelles shown to be present on the endometrial wall during the implantation phase. They have been detected by electron microscopy and are specific markers for uterine receptivity. Progesterone dependent, pinopodes are present 20-21 days into the luteal cycle. [Cavagna & Mantese, 2003] Their function has not fully been established, but pinopodes are thought to play a role in protecting the blastocyst from being swept by the cilia on the endometrial wallpromoting withdrawal of uterine fluid and facilitating molecular adhesion of the pinopodes with the blastocyst. The life span of fully developed pinopodes lasts no more than 48 hours suggesting a transient cell state. Following ovarian stimulation with clomiphene citrate and human chorionic gonadotropin (hCG), pinopodes formed a little earlier, on days 17 or 18 than in the natural state.. [Cavagna & Mantese, 2003] It is thus possible that ovarian stimulation and early pinopode formation may have a role in shifting the window of receptivity resulting in asynchrony between the endometrium and blastocyst thereby negatively influencing implantation rates with IVF.

Integrins

Integrins are a family of transmembrane glycoproteins, formed by the interaction of two different, non-covalently linked α and β subunits. [Achache & Revel, 2006] They are adhesion molecules which participate in cell-adhesions and have also shown to play part in adhesions between cells and extracellular components. [Ceydell, 2006] In addition, integrins participate in many physiologically important processes including embryological development, haemostasis, thrombosis, wound healing, immune and non-immune defense mechanisms and oncogenic transformation. Specifically, the αvβ3 integrin as well as its ligand osteoponin was positively detected by immunohistochemistry on the endometrial luminal epithelial surface, which first interacts with the trophoblast. [Achache & Revel, 2006; Apparao ET AL., 2001] The expression of the endometrial stromal integrins may be modulated by several factors and the expression of the αvβ3 integrin in the endometrial stroma was demonstrated to be stimulated by IL- α, IL- β and TNF-α. [Ceydell, 2006] Integrins have been proposed as markers for endometrial receptivity, and the αvβ3 glycoprotein particularly has been directly associated with implantation.

L-selectin

Selectins are lectin like proteins and include E-, L-, and P-selectins, all of which were originally thought o be expressed solely by hemangioblast descendants. P- selectins are expressed on the surface of platelets, E- selectins are expressed on activated endothelial cells, and L-selectins are expressed on lymphocytes. Glycoproteins carrying oligosaccharide formations including CD34, GlyCAM-1, PSGL-1, podocalyxin, and endoglycan, are recognized by the selectin molecules. [Foulk et al., 2007] Selectins are responsible for the tether and roll mechanism on endothelial surfaces. Once leucocytes slow down and subsequently arrest, integrin activation triggers adhesion and transmigration through the vascular endothelium. [Torry et al., 2007] Recently, Genbacec et al. [Genbacev et al., 2003] have shown that hatched blastocysts expressed L-selectin and used this molecule to mediate its attachment to the luminal epithelial surface via MECA-79, its carbohydrate ligands, and related epitopes. [Foulk et al., 2007] Also, Foulk and Zdravkovic have shown that lack of expression of the L-selectin ligand MECA-79 in mid-luteal endometrial biopsies were indicative or low or no chance of pregnancy.

Heparin binding-epidermal growth factor

Heparin binding-epidermal growth factor (HB-EGF) interacts with the EGF receptor and belongs to the epidermal growth factor family. It has been shown that HB-EGF expression is low during the proliferative endometrial phase, attaining its highest measure immediately prior to the implantation window, suggesting that it may have a role during the blastocyst implantation process. [Cavagna & Mantese, 2003; Lessey et al., 2002] It has been suggested that HB-EGF promotes implantation and trophoblast invasion through paracrine/autocrine signaling as cells penetrate the stroma. HB-EGF has also been shown to inhibit apoptosis and induces an invasive trophoblast phenotype. The co-existence of HB-EGF and pinopodes has been investigated with electron microscopy and immunochemistry, and shows that the expression of HB-EGF is highest when fully developed pinopodes are present, supporting the role of HB-EGF in the implantation process. [Cavagna & Mantese, 2003, Stavreus et al., 2001]

Chorionic gonadotropin and Notch 1

Chorionic gonadotropin is one of the early embryonic secretions from the trophoblast cells of the pre-implantation embryo. This helps maintain the corpus luteum of pregnancy, and leads to the modifications in morphology and endometrial gene expression preparing for implantation.

The notch family of receptors mediates a highly conserved pathway that regulated differentiation and pro-survival signals from humans to varied species of invertebrates. [Afshar et al., 2007; Paria et al., 2002] Notch proteins are ligand-dependant transmembrane receptors that transduce extracellular signals responsible for cell-fate and differentiation throughout development. Notch signaling often restricts the differentiation fates of a cell, directing it to a specific cell fate in cooperation with other signals, while at the same time inhibiting differentiation toward an alternate fate and promoting survival. Evidence indicates that Notch signaling regulates all three branches of the fate cell decision tree; differentiation, cell cycle progression and apoptotic cell death. Recently Afshar et al. have shown the co-expression of αSMA and Notch 1, both arising from CG signaling, inhibits apoptosis of stromal cells during the establishment of pregnancy. Shedding of the uterine lining and the inability of the uterus to accept an embryo can be correlated with low expression of Notch 1. Survival of the uterine lining can be mediated by (h)CG supplementation or progesterone as they will induce the expression of Notch 1. [Afshar et al., 2007]

Mucins

Mucins are glycoproteins high in molecular weight, which contain at least 50% of carbohydrate O-linked to a theonine/serine rich peptide core. [Gendler et al., 1990] MUC-1 is a large glycoprotein with a molecular weight >250 kDa. [Achache & Revel, 2006] When highly expressed on a cell surface, MUC-1 produces a steric hindrance phenomenon interfering with cellular adhesion. Cell-cell and cell-matrix adhesions are inhibited in direct correlation to the length of the MUC-1 ectodomain. [Hilkens et al, 1992] The apical surface of most epithelial cells is protected by a thick glycocalyx composed mostly of mucins that are believed to protect the cell surface from pathological processes. In the endometrium, MUC-1 is probably the first molecule the blastocyst encounters on the endometrial wall before implantation. This interaction would seem to indicate the blastocyst might be deterred from the endometrial wall until a proper location is encountered for implantation. In mice, rats, and pigs it has been shown that MUC-1 is down-regulated during the window of receptivity and thus optimizing the interaction between blastocyst and uterine wall. Paradoxically in humans, it has been shown that MUC-1 is up-regulated during the pre-implantation period. Therefore, it was suggested that humans must have a mechanism to induce inhibitory factors to down-regulate the MUC-1 barrier. High progesterone levels apparently reduce MUC-1 levels, thus unmasking intracellular adhesion molecules (CAM) on the surface of the endometrium and increasing uterine receptivity. [Bowen et al., 1996] Immunohistochemistry and scanning electron microscopy have shown that the MUC1 epitope corresponds only to ciliated cells. But the surface of non-ciliated cells such as pinopods has not been correlated to MUC-1. It has been suggested that pinopodes are important in providing a MUC-1 free area for blastocyst implantation. It seems that even though MUC-1 appears to have negative effects on implantation, its upregulation and extension beyond the glycocalyx covering the endometrium suggest it may have a temporary role in directing the embryo to effective implantation. [Achache & Revel, 2006]

Calcitonin

Parafollicular cells of the thyroid release calcitonin in response to hypercalcemia to reduce calcium levels. Though its role remains to be determined, calcitonin is expressed in the human endometrium during the secretory phase with highest concentrations on luteal cycle days 19-21, coinciding with the implantation period. It has also been demonstrated progesterone induces calcitonin gene expression in the endometrium. [Cavagna & Mantese, 2003; Kumar, 1998] By immunoreactivity for calcitonin mRNA,calcitonin seems to be absent during the proliferative and ovulatory phase. This finding may be another reason to suspect that calcitonin may be a marker for uterine receptivity. Calcitonin controls calcium homeostasis by binding to specific receptors identifeied as CR1a and CR1b. [Sexton et al., 1993; Wang, 1998] CR1a receptors have been found to be present in murine oocytes and zygotes in low concentrations, but significant increase of this receptor was found in embryos between the 8 cell and blastocyst stage. Wang et al. have also shown blastocysts differentiate in vitro at an accelerated rate when treated with 10 nM calcitonin for 30 minutes. [Cavagna & Mantese, 2003; Wang, 1998] Though this seems to demonstrate the role of calcitonin in embryonic development, further studies will need to be conducted to show the definitive role of calcitonin during implantation and development of the embryo.

Prostaglandins

As implantation takes place, the blastocyst needs access and connection to the maternal vascular system. For this to occur there needs to be an increase of vascular permeability at the site of implantation. [Chakraborty et al., 1996] Prostaglandins (PGs) are known to possess vasoactive factors,play a definitive role in ovulation, fertilization, and labor, and recently have shown to be crucial during the implantation process. [Achache & Revel, 2006, Song et al., 2006]

Prostaglandins are eicosanoids consisting of four members, PGD2, PGE2, PGF2α, and prostacyclin (PGI2). These are generated by the action of two enzymes, cytosolic phospholipase A2 (cPLA2), and cyclooxygenase (COX). Song et al. have demonstrated female mice lacking the cPLA2 and COX enzymes are not able to produce PG, leading to significant implantation defects. cPLA2 knockout mice also exhibited pregnancy failures and small litter size, secondary to delayed implantation. Exogenous administration of PG was able to restore embryo implantation at the correct time. It is not clear whether diminished expression of PG prevents human fertility because mice lacking PG will be fertile but present with fine tuning details. Thus it is postulated a similar process in humans leading to delayed implantation could lead to early pregnancy loss. Further investigation on the role of PGs at the time of human implantation and its possible role in late-pregnancy abnormalities needs to be further explored. [Achache & Revel, 2006, Song et al., 2006]

HOX genes

Homeobox genes HOXA-10 and HOXA-11 have been linked with endometrial receptivity. Mutations in these genes have lead to failure to achieve normal implantation in mice. [Cavagna & Mantese, 2003; Daftary & Taylor, 2001] Growth and development of the human endometrium have been linked with these genes, and shown to have significant up-regulation in the mid-secretory phase correlating with the implantation window. Female mice with homozygous mutations in the HOXA-10 or HOXA-11 have been shown to be infertile due to endometrial factors. [Satokata et al., 1995] According to Benson et al., the HOXA-10 gene may be important during morphogenesis for proper patterning of the reproductive tract and in adult endometrium for adequate implantation events.

In women with endometriosis, Taylor et al. observed HOX gene expression is altered resulting in endometrial molecular alterations resulting in decreased endometrial receptivity. These observations further support the importance HOX gene expression may have during implantation process.

Angiogenesis

Vascular development at the maternal fetal interface is an essential component for successful implantation and development. Trophoblasts, natural killer cells, and other cell types are responsible for this development. Trophoblasts are well known to produce angiogenic growth factors. [Cross et al., 2002; Torry et al., 2007] Ungranulated uterine natural killer cells (uNK) precursors are recruited to the endometrium during the transition of the endometrium to the secretory phase. Progesterone allows the development of the pre-uNK into large granulated uNK cells. These appear to be present during the implantation phase and have a role in releasing cytokines responsible for angiogenesis in early pregnancy, and development of spiral arteriole formation as the pregnancy progresses. [Leonard et al., 2006] In vitro models of mice have suggested that progesterone serves to up-regulate decidua IL-15, in turn serving as a main activator of uNK population. [Leede-Bataille et al., 2005]

Other cells such as B and T lymphocytes have also been implicated in angiogenesis during the early phases of pregnancy. B lymphocytes have been shown to express the c-Myc oncogene, which can induce angiogenesis by producing VEGF. [Ruddell et al., 2003] Vascular endothelial growth factor (VEGF) is a known angiogenic substance involved in the process of vascular proliferation. [Tammela et al., 2005] During the peri-implantation phases, certain VEGF receptors appear to be expressed and function to optimize blastocyst implantation by mediating vascular permeability. These are VEGFR-1, VEGFR-2, and NRP-1. [Halder et al., 2000; Torry et al., 2007] The function and expression of VEGF have shown to be pivotal for angiogenesis during the implantation process and early placental development. Disturbance of this process could lead to implantation failure and early pregnancy loss.

Insulin like growth factor-II (IGF-II)

Insulin-like growth factors along with their binding proteins are thought to be responsible for differentiation, endometrial growth, angiogenesis, and apoptosis. [Cavagna & Mantese, 2003] IGF-II in particular is a known mediator of trophoblast function and is required for suitable placental growth and transport function. [Herr et al., 2003] Trophoblasts havebeen shown to express IGF-II while vessels near the implantation site have similarly been shown to expresses IGF-II receptors indicating IGF-II may directly act as an angiogenic growth factor. [Torry et al., 2007] In mice, IGF-II has demonstrated its vessel proliferation potential by inducing angiogenic growth factors such as VEGF and proliferin. Insulin like growth factors are regulated by insulin-like growth factor binding proteins (IGFBP). [Cavagna & Mantese, 2003] Litcht et al. have shown that secretion of IGFBP-1 by the endometrium occurs approximately 10 days after the LH surge, correlating with the implantation window. [Licht et al., 2002] With IGFBP-1 being the predominant regulatory factor for IGF-II, it may play an important role in endometrial receptivity and implantation.

Leukemia Inhibitory Factor (LIF)

In 1992, Hilton demonstrated LIF to be a haemapoietic factor by its capability to stimulate macrophage differentiation of the mouse myeloid leukemia cell line. [Achache & Revel,

2006; Hilton, 1992] Proliferation, cell survival, and differentiation, are some of the autocrine and paracrine effects of LIF, and have led researchers into investigating its function in blastocyst development and implantation. A study by Stewart [Stewart, 1994] showed that female mice expressing homozygous LIF gene deficiency displayed failed embryo implantation. Further evidence of the importance of LIF was observed as LIF supplementation rescued embryo implantation in the previously affected mice. LIF expression was observed to reach maximum concentrations in the mid- to late-secretory phase. Endometrial biopsies have shown LIF mRNA expression on days 18 to 28 of the menstrual cycle with maximum expression on day 20. [Charnock-Jones et al., 1994] Infertile patients and those with repeated implantation failureshave been shown to have abnormal levels of LIF supporting the role of LIF as a fundamental element in the implantation process. [Achache & Revel, 2006] Preclinical and clinical trials have investigated the effects of recombinant human LIF (r-hLIF) in improving endometrial receptivity. [Brinsden et al., 2003] In light of the importance of LIF in the implantation process, r-hLIF could be an important tool in the near future to optimize endometrial receptivity.

Serum-and Glucocorticoid-Regulated Kinase 1 (SGK1)

Recently, Feroze-Zaidi el al. demonstrated that women with unexplained fertility or recurrent implantation failure after IVF showed an abnormal expression of the SGK1 gene in the luminal epithelial cells during the midsecretory receptive phase corresponding with the implantation window. [Fakhera et al., 2007] Regulation of epithelial Na+ channels (ENaCs) is known to be controlled by SGK1. Uterine fluid homeostasis could thus be directly influenced by SGK1 leading to decreased uterine receptivity and disruption of successful implantation. Differentiating human endometrial stromal cells (HESCs) also activate SGK1, which stimulates the expression of prolactin (PRL), a most important decidual marker gene. [Brosens & Gellersen, 2003, 2006]

FOXO proteins are known to be able to regulate genes involved in proaptotic properties, and also genes involved in differentiation, cell cycle arrest, DNA repair, and oxidative defenses. [Fakhera et al., 2007; Sunters et al., 2003] Phosphorylation of transcription factors regulating expression of FOXO proteins, are targeted by kinases including SGK1 which serve to inactivate such proteins. [Brunet et al., 2001; Rena et al., 2003] Increased activity of SKG1 in the midsecretory phase may disrupt implantation by disrupting normal activity of ENAC-mediated Na+ and water transport or by interrupting focal apoptosis.

Interleukin-6 (IL-6)

IL-6 is a cytokine classically known to induce immunoglobulin production in activated B cells, but also found to display a wide variety of functions outside the B-lymphocyte system. IL-6 expression in the human endometrium has been detected with the highest levels corresponding to the luteal phase. [Achache & Revel, 2006] mRNA expression of IL-6 steadily increases during the mid- to late-secretory phase and then decreases again in the late-secretory phase. During the crucial window of implantation, immunoreactivity for IL-6 becomes markedly detectable. The epithelial and glandular cells are the areas where the protein is mostly pronounced, compared to the stroma. During the window of implantation, receptors for IL-6 can be found not only in the endometrium, but are also expressed in the blastocyst, suggesting the paracrine/autocrine role of IL-6 during the peri-implantation period. Experiments performed using mice with disrupted IL-6 genes have shown despite implantation , the growth and development of the blastocyst becomes compromised. [Achache & Revel, 2006; Salamonsen et al., 2000] This suggests that even though IL-6 may not be an essential element for implantation, the lack of its presence could still explain infertility in some cases. Recent findings of patients with recurrent abortions have shown that IL-6 endometrial m-RNA is suppressed in the mid-secretory phase, thus supporting the role and importance of IL-6 in infertility.

Interleukin-1 (IL-1)

IL-1α, IL-1β, and IL-1 receptor antagonist (IL-1ra) are all included in the family of IL-1, and serve as pivotal mediators of the immunologic and inflammatory response. In past experiments with mice, knockout mice for IL-1 were still able to proceed with implantation, but of interest, mice who received intraperitoneal injections of the IL-1ra displayed blastocysts unable to implant on the endometrial wall. Simon attributed this to the down regulation of crucial integrins at the luminal epithelial surfaces by the IL-1ra. In humans, it has been observed that administration of IL-1 causes an increase of β3 expression in the culture media of EECs thereby optimizing blastocyst implantation. [Achache & Revel, 2006] Leptin has also been shown to increase integrin β3 expression. Interestingly enough, IL-1β acts in stimulating leptin secretion and up-regulating its Ob-R receptor in EECs. IL-1 RtI mRNA and protein have shown to be present in maximal levels during the luteal phase in the human epithelial endometrium, and expression of the IL-1 antagonist has been shown to be reduced during the period of the implantation window. This finding suggests that suppression of the IL-1 antagonist during this crucial period of implantation maximizes successful implantation. [Boucher et al., 2001]

In women with endometriosis, the levels of IL-1ra and IL-1α were found to be markedly increased when compared to control groups in the PF and serum, and may serve as an explanation of the pathogenesis and infertility in such patients. [Kondera-Anasz et al. 2005]

Leptin

Acting both at the endocrine and paracrine level, leptin has been associated with regulation of body weight and reproductive function. [Cervero et al., 2004] Leptin is the product of the OB gene. Studies with rodents have determined this ligand-receptor system to be necessary for implantation. Receptors associated with leptin include total leptin receptor (OB-RT), the long form (OB-RL), and HuB219.1 and HuB219.3 short isoforms found in the endometrium. Studies with mice expressing ob/ob mutations resulted in phenotypically obese and sterile mice. Exogenous leptin treatment was able to restore sterility in these mice, but food restriction was not, implicating leptin as a requirement for normal reproductive functioning. [Cervero et al., 2004] Additionally, leptin has also been shown to increase integrin β3 expression, an important ligand protein essential for endometrial receptivity and implantation. The leptin receptors OB-RT, OB-RL, HuB219.1, and HuB219.3 have all demonstrated maximal expression in the late luteal phase. [Achache & Revel, 2006]

Cadherins

Cadherins are responsible for calcium-dependent cell-to-cell adhesion mechanisms and belong to a group of glycoproteins divided into N-, P-, and E-cadherins, all displaying specific functions and tissue distributions. Of all the cadherins, E-cadherin is the most studied pertaining to implantation, is ubiquitous, and is believed to be responsible for maintainance of adherens junctions in epithelial cells. [Singh & Aplin, 2009] E-cadherin suppression is responsible for cell-cell adhesion dysfunction. Riethmacher et al. demonstrated that targeted mutation of the E-cadherin gene resulted in defective pre-implantation development in mice.

During the luteal phase, E-cadherin mRNA levels are significantly elevated and regulation seems to be mainly controlled by intracellular calcium levels. E-cadherin cytoskeletal organization and disassembly at the adherens junction are mediated by rising levels of calcium which work by acting on signaling pathways. In vitro studies have shown that calcitonin produces a transient rise in intracellular calcium levels, suppressing E-cadherin at cellular contact sites. These experiments were performed by Li et al. on cultured Ishikawa cells.

Calcitonin appears to be an important regulator of implantation. Progesterone acts to increase calcitonin levels, which in-turn acts to increase intracellular calcium thus regulating E-cadherin expression. E-cadherin then seems to serve two main functions of uterine receptivity: adhesiveness in the preliminary phases; and inactivation by the actions of progesterone and calcitonin in the secretory phase to allow epithelial cell disassociation and implantation. [Achache & Revel, 2006]

Cyclin E and p27

Cyclins are known to control mitotic phase progression in cells. The G1 to S phase transition is controlled by the rate limiting step of Cyclin E, whereas prevention of the cell cycle progression is controlled by the p27 cyclin-dependent kinase inhibitor. [Kliman et al., 2006] While the plausible role of cyclin E involves proliferation, p27 is mostly responsible for differentiation. [Dubowy et al., 2003] Conbsistent with these actions, estrogen has positive regulatory effects on Cyclin E andprogesterone seems to induce a dominant p27 state. Cyclin E activity is present in the cytoplasm of epithelial cells whereas p27 activity is exclusively active in the nucleus. While present in the early phases of the mestrual cycle, Cyclin E reactivity seems to rapidly decrease after cycle day 19; this could be explained by its subsequent movement towards the nucleus where it binds to p27 thereby becoming inactivated.

The Endometrial Function Test (EFT) is a means to assess Cyclin E by immunohistochemically staining endometrial biopsies using antibodies against Cyclin E; and also as a means to identify an abnormally developing endometrium. [Dubowy et al., 2003] EFT showing a persistence of Cyclin E was associated with glandular developmental arrest (GDA), and observed in women with infertility. The overexpression of Cyclin E seemed to indicate that cells were arrested at an earlier phase of the menstrual cycle, possibly due to a premature expression of p27. [Kliman et al., 2006] The development of the EFT associated with cyclin markers and their correlation to estrogen and progesterone could serve as an important tool in the near future to assess endometrial receptivity and the effects of exogenous hormone administration in infertile patients. [Kliman et al., 2006]

Colony Stimulating Factor-1 (CSF-1)

CSF-1 is a haemopoietic growth factor inducing proliferation and differentiation of cells belonging to the mononuclear phagocytic lineage. Pollard et al. have demonstrated that op/op mice with mutations in CSF gene displayed multiple skeletal defects and decreased implantation rates. Other studies have shown CSF-1 to also be an important factor when it comes to ovulation. Op/op mice compared to wild type mice showed significant lower follicular development and ovulation rates. It has been shown that women with lower preconceptional CSF-1 levels are more prone to recurrent abortions compared to women with higher preconceptional CSF-1 levels. [Cavagna & Mantese, 2003]

2. Clinical implications

Continuing investigation into understanding and exploring new markers of endometrial receptivity remain a high priority in reproductive endocrinology. Recent studies performed by Haouzi and associates have found new genes expressed during the implantation window by the human endometrium. [Haouzi et al., 2009] This information along with knowledge of previously discussed biomarkers can lead investigators to a more thorough approach when performing endometrial biopsies during a natural cycle especially in patients who have had unsuccessful IVF cycles. The goal of such investigation is to better understand the requirements of a hospitable environment for blastocyst implantation. Such knowledge may decrease unsuccessful implantation and facilitate a single embryo transfer in a well known receptive environment during an IVF cycle.

3. Future applications

With recent significant attention given to endometrial receptivity, it is with no surprise that new methods of investigating the endometrial factor are under investigation and may soon become routine when exploring causes for infertility. Recently performed studies have now started to analyze endometrial secretions prior to embryo transfers in IVF and IUI patients. [Boomsma et al., 2009] Recent research conducted by Boomsma and associates evaluated secretions of different cytokines including interleukins, tumor necrosis factor-α, macrophage migration inhibitory factor, eotaxin, monocyte chemotactic protein-1, and heparin-binding epidermal growth factor. [Boomsma et al., 2009] Such novel modalities may soon elucidate new therapies and treatments of defective endometrial receptivity.

4. Conclusion

With the precisely timed roles of different cytokines, hormones, and immune regulatory mechanisms, implantation is an intricate process requiring the collaboration of synchronized timed events and chemical interactions. As previously discussed, the "window of implantation" corresponds to a short period of time between days 20 and 24 of the menstrual cycle when the endometrium becomes receptive to the oncoming blastocyst. During the first part of the menstrual cycle, estrogen is present as the predominant hormone causing endometrial cell proliferation. Progesterone secreted by luteinized follicles after ovulation in the latter phase of the menstrual cycle serves to induce cell differentiation.

Approximately five-six days after ovulation, the blastocyst will enter the uterine cavity in search of a well prepared endometrium for implantation. Biomarkers such as the ones previously discussed are vital to ensure this process is successful. Selectins and mucins play a role in leading the blastocyst to a receptive endometrium , while integrins and cadherins serve as adhesion molecules for nidation. This fine orchestration of biomarkers and timed events has lead scientists toward improved understanding of the endometrium and its role during implantation. During the last decades, many advances have been made to improve ovulation and the quality of embryos. While remarkable advances such as IVF and other ART have been achieved, scientists are starting to realize the importance of a "fertile ground" at the embryo-uterus interface. Current research leading to the better understanding of biomarkers and endometrial receptivity may lead to optimization of embryo implantation in the future. Screening for receptivity markers and treating patients accordingly may allow for increasing use of a single embryo transfer with IVF leading to fewer complications encountered from multiple gestations. Patients will in tandem benefit by avoiding high costs of recurrent ART treatments and emotional despair from failed procedures. Some physicians are already taking proactive approaches in assessing endometrial receptivity by assessing biomarkes such as integrins, cyclin E, p27, and recently, even genes from endometrial biopsies. Such screenings may be standard in the near future and may lead to favorable treatments with subsequent higher rates of successful implantation.

5. References

[1] Foulk RA, Zdravkovic T, Genbavec O, Prokobphol A. Expression of L-selectin ligand MECA-79 as a predictive marker of human uterine receptivity. J Assist Reprod Genet 2007;24:316-321.

[2] Torry DS, Leavenworth J, Chang M, Maheshwari V, Groesch K, Ball ER, Torry RJ. Angiogenesis in implantation. J Assist Reprod Genet 2007;24:303-315.

[3] Roussev RG, Coulam CB. HLA-G and its role in implantation (review). J Assist Reprod Genet 2007;24:288-295.

[4] Meyer WR, Castlebaum AJ, Somkutti S, Sagoskin AW, Doyle M, Harris JE, Lessey BA. Hydrosalpinges adversely affect markers of endometrial receptivity. Human Reproduction 1997;12:1393-1398.

[5] Cheung W, Ng EH, Chung P. A randomized double-blind comparison of perifollicular vascularity and endometrial receptivity in ovulatory women taking clomiphene citrate at two different times. Human Reproduction 2002;17:2881-2884.

[6] Fakhera F, Fusi L, Takano M, Higham J, Salker M, Goto T. Role and regulation of the serum - and glucocorticoid-regulated kinase 1 in fertile and infertile human endometrium. Endocrinology 2007;148:5020-5029.

[7] Achache H, Revel A. Endometrial receptivity markers, the journey to successful embryo implantation. Human Reproduction Update 2006;6:731-746.

[8] Diedrich K, Devroey P, Griesinger G. The role of the endometrium and embryo in human implantation. Human Reproduction Update 2007;13:365-377.

[9] Afshar Y, Stanculescu A, Miele L, Fazleabas AT. The role of chorionic gonadotropin and Notch 1 in implantation. J Assist Reprod Genet 2007;24:296-302.

[10] Nikas G, Toner J, Jones H. Endometrial pinopodes indicate a shift in the window of receptivity in IVF cycles. Human Reproduction 1999;14:787-792.

[11] Damario MA, Lesnick TG, Lessey BA, Mandelin E, Rosenwalks Z. Endometrial markers of uterine receptivity utilizing the donor oocyte model. Human Reproduction 2001;16:1893-1899.
[12] Cavagna M, Mantese JC. Biomarkers of endometrial receptivity - a review. Placenta 2003;24:39-47.
[13] Strowitzki T, Germeyer A, Popovici R, Wolf M. The human endometrium as a fertility-determining factor. Human Reproduction Update 2006;5:617-630.
[14] Cittadini E. Human implantation: the new frontiers of human assisted reproductive technologies. Reproductive BioMedicine Online 2007;1;1-3
[15] Boomsma CM, Macklon MS. What can the clinician do to improve implantation? Reproductive BioMedicine Online 2006;13:845-855.
[16] Horcajadas JA, Pellicer A, Simón C. Wide genomic analysis of human endometrial receptivity: new times, new opportunities. Human Reproduction Update 2007;13:77-86.
[17] Ceydell N, Kaleli S, Calay Z, Akbas F. Difference in $\alpha v\beta 3$ integrin expression in endometrial stromal cell in subgroups of women with unexplained infertility. European Journal of Obstetrics & Gynecology and Reproductive Biology 2006;126:206-211.
[18] Goiran D, Mignot TM. Embryo-maternal interactions at the implantation site: a delicate equilibrium. Eur J Obstet Gynecol Reprod Biol 1999;83:85-100.
[19] Lessey BA, Gui Y, Aparao SL. Regulated-expression of heparin binding EGF-like growth factor (HB-EGF) in the human endometrium: a potential paracrine role during implantation. Mol Reprod Dev 2002;62:446-455.
[20] Zhu LJ, Polihronis M, Bagchi MK. Calcitonin is a progesterone-regulated marker that forecasts the receptive state of endometrium during implantation. Endocrinology 1998;139:3923-3935.
[21] Fournel S, Huc X, Alam A. Cutting edge: soluble HLA-G1 triggers CD95/CD95 ligand-mediated apoptosis in activated CD8+ cells interacting with CD8. J Immunol 2000;164:6100-6104.
[22] Martel D, Frydman R, Glissant M. Scanning electron microscopy of postovulatory human endometrium in spontaneous cycles and cycles stimulated by hormone treatment. J Endocronl 1987;114:319-324.
[23] Apparao KB, Murray MJ, Fritz MA, Meyer WR. Osteoponin and its receptor alphavbeta(3) integrin are coexpressed in the human endometrium during the mestrual cycle but regulated differentially. J lin Endocrinol Metab 2001;86:4991-5000.
[24] Alon R, Feigelson S. From rolling to arrest on blood vessels: leukocyte tap dancing on endothelial integrin ligands and chemokines at sub-second contacts. Semin Immunol 2002;14:93-104.
[25] Genbacev OD, Prakobphol A, Foulk RA, Krtolica A, Ilic D, Singer MS, et al. Trophoblast L-selectin mediated adhesion at the maternal-fetal interface. Science 2003;299:405-408.

[26] Yoo, Barlow, Mardon. Temporal ansd special regulation of expression of heparin-binding epidermal growth factor-like rowth factor in the human endometrium: a possible role in blastocyst implantation. Dev Genet 1997;21:102-108.

[27] Stavreus E, Nikas G, Sahlin L, Eriksson H. Formation of pinopodes in human endometrium is associated with the concentrations of progesterone and progesterone receptors. Fertil Steril 2001;76:782-791.

[28] Paria BC, Reese J, Das SK, Dey SK. Deciphering the cross-talk of implantation: advances and challenges. Science 2002;296:2185-2188.

[29] Artavanis-Tsakonas S, Matsuno K, Fortini ME. Notch signaling. Science 1995;268:225-232.

[30] Artavanis-Tsakonas S, Rand MD, Lake RJ. Notch signaling: cell fate control and signal integration in development. Science 1999;284:770-776.

[31] Gendler SJ, Lancaster CA, Taylor-Papadimitriou, Duhig J, Peat N, Lalani EN. Molecular cloning and expression of human tumor-associated polymorphic epithelial mucin. J Biol Chem 1990;265:15286-15293.

[32] Hilkens J, Ligtenberg MJ, Vos HL, Litvinov SV. Cell membrane associated mucins and their adhesion-modulating property. Trends Biochem Sci 1992;17:359-363.

[33] Hey NA, Li TC, Devine PL, Graham RA. MUC1 in secretory phase endometrium: expression in precisely dated biopsies in flushings from normal and recurrent miscarriage patients. Hum Reprod 1995;10:2655-2662.

[34] Bowen JA, Bazer FW, Burghardt RC. Spacial and temporal analyses of intergrin and Muc-1 expression in porcine uterine epithelium and trophectoderm in vivo. Biol Reprod 1996;55:1098-1106.

[35] Kumar S, Zhu LJ, Polihronis M, Cameron ST, Baird ST, Dua A. Progesterone induces calcitonin gene expression in human endometrium within the putative window of implantation. J Clin Endocrinol Metab 1998;83:4443-4450.

[36] Sexton PM, Houssami S, Hilton JM, Center RJ. Identification of brian isoforms of the rat calcitonin receptor. Mol Endocrinol 1993;7:815-821.

[37] Wang UK, Rout UK, Bagchi IC, Armant DR. Expression of calcitonin receptors in mouse preimplantation embryos and their function in regulationnof blastocyst differentiation by calcitonin. Development 1998;125:4293-4302.

[38] Chakraborty I, Das SK, Wang J. Developmental expression of the cyclo-oxygenase-1 and cyclo-oxygenase-2 genes in peri-implantation mouse uterus and their differential regulation by the blastocyst and ovarian steroids. J Mol Endicronlol 1996;16:107-122.

[39] Song H, Lim H, Paria BC, Matsumoto H, Swift LL, Morrow J, Bonventre JV, Dey SK. Cytosolic phospholipase A2alpha is crucial [correction of A2alpha deficiency is crucial] for 'on-time' embryo implantation that directs subsequent development. Development 2002;129:2879–2889.

[40] Wilcox AJ, Baird DD, Weinberg CR. Time of implantation of the conceptus and loss of pregnancy. N Engl J Med 1999;340:1796–1799.

[41] Ma L, Benson GV, Lim H, Dey SK, Maas RL. Abdominal B (AbdB) Hoxa genes: regulation in adult uterus by estrogen and progesterone and repression in

mullerian duct by the synthetic estrogen diethylstilbestrol (DES). Dev Biol 1998;197:141–154.
[42] Daftary GS, Taylor HS. Molecular markers of implantation: clinical implications. Curr Opin Obstet Gynecol 2001;13:269–274.
[43] Satokata I, Benson G, Maas R. Sexually dimorphic sterility phenotypes in Hoxa 10 deficient mice. Nature 1995;374:460–463.
[44] Benson GV, Lim H, Paria BC, Satokata I, Dey SK, Maas RL. Mechanisms of reduced fertility in Hoxa-10 mutant mice: uterine homeosis and loss of maternal Hoxa-10 expression. Development 1996;12:2687–2696.
[45] Cross JC, Hemberger L, Lu Y, Nozaki T, Masutami M. Trophoblast functions, angiogenesis and remodeling of the maternal vasculature in the placenta. Mol Cell Endocrinol 2002;187:207-212.
[46] Leonard S, Murrant C, Tayade C, Heuvel M, Watering R, Croy BA. Mechanisms regulating immune cell contributions to spiral artery modification-Facts and hypotheses-a review. Placenta 2006;27:S40-6.
[47] Leede-Bataille N, Bonnet-Chea K, Hosny G, Dubanchet S, Frydman R, Chaouat G. Role of the endometrial tripod interleukin-18, -15, and -12 in inadequate uterine receptivity in patients with a history of repeated in vitro fertilization- embryo transfer failure. Fertil Steril 2005;83:598-605.
[48] Ruddell A, Mezquita P, Brandvold KA, Farr A, Iritani BM. B-lymphocyte-specific c-Myc expression stimulates early and functional expansion of the vasculature and lymphatics during lymphomagenesis. Am J Pathol 2003;163:2233-45.
[49] Tammela T, Enholm B, Alitalo K, Paavonen K. The biology of vascular endothelial growth factors. Cardiovasc Res 2005;65:550-63.
[50] Halder JB, Zhao X, Soker S, Paria BC, Klagsbrun M, Das SK. Differentail expression of VEGF (164)-specific receptor neuropilin-1 in the mouse uterus suggests a role for VEGF (164) in vascular permeability and angiogenesis during implantation. Genesis 2000;26:213-24.
[51] Herr F, Liang OD, Herrero J, Lang U, Preissner KT, Han VK, et al. Possible angiogenic roles of insulin-like growth factor II and its receptors in uterine vascular adaptation to pregnancy. J Clin Endocrinol Metab 2003;88:4811–7.
[52] Volpert O, Jackson D, Bouck N, Linzer DI. The insulin-like growth factor II/mannose 6-phosphate receptor is required for proliferin-induced angiogenesis. Endocrinology 1996;137:3871–6.
[53] Licht P, Russu V, Lehmeyer J, Moll J, Wildt L. Intrauterine microdyalisis reveals cycle-dependent regulation of endometrial insulin-like growth factor binding protein-1 secretion by human chorionic gonadotropin. Fertil Steril 2002;78:252-258.
[54] Hilton DJ. LIF: lots of interesting functions. Trends Biochem Sci 1992;17:72–76.
[55] Stewart CL. Leukaemia inhibitory factor and the regulation of pre-implantation development of the mammalian embryo. Mol Reprod Dev 1994;39:233–238.
[56] Charnock-Jones DS, Sharkey AM, Fenwick P and Smith SK. Leukaemia inhibitory factor mRNA concentration peaks in human endometrium at the time of implantation and the blastocyst contains mRNA for the receptor at this time. J Reprod Fertil 1994;101:421–426.

[57] Brinsden PR, Ndukwe G, Engrand P, Pinkstone S, Lancaster S, Macnamee MC and De Moustier B. Does recombinant leukemia inhibitory factor improve implantation in women with recurrent failure of assisted reproduction treatment? O-050 ESHRE Annual Meeting, 2003; Madrid, Spain.
[58] Brosens JJ, Gellersen B. Death or survival: progesterone-dependent cell fate decisions in the human endometrial stroma. J Mol Endocrinol 2006;36:389–398.
[59] Gellersen B, Brosens J. Cyclic AMP and progesterone receptor cross-talk in human endometrium: a decidualizing affair. J Endocrinol 2003;178:357–372.
[60] Sunters A, Fernandez de Mattos S, Stahl M, Brosens JJ, Zoumpoulidou G, Saunders CA, Coffer PJ, Medema RH, Coombes RC, Lam EW. FoxO3a transcriptional regulation of Bim controls apoptosis in paclitaxel-treated breast cancer cell lines. J Biol Chem 2003;278:49795–49805.\
[61] Dijkers PF, Medema RH, Pals C, Banerji L, Thomas NS, Lam EW, Burgering BM, Raaijmakers JA, Lammers JW, Koenderman L, Coffer PJ. Forkhead transcription factor FKHR-L1 modulates cytokine-dependent transcriptional regulation of p27(KIP1). Mol Cell Biol 2000;20:9138–9148.
[62] Brunet A, Park J, Tran H, Hu LS, Hemmings BA, Greenberg ME. Protein kinase SGK mediates survival signals by phosphorylating the forkhead transcription factor FKHRL1 (FOXO3a). Mol Cell Biol 2001;21:952–965.
[63] Rena G, Woods YL, Prescott AR, Peggie M, Unterman TG, Williams MR, Cohen P. Two novel phosphorylation sites on FKHR that are critical for its nuclear exclusion. EMBO J 2002;21:2263–2271.
[64] Woods YL, Rena G, Morrice N, Barthel A, Becker W, Guo S, Unterman TG, Cohen P. The kinase DYRK1A phosphorylates the transcription factor FKHR at Ser329 in vitro, a novel in vivo phosphorylation site. Biochem J 2001;355:597–607.
[65] Revel A, Helman A, Koler M, Shushan A, Goldshmidt O, Zcharia E, Aingorn H, Vlodavsky I. Heparanase improves mouse embryo implantation. Fertil Steril 2005;83,580–586.
[66] Akira S, Taga T, Kishimoto T. Interleukin-6 in biology and medicine. Adv Immunol 1993;54,1–78.
[67] Vandermolen DT, Gu Y. Human endometrial interleukin-6 (IL-6): in vivo messenger ribonucleic acid expression, in vitro protein production, and stimulation thereof by IL-1 beta. Fertil Steril 1996;66,741–747.
[68] von Wolff M, Thaler CJ, Zepf C, Becker V, Beier HM, Strowitzki T. Endometrial expression and secretion of interleukin-6 throughout the menstrual cycle. Gynecol Endocrinol 2002;16,121–129.
[69] Tabibzadeh S, Kong QF, Babaknia A, May LT. Progressive rise in the expression of interleukin-6 in human endometrium during menstrual cycle is initiated during the implantation window. Hum Reprod 1995;10,2793–2799.
[70] Kopf M, Baumann H, Freer G, Freudenberg M, Lamers M, Kishimoto T, Zinkernagel R, Bluethmann H, Kohler G. Impaired immune and acute-phase responses in interleukin-6-deficient mice. Nature 1994;368,339–342.
[71] Salamonsen LA, Dimitriadis E, Robb L. Cytokines in implantation. Semin Reprod Med 2000;18,299–310.

[72] Lim KJ, Odukoya OA, Ajjan RA, Li TC, Weetman AP, Cooke ID. The role of T-helper cytokines in human reproduction. Fertil Steril 2000;73,136–142.

[73] Dinarello CA. Biology of interleukin 1. FASEB J 1998;2,108–115.

[74] Simon C, Frances A, Piquette GN, el Danasouri I, Zurawski G, Dang W, Polan ML. Embryonic implantation in mice is blocked by interleukin-1 receptor antagonist. Endocrinology 1994;134,521–528.

[75] Simon C, Gimeno MJ, Mercader A, O'Connor JE, Remohi J, Polan ML, Pellicer A. Embryonic regulation of integrins beta 3, alpha 4, and alpha 1 in human endometrial epithelial cells in vitro. J Clin Endocrinol Metab 1997;82,2607–2616.

[76] Gonzalez RR, Leavis P. Leptin upregulates beta3-integrin expression and interleukin-1beta, upregulates leptin and leptin receptor expression in human endometrial epithelial cell cultures. Endocrine 2001;16,21–28.

[77] Simon C, Piquette GN, Frances A, Polan ML. Localization of interleukin-1 type I receptor and interleukin-1 beta in human endometrium throughout the menstrual cycle. J Clin Endocrinol Metab 1993;77,549–555.

[78] Boucher A, Kharfi A, Al-Akoum M, Bossu P, Akoum A. Cycle-dependent expression of interleukin-1 receptor type II in the human endometrium. Biol Reprod 2001;65,890–898.

[79] Kondera-Anasz Z, Sikora J, Mielczarek-Palacz A, Jonca M. Concentrations of interleukin (IL)-1alpha, IL-1 soluble receptor type II (IL-1 sRII) and IL-1 receptor antagonist (IL-1 Ra) in the peritoneal fluid and serum of infertile women with endometriosis. Eur J Obstet Gynecol Reprod Biol 2005;123,198–203.

[80] Cervero A, Horcajadas JA, Martin J, Pellicer A, Simon C. The leptin system during human endometrial receptivity and preimplantation development. J of Clin Endocrinol Metab 2004;89:2442-2451.

[81] Houseknecht KL, Baile CA, Matteri RL, Spurlock ME. The biology of leptin: a review. J Anim Sci 1998;76:1405–1420.

[82] Holness MJ, Munns MJ, Sugden MC. Current concepts concerning the role of leptin in reproductive function. Mol Cell Endocrinol 1999;157:11–20.

[83] Zhang Y, Proenca R, Maffei M, Barone M, Leopold L, Friedman JM. Positional cloning of the mouse obese gene and its human homologue. Nature 1994;372:425–432.

[84] Chehab FF, Lim ME, Lu R. Correction of the sterility defect in homozygous obese female mice by treatment with the human recombinant leptin. Nat Genet 1996;12:318–320.

[85] Mounzih K, Lu R, Chehab FF. Leptin treatment rescues the sterility of genetically obese ob/ob males. Endocrinology 1997;138:1190–1193.

[86] Gumbiner BM. Cell adhesion: the molecular basis of tissue architecture and morphogenesis. Cell 1996;84,345–357.

[87] Huber O, Bierkamp C, Kemler R. Cadherins and catenins in development. Curr Opin Cell Biol 1996;8,685–691.

[88] Riethmacher D, Brinkmann V and Birchmeier C. A targeted mutation in the mouse E-cadherin gene results in defective preimplantation development. Proc Natl Acad Sci USA 1995;92,855–859.

[89] Fujimoto J, Ichigo S, Hori M, Tamaya T. Alteration of E-cadherin, alpha- and beta-catenin mRNA expression in human uterine endometrium during the menstrual cycle. Gynecol Endocrinol 1996;10,187-191.

[90] Gumbiner BM. Cell adhesion: the molecular basis of tissue architecture and morphogenesis. Cell 1996;84,345-357.

[91] Li Q, Wang J, Armant DR, Bagchi MK, Bagchi IC. Calcitonin down-regulates E-cadherin expression in rodent uterine epithelium during implantation. J Biol Chem 2002;277,46447-46455.

[92] Kliman HJ, Honig S, Walls D, Luna M, Mc Sweet JC, Copperman AB. Optimization of endometrial preparation results in a normal endometrial test (EFT) and good reproductive outcome in donor ovum recipients. Physiology 2006;23:299-303.

[93] Dubowy R, Feinberg R, Keefe D, Doncel G, Williams S, McSweet J, Kliman HJ. Improved endometrial assessment using cyclin E and p27. Fertil Steril 2003;80:146-56.

[94] Kliman HJ. The soil test for your endometrium: the endometrial function test (EFT). Fertility today 2006;spring:108-111.

[95] Stanley ER, Guilbert LJ, Tushinski RJ, Bartelmez SH. CSF-1-a mononuclear phagocyte lineage specific haemopoietic growth factor. J Cell Biochem 1983;21:151-159.

[96] Pollard JW, Hunt JS, Wiktor-Jedrzejczak WQ, Stanley ER. A pregnancy defect in the osteopetrotic (op/op) mouse demonstrates the requirement for CSF-1 in female fertility. Dev Biol 1991:148:273-283.

[97] Cohen E, Zhu L, Pollard JW. Absence of colony stimulating factor-1 in osteopetrotic (cs fmop/cs fmop) mice disrupts estrous cycles and ovulation. Biol Reprod 1997;56:110-118.

[98] Daiter E, Pampfer S, Yeung YG, Barad G, Stanley ER, Pollard JW. Expression of colony stimulating factor-1 in the human uterus and placenta. J Clin Endocrinol Metab 1992:74:850-858.

[99] Katano K, Matsumoto Y, Ogasawara M, Aoyama T, Ozaki Y, Kajiura S, Aoki. Low serum M-CSF levels are associated with unexplained recurrent abortion. Am J Reprod Immunol 1997;38:1-5.

[100] Shinetugs B, Runesson E, Bonello NP, Brannstrom M, Norman RJ, Colony stimulating factor-1 concentrations in blood and follicular fluid during the human menstrual cycle and ovarian stimulation: possible role in the ovulatory process. Hum Reprod 1999;14:1302-1306.

[101] Simon C, Martin JC and Pellicer A. Paracrine regulators of implantation. Baillieres Best Pract Res Clin Obstet Gynaecol 2000;14:815-826.

[102] Enders A. A morphological analysis of the early implantation stages in the rat. Am J Anat 1967;125:1-29.

[103] Ledee-Bataille N, Lapree-Delage G, Taupin JL, Dubanchet S, Frydman R and Chaouat G. Concentration of leukaemia inhibitory factor (LIF) in uterine flushing fluid is highly predictive of embryo implantation. Hum Reprod 2002;17:213-218.

[104] Ganong WF. Review of Medical Physiology. 22nd Edition 2005:411-467.

[105] Boomsma, CM, Kavelaars A, Eijkemans MJC, Amarouchi K, Teklenburg G, Gutknecht D. Cytokine profiling in endometrial secretions: a non-invasive window on endometrial receptivity. Reproductive BioMedicine Online 2009;18,85-94.
[106] Haouzi D, Mahmoud K, Fourar M, Bendhaou K, Dechaud H, Reme T, Dewailly D, Hamamah S. Identification of new biomarkers of human endometrial receptivity in the natural cycle. Human Reproduction 2009; 24,198-205.
[107] Singh H, Aplin J. Adhesion molecules in endometrial epithelium: tissue integrity and embryo implantation. Journal of Anatomy 2009; 215, 3-13.
[108] Aghajanova L, Hamilton AE, Giudice LC. Uterine Receptivity to Human Embryonic Implantation: Histology, Biomarkers, and Transcriptonics. Semin Cell Dev Biol. 2008; 19:204-211.

16

Fertility Cryopreservation

Francesca Ciani[1], Natascia Cocchia[2], Luigi Esposito[3] and Luigi Avallone[1]
[1]*Department of Biological Structures, Functions and Technology*
[2]*Department of Veterinarian Clinical Sciences*
[3]*Department of Animal Sciences and Inspection of Food of Animal Origin*
University of Naples Federico II
Italy

1. Introduction

The cryobiology is the science of low temperature biology. Fertility cryopreservation is a vital branch of reproductive science and involves the preservation of gametes (sperm and oocytes), embryos, and reproductive tissues (ovarian and testicular tissues) for use in assisted reproduction techniques (ART). The cryopreservation of reproductive cells is the process of freezing, storage, and thawing of spermatozoa or oocytes. It involves an initial exposure to cryoprotectants, cooling to subzero temperature, storage, thawing, and finally, dilution and removal of the cryoprotectants, when used, with a return to a physiological environment that will allow subsequent development. Proper management of the osmotic pressure to avoid damage due to intracellular ice formation is crucial for successful freezing and thawing procedure.

Management of non-cryopreserved reproductive cells (i.e., spermatozoa or oocytes) and tissues (i.e., testicular tissue or ovarian tissue) is problematic due to difficulties in donor-recipient synchronization and the potential for transmission of infectious pathogens, which cumulatively limits widespread application of these techniques. Cryopreserved cells and tissues can endure storage for centuries with almost no change in functionality or genetic information, making this storage a method highly attractive. Cryopreservation procedures are established on the basis of cellular physical characteristics in order to maintain viability and limit membrane damage that may occur during exposure to such non-physiological conditions as sub-zero temperatures, ice format, ion and high solute concentrations. Afterwards, there is a pressing need for the development of optimum cryopreservation methods for reproductive cells and tissues from many species. There are two major techniques for cryopreservation: freeze-thaw processes and vitrification. The major difference between them is the total avoidance of ice formation in vitrification. However, the biotechnology of the reproduction, although widely implemented, has generated protocols currently used to cryopreserve bovine sperm or oocytes, for example, that are still suboptimal, and cannot readily be extrapolated to other species' gametes.

ART provide an ensemble of strategies for preserving fertility in patients and commercially valuable or endangered species. Nevertheless, it is very difficult to successfully cryopreserve. Currently, there is a growing interest to understand the underlying cryobiological fundamentals responsible for low survival rates in an effort to develop better cryopreservation.

The key factors that affect the life-span of spermatozoa are the combinations of storage temperature, cooling rate, chemical composition of the extender, cryoprotectant concentration, reactive oxygen species (ROS), seminal plasma composition and hygienic control. Sperm preservation protocols vary among animal species owing to their inherent particularities that change extenders used for refrigeration and freezing.

On the other hand, oocytes are available only in limited number as compared to spermatozoa, therefore, a cryopreservation protocol must allow a high rate of viability maintenance when they are employed in practical application in ART programs. One of the key factors that influence the freezing process is the ratio of surface area to volume. The oocytes require a longer time to reach osmotic balance with the cryoprotectant solution than the spermatozoa, due to their bigger volume. Then, during cooling of oocytes, various forms of cellular damage may occur, including cytoskeleton disorganization, chromosome and DNA abnormalities, spindle disintegration, plasma membrane disruption and premature cortical granule exocytosis with its related hardening of the zona pellucida.

Currently, there is an increasing research effort directed towards the utilization of cryopreserved testicular tissue containing abundant numbers of germ cells at various developmental stages. Advanced stage (i.e., spermatids, spermatozoa) germ cells can be successfully retrieved from cryopreserved testicular tissue following mechanical extraction or enzymatic digestion, and it is now possible to harvest these cells at earlier stages of development (i.e., spermatogonia) for further maturation *in vivo*.

The ovarian cortex contains many thousands of primordial follicles composed of early stage oocytes surrounded by a single layer of granulosa cells. These cells may be less sensitive to cryopreservation damage because they are small and without a zona pellucida. Therefore, animal gametes have been shown to survive storage at low temperatures, and recent results are very encouraging, although reproducible methods have yet to be obtained in many species.

2. History

The idea of cryopreserving human sperm dates back to 1776, when Lazaro Spallanzani, member of the italian clergy and scientist reported that sperm became motionless when cooled by snow. In 1866, Mantegazza was the first to suggest posthumous reproduction for soldiers about to die in combat by shipping their frozen sperm back home.

The technology behind reproductive cell and tissue cryopreservation has been derived from basic scientific principles, developed over the last 50 years. The use of theoretical techniques combined with experimental research has led to many exciting improvements and provided insight into optimal methods of cryopreservation. The fertility cryopreservation has been an ever increasing field since Polge et al., (1949), in United Kingdom, produced the first chicks from cryopreserved fowl sperm, in which, partly by error, a sample was frozen with additional glycerol. Afterwards, Bunge & Sherman (1953) found that human spermatozoa treated with 10% glycerol and freezed with 'dry ice' survived in high precentage. Edwards et al. (1969) fertilized the first human egg *in vitro*. In the subsequent decades, assisted fertility clinics and commercial animal breeders have been using cryopreserved sperm successfully for artificial insemination. Although it had been shown that sperm could survive freezing and storage at low as -196° C, the functional ability of previously frozen sperm did not become apparent until the introduction of cryoprotectants. Sherman (1964) was the first to demonstrate the functional capacity of previously frozen sperm to fertilize an oocyte. The first successful human pregnancy as a result of frozen sperm was in 1969 and following this, the freezing of human sperm was largely done until the first sperm bank was opened in California in 1977. The birth of the first child to *in vitro* fertilization heralded the onset of a global expansion in the use of ART to treat infertile couples. This renewed the interest in cryobiological technology in an effort to preserve surplus embryo for future use (Kelly et al., 2003). Afterwards, methods of fertility recovery widened from sperm cryopreservation to oocytes and embryo cryopreservation.

3. Cryobiology fundaments

Cryopreservation holds tissues at temperature between -140 and -200° C, at this range no biological activity can occur, producing a state of "suspended animation" of tissue that can be maintained indefinitively (Fuller & Paynter, 2004). Cryopreserved cells and tissues can endure storage for centuries with almost no change in functionality or genetic information, making this storage a method highly attractive. Cryopreservation is the process of cooling and warming, cryo-storage that harms cells or tissue (Mullen & Critser, 2007; Barrett & Woodruff, 2010).

Freezing is the separation of pure water as ice, which concentrates any solutes present in the remaining liquid phase. This raises the possibility of two sources of freezing injury, ice itself and the altered liquid phase. Water is everywhere in the cell, it is important for the functions of the macromolecules and other cell structures such as lipid membranes. It is the universal biocompatible solvent, but also possesses unique properties for stability of living cells. Low temperatures have defined effects on cell structure and function and it is the phase transition of water to ice that is the most profound challenge for survival (Fuller & Painter, 2004). Some effects of cooling are frankly harmful: for example, cooling switches off the Na-pump, which is responsible for the regulation of cell volume, and as a result cooled cells swell (Leaf, 1959); membrane lipids undergo phase changes which may in themselves be harmful, and which also have dramatic effects on the reaction rates of membrane-bound enzymes (Lyons, 1972); poorly soluble materials may precipitate, and dissociation constants change, resulting in changes in the composition and pH of solutions (van den Berg, 1959; van den Berg and Rose, 1959); some cells are damaged or even killed by a reduction in temperature *per se*, especially if cooling is rapid, a phenomenon known as thermal shock (Lovelock, 1955).

An implicit assumption is that the conditions leading to the formation of large ice crystals inside the cell is lethal (Mazur, 1977), then to preserve structurally intact living cells and tissue, the techniques of cryopreservation focus attention on the mechanisms of damage and protection in living cells and tissues at low temperatures in attempts to preserve the viability of tissues (Muldrew & McGann, 1990). Several approaches are being taken to understand and avoid potential damaging conditions during cooling by reducing the total amount of ice formed (Farrant et al., 1977), or by preventing the formation of ice (Mazur, 1963).

The formation of ice in the environment of the cell induces changes to which the cell must respond. The morphology of ice crystals formed during freezing depends on many factors, including the composition of solution, the cooling rate, and the temperature. When a cell suspension is cooled below its freezing point, water is removed from the isotonic solution in the form of ice, increasing the concentration of solutes (e.g., salt), which remain in the unfrozen fraction and hence increasing the osmotic pressure of the remaining unfrozen solution which not only helps to reduce ice formation inside the cell but also severely dehydrates cells and can cause cell damage and death. The isotonic salt solution (0.15 M) is cooled at -0.56° C. As the cooling is continued, and further ice separates, the salt, in the remaining liquid, is more concentrated. The remaining solution is progressively diminished in volume and increased in strength until at -21.1° C the saline has reached a concentration of 5.3 M; at this temperature, eutetic point, the remaining solution solidifies. Therefore, when cells are suspended in isotonic saline that is frozen, they are subjected to a 32-fold increase in sodium chloride concentration. In the mixed solute systems that occur in practice, similar changes in osmolality occur, but in addition there are changes in composition brought about by differing solubility characteristics of the various solutes (Pegg, 1976; 2007). The dynamics of cell volume change are important in relation to possible membrane damage by mechanical means such as plasma membrane stretching and even rupture (Leibo et al., 1978; Mazur & Schneider, 1986).

The formation of ice is normally entirely extracellular. There are several reasons for this. In the first place, when heat is removed by conduction from the external surface of the specimen, the coldest point will always be in the extracellular fluid. Secondly, the extracellular fluid forms one large compartment, whereas the intracellular space consists of very many small compartments: the probability of ice nucleation occurring in any given compartment is directly related to its size, and this makes it inevitable that nucleation will occur in the extracellular fluid before a significant number of cells have frozen internally. Once ice has started to form, it will propagate throughout that compartment until equilibrium is reached. Hence, even if a few cells should freeze internally before extracellular freezing starts, once extracellular ice has formed it will continue to grow in that space, and since cell membranes are impermeable to the main solutes present, water will be withdrawn from the cells by the increased external osmolality. Hence the cells will shrink, and so long as cooling is slow enough to allow water to leave the cells to maintain equilibrium, no further intracellular freezing will occur. Thus, it is important to understand how cooling can be used to produce stable conditions that preserve life.

Although many cells and tissues can be successfully cryopreserved, without intracellular ice formation, and can be stored in liquid nitrogen indefinitely, there could be the risk of ice formation during the thawing process, if conducted improperly. If samples are thawing slowly, ice crystals can form and/or grow causing more damage; however, if samples are thawed rapidly enough, there is little time for ice nucleation and growth to occur (Fabbri, 2006; Fabbri et al., 2006).

The phenomenon of recrystallization in frozen samples occurs as smaller ice crystals with higher surface energy dissolve and larger crystals grow; the rate of recrystallization increases with increasing temperature (Mazur & Schmidt, 1968). Recrystallization of both intracellular and extracellular ice occurs during warming although the total amount of ice decreases as the temperature increases. It has been suggested that cells cooled under conditions resulting in little intracellular ice formation may be recovered undamaged if the warming rate is rapid, but would be irreparably damaged by the recrystallization of the intracellular ice on slow warming. This suggests that membrane damage caused by the osmotic pressure gradient may be resealed if the warming conditions prevent the recrystallization of ice crystals traversing the membrane (Mazur et al., 1972; McGann & Farrant, 1976). A similar resealing repair mechanism for freeze-thaw damaged cells was proposed by Law et al. (1980) which could also explain the 6% of cells that retained their barrier properties after forming intracellular ice. After thawing, there is further risk of damage during the course of removing cryoprotectants. If cells are immediately put into a significantly lower concentration of cryoprotectant, water will rapidly move into the cell and the cells can swell and burst. Therefore, it is usually advised that a series of decreasing concentrations of cryoprotectant is used to slowly remove the cryoprotectants and gently rehydrate cells. As an alternative, it can also be very effective to use a non-penetrating cryoprotectant such as sucrose to reduce osmotic shock during the step-down process (Shaw, 2000).

4. Cryopreservation methods

Two are the most utilized methods for gamete cryopreservation: slow freezing and vitrification. Slow freezing uses low concentrations of cryoprotectants which are associated with chemical toxicity and osmotic shock. Vitrification is a rapid method that decreases cold shock, without the risks of solution effects or crystallization, and uses high cooling rates in combination with a high concentration of cryoprotectant (Arav et al., 2002).

4.1 Slow freezing

Slow freezing is a conventional cryopreservation process in which a relatively low concentratiton of cryoprotectant is used (1.5 M), it shows little toxicity to cells or tissue and requires expensive equipment. As the cryoprotectant is added to cells, it results in initial cellular dehydration followed by a return to isotonic volume with the permeation of cryoprotctant and water. Generally, cells are cooled slowly using a controlled rate freezing machine, which allows samples to be cooled at various rates; ovarian tissue is generally cryopreserved at 2° C/min prior to ice seeding and 0.3° C/min after crystallization to ensure the tissue is dehydrated before intracellular ice formation occurs. Optimal rates to minimize intracellular rates formation vary among cells and tissue types (Fuller & Painter, 2007).

It is generally believed that cell injury at low cooling rates is principally due to the concentration of both intracellular and extracellular electrolytes and that cryoprotectants act by reducing this build-up. Experimental data support this explanation, in fact the extent of damage to human red blood cells during freezing in solutions of sodium chloride/glycerol/water can be quantitatively accounted for by the increase in solute concentration. Furthermore, a given degree of damage occurs at lower concentrations of solute in the presence of higher concentrations of glycerol; it appears that glycerol contributes as element of damage itself (Barbas & Mascarenhas, 2009).

4.2 Vitrification

Whereas in conventional cryopreservation the concentration of the cryoprotectant is low and the cooling rate is very slow to avoid ice crystallization, vitrification is an ultrarapid cooling technique that requires a high concentration of cryoprotectant. In 1985, vitrification was first reported with mouse embryos (Rall & Fahy, 1985) and was then further developed in animal reproduction (Ali & Shelton, 1993). In 1999 the first successful pregnancies and deliveries after vitrification of human oocytes were reported (Kuleshova et al., 1999). Since then, scientific interest on vitrification has risen significantly (Liebermann et al., 2002; 2003). The physical definition of vitrification is the solidification of a solution at low temperature, not by ice crystallization but by extreme elevation in viscosity during cooling, such that the cells or the tissues are placed into the cryoprotectant and then plunged directly into liquid nitrogen. Water is largely replaced by the cryoprotectant. The cooling rate achieved is between 15.000 to 30.000° C/min, and water is transformed directly from the liquid phase to a glassy, vitrified state. With this method no ice crystals form that can damage the cells or the tissues. This approach is attractive from a technical standpoint; unfortunately, cyroprotectant solutions are toxic to cells at very high concentrations. Solute toxicity is a major drawback of using vitrification for preservation, even with high cooling rates. To reduce toxicity, concentrations of cryoprotectants can be lowered as long as cooling is fast enough to preclude ice formation (Herrero et al., 2011).

5. Cryoprotectants

Intracellular freezing is generally lethal but can be avoided by sufficiently slow cooling, and under usual conditions solute damage dominates. However, extracellular ice plays a major role in cells and tissues. Cryoprotectants are defined functionally as any compound that increases cell survivability when used in a cryopreservation method and act primarily by reducing the amount of ice that is formed at any given subzero temperature. If sufficient cryoprotectant could be introduced, freezing would be avoided altogether and a glassy or vitreous state could be produced, but osmotic and toxic damage caused by the high concentrations of cryoprotectant that are required then become critical problems. The transport of cryoprotectants into and out of cells and tissues is sufficiently well understood to make optimization by calculation a practical possibility but direct experiment remains crucial to the development of other aspects of the cryopreservation process.

Cryoprotectants are included in cryopreservation medium to reduce the physical and chemical stresses derived from cooling, freezing and thawing of sperm cells (Gao et al., 1997; Purdy, 2006). Cryoprotectants are classified as either penetrating or non penetrating. Penetrating cryoprotectants (glycerol, dimethyl sulfoxide, ethylene glycol, propylene glycol) cause membrane lipid and protein rearrangement, resulting in increased membrane fluidity, greater dehydration at lower temperatures, reduced intracellular ice formation, and increased survival to cryopreservation (Holt, 2000). Additionally, penetrating cryoprotectants are solvents that dissolve sugars and salts in the cryopreservation medium (Purdy, 2006). A non penetrating cryoprotectant (egg yolk, nonfat skimmed milk, trehalose, aminoacids, dextrans, sucrose) doesn't cross plasma membrane and only acts extracellularly (Aisen et al. 2000). Therefore, non penetrating cryoprotectant may alter the plasma membrane, or act as a solute, lowering the freezing temperature of the medium and decreasing the extracellular ice formation (Amann, 1999; Kundu et al. 2002).

The historic discovery of the cryoprotective effect of glycerol was made in 1948 when Polge et al. (1949) found that fowl spermatozoa had been cooled to -76° C in 1.1 M glycerol recovered with little damage after thawing. Many commonly used cryoprotective agents penetrate cell membranes actually produces some problems and is certainly not a necessary property for cryoprotection. Penetrating cryoprotective agents like glycerol and dimethylsulphoxide (DMSO) permeate a good deal more slowly than water and consequently they all produce osmotic transients, the severity and duration of which vary with the compound and the cell in question. In general, osmotic disturbances have more severe effects during thawing and resuspension of the cells in cryoprotectant-free medium (when the solute is leaving the cells) than during initial equilibration and cooling (when it is entering the cells). This is due to the greater sensitivity of cells to swelling than to shrinkage. It is certainly very important to minimize osmotic disturbances during thawing and subsequent manipulations since they can contribute very significantly to the damage suffered by stored cells and tissues.

The most used cryoprotectant for sperm is glycerol. Similar to nonpermeating cryoprotectants, glycerol exerts an extracellular effect by osmotic stimulation of cell dehydration, thus decreasing the volume of intracellular water available for freezing. An intracellular effect of glycerol, exerted through its ability to permeate the cell membrane, is a decrease of intracellular osmotic stress effect of dehydration. This occurs by replacing intracellular water necessary for the maintenance of cellular volume, interaction with ions and macromolecules, and depressing the freezing point of water. Permeating cryoprotectants, depending on the concentration used, are toxic and can induce membrane damage and decrease sperm motility. Important cellular features for determining the most appropriate freezing rates as well as types and concentrations of cryoprotectant used are surface to volume ratio, membrane permeability to water, and cryoprotectants (and the corresponding activation temperatures) and membrane liability to physical stress. Spermatozoa from different species require different protocols for successful cryopreservation because of inherited particularities in cell shape, cell volume, organelles size, and composition (Medeiros et al., 2002).

Currently, three are the widely used permeating cryoprotectants in fertility cryopreservation: dimethyl sulfoxide (DMSO), ethylene glycol (EG), and propylene glycol (PG). These cryoprotectants have similar properties: solubility in water at low temperatures, cell permeability, and relatively low toxicity. However, each of these CPAs also has different degrees of membrane permeability, as has been shown with mammalian oocytes.

The transport of cryoprotectants into and out of cells and tissues is sufficiently well understood to make optimization by calculation a practical possibility but direct experiment remains crucial to the development of other aspects of the cryopreservation process.

6. Germplasm cryopreservation

6.1 Why cryopreserve genetic material?

Assisted reproductive technologies (ART) provide an ensemble of strategies for preserving fertility in patients and commercially valuable or endangered species. Cryopreservation is a way of preserving germplasm that have applications in agriculture, aquaculture, biotechnology and conservation of threatened species (Holt, 1997; Andrabi & Maxwell, 2007).

Fertility cryopreservation is an emerging field that encompasses a variety of fertility therapies for patients anticipating medical treatment that could affect future reproductive outcomes. Although most frequently associated with cancer treatment, fertility preservation has also been used for medical conditions like lupus, glomerulonephritis, and myelodysplasia, as well as in adolescent females with conditions known to be associated with premature ovarian failure (Jensen et al., 2011).

Current indications for sperm storage are quite broad and include every case and circumstance in which a future damage to the male reproductive system is suspected. It is known that sperm cryopreservation mainly affects its motility (Donnelly et al., 2001). The indications for spermcryobanking have been greatly expanded since oocytes can be fertilized even by one viable spermatozoon through intracytoplasmic sperm injection (ICSI) (Palermo et al., 1992). Although intrauterine insemination with thawed sperm is less successful that with fresh sperm (Sherman, 1973), ICSI with thawed sperm is successful as long as viable spermatozoa are injected (Kuczynski et al., 2001). This procedure has enabled men who have few surviving seminal or even testicular spermatozoa to fertilize their partner's oocytes. ICSI provides a realistic chance to achieve pregnancies and births when the sperm quantity and quality is extremely low, and in cases in which the sperm source is not renewable.

Concerning threatened species, cryopreservation of genetic material is used to the genetic management programmes of those species and genetic resource banking (Holt, 1997). Semen banks are currently more developed for rare domestic breeds (cattle, sheep, goats and pigs) than for non-domestic species, but the concept of using them to facilitate the management and conservation of endangered species is being promoted extensively (Roth et al., 1997). In order to maximize genetic diversity, a rare animal from the family bovidae could be saved with 1000 sperm doses collected from 25 different males (Comizzoli et al., 2000).

Nowadays, semen cryopreservation has other biotechnological applications. It can also be used to solve problems of preservation of semen and DNA from endangered species and, therefore, conservation of biodiversity. Cryopreservation of gametes is an important tool in assisted reproduction programmes; long-term storage of oocytes or spermatozoa is necessary when *in vitro* fertilization (IVF) or artificial insemination is to be performed at a future date or when geographical or temporal distance between donors result in non-simultaneous availability of male and female gametes, conservation by cryopreservation is the only option (Luvoni & Pellizzari, 2000). Cryopreservation of spermatozoa, oocytes, and embryo offer a potential tool for rescuing genetic material from alive or dead males or females of endangered populations, both if they are (Ciani et al., 2008; Cocchia et al., 2009; 2010).

Cryopreservation of testicular tissue would benefit at least two groups of patients: prepubertal boys who are undergoing chemotherapy or radiotherapy and infertile men who are undergoing testicular biopsy. In spite of attempts to protect seminiferous epithelium by hormone treatments (Meistrich et al., 1996; Thomson et al., 2002), prepubertal boys often lose their sperm production during cancer treatment. Especially in connection with bone marrow transplantation, the destruction of spermatogonia is often inevitable, and also the Leydig cells probably undergo damage (Siimes & Rautonen, 1990). In postpubertal boys and men, cryopreservation of semen is clinically well established and widely used, but also in them, restoration of natural fertility after cancer treatment would be a great benefit (Song et al., 2010).

Management of non-cryopreserved reproductive cells (i.e., spermatozoa or oocytes) and tissues (i.e., testicular tissue or ovarian tissue) is problematic due to difficulties in donor–

recipient synchronization and the potential for transmission of infectious pathogens, which cumulatively limits widespread application of these techniques (Woods et al., 2004). Paralleling the introduction of cryobiology to assisted reproduction has been the realization of a number of moral and ethical issues to gamete and/or embryo storage (Kelly et al., 2003).

6.2 Sperm cryopreservation

The most broadly practiced mammalian spermatozoa cryopreservation methods consist of a series of non-physiological steps that involve hypertonic cryoprotectant addition, cooling, warming, and cryoprotectant removal. Several studies have focused on the fundamental biophysical conditions that determine optimal cryoprotectant addition and removal, and cooling and warming rates (Morris et al., 1999). With this type of approach, it becomes theoretically possible to calculate the minimal number of cryoprotectanct. Sperm cryopreservation has been most successfully associated with human and bovine reproductive technologies. The most successful cryopreservation methods for spermatozoa from these species use slow initial cooling rates (1-5° C/min) starting from room temperature to a seeding temperature, followed by faster cooling rates after initial ice formation (100-200° C/min) in the presence of glycerol buffered with egg yolk-citrate medium.

Mammalian sperm are very sensitive to cooling from body temperature to near the freezing point of water. Damage to sperm, known as cold shock, is observed as an irreversible loss of motility upon rewarming. Cold shock effects on other cellular functions, such as loss of selectivity in membrane permeability, can be observed as intracellular staining with dyes that are not permeable to the intact plasma membrane. Ultrastructurally, cold shock is manifested most clearly by a disruption of the acrosomal membranes.

Membrane permeability is increased after cooling and this may be a consequence of increased membrane leakiness of specific protein channels. Calcium regulation is affected by cooling and this has severe consequences in cell function, inclusively cell death. The uptake of calcium during cooling influences capacitation changes and fusion events between plasma membrane and acrosomal membrane. Sperm membrane is a structure that undergoes reorganization during capacitation, and cryopreservation results in sperm being more reactive to their environment (Bailey et al., 2000). Cold shock reduces membrane permeability to water and solutes and injures acrosomal membranes (Purdy, 2006). The main changes that occurs during freezing are mainly ultrastructural, biochemical and functional, which impairs sperm transport and survival in the female reproductive tract and reduces fertility in domestic species (Salamon & Maxwell, 2006). The ultra structural damage is greater in ram than bull spermatozoa. Greater damages have been detected in plasma and acrosome membranes, mitochondrial sheath and axoneme (Salamon & Maxwell, 2006; Barbas & Mascarenhas, 2009).

There are only few studies dealing with sperm vitrification. Classical vitrification technique with high concentration of permeable cryoprotectants (30 to 50%) cannot be performed to cryopreserve human spermatozoa because of the lethal effect of osmotic shock. This is why vitrification had been performed mostly with oocytes and embryos. An alternative could be to use very rapid cooling and warming rates on a very small sample size. It has been shown that vitrification of human spermatozoa using cryoloops without cryoprotectants is possible Nawroth et al., 2005). Furthermore, why can vitrification be successful in the absence of cryoprotectants? Probably it depends on the size and the more stability of human spermatozoa respect to other mammals (boar, bull, ram, rabbit, cat, dog, and horse). Furthermore, the amount of osmotically inactive water is higher in spermatozoa, and is bound to several macromolecular structures such as DNA, histones, hyaluronidase, etc. (Thurston et al., 2002). Therefore, the amount of high molecular weight components can be 6–16 times higher than in embryos, resulting in enhanced viscosity and glass transition temperature The DNA integrity of vitrified sperm is comparable with that of slowly frozen/thawed spermatozoa. Such findings suggest that a wide range of cooling rates for spermatozoa can be acceptable (Isachenko et al., 2003; 2004a; 2004b; Nawroth et al., 2005).

Cryopreservation of testicular tissue is offered in some centres but is still considered experimental; potential future uses include *in vitro* maturation of spermatogonia into spermatocytes or germ-cell transplant into native testicular tissue.

7. Female germplasm cryopreservation

7.1 Introduction

During the course of the last 55 years, the science of reproductive biology, namely *in vitro* fertilization (IVF), has coincided with the ability to preserve embryos and oocytes (Fuller & Paynter, 2004). Currently, embryo and oocyte cryopreservation is the sole approved technology for human female patients wanting to preserve genetic material for future use.

Preservation of female genetics can be done through the preservation of germplasm (oocytes and embryos). It can also be done by preservation of ovarian tissue or entire ovary for transplantation, followed by oocyte harvesting or natural fertilization.

For most of the species on Earth, with current knowledge in cryopreservation, probably only male gametes can be preserved, whereas oocytes or embryos at any stage of development cannot. The culprits are in the vast differences in size, composition, and associated structures. As such, the issue of intracellular ice formation becomes a major concern, even at relatively slow cooling rates.

Embryo cryopreservation has been a proven method to preserve fertility. The first report on successful embryo cryopreservation was published in Whittingham (1977), Whittingham et al. (1972), Wilmut (1972) and Wilmut & Rowson (1973), more than two decades after Polge et al. (1949), that reported their success in freezing spermatozoa. The modification of cooling rate that came a few years later (Willadsen et al,. 1976; 1978) resulted in a basic protocol that is still in large use today. Thus, cryobanking of embryos can help in establishing founder populations with the aim of eventual reintroduction into the wild (Ptak et al,. 2002). However, evolution made each species unique in many aspects, one of which is the development of highly specialized reproductive adaptation, a specialization that is part of the definition of a species. While thousands and thousands of offspring were born following the transfer of frozen-thawed embryos in humans, cattle, sheep, and mice, success is very limited in many other, even closely, related species (Abe et al., 2011; Aller et al., 2002).

To date, the number of species in which embryo cryopreservation has been reported stands only at about 40 including humans and domestic and laboratory animals. In wild animals, especially with endangered species, this is often almost impossible, and the opportunity to collect oocytes or embryos is very rare. To overcome this limitation, researchers find imperative to use laboratory, farm, or companion animals as models during the process of developing of the necessary reproductive techniques associated with embryo cryopreservation. In some instances, appropriate model species were found. For example, studies on the domestic cat helped to develop various technologies, which were later applied to nondomestic cats (Dresser et al. 1988; Pope et al., 1984; Pope, 2000; Cocchia et al., 2010) or cattle served as a model for other ungulates (Loskutoff et al., 1995). Unfortunately, for many species (e.g. elephant, rhinoceros), no suitable model can be located, and studies should be conducted with the limited available resources with relying on the already available knowledge from research on other species (Bilton & Moore, 1976; Breed et al., 1994).

Cryopreservation of embryos in the few mammalian species in which it was attempted shows some, though often very limited, success. When considered from conservation standpoint, embryo freezing has the advantage of preserving the entire genetic complement of both parents, but it is not always possible to obtain embryos for the female valuable genetic material preservation. In many situations, then, oocyte and ovarian tissue cryopreservation represent an attractive potential means of preserving female germ cells for subsequent use in assisted reproduction (Vajta & Nagy, 2006; Abir et al., 2006; Whittingham & Adams, 1974).

In Human Chemotherapy and/or radiotherapy can induce premature ovarian failure in most of female cancer patients. Some patients may be too sick or too young to undergo fertility treatments or have hormone sensitive cancers that preclude standard approaches. As current cancer treatments improve, the survival rate of young female cancer patients has steadily increased. However, ionizing radiation and most of alkylating agents (e.g., busulfan, carboplatin, chlorambucil, cisplatin, cyclophosphamide, dacarbazine, ifosfamide, thiotepa) that used for gonadotoxic chemotherapy regimens can often induce premature ovarian failure, rendering the patient infertile. In addition, bone marrow transplantation, which is used in the treatment of cancerous and noncancerous hematologic diseases, also results in ovarian failure because heavy chemotherapy and radiotherapy is utilized to destroy the pre-existing bone marrow. Also, in nearly all cancers, with the possible exception of breast cancer, chemotherapy is initiated soon after diagnosis. Because preparation and stimulation for oocyte retrieval usually requires 2 to 3 weeks or longer, it is generally not feasible to freeze embryos from an adult female cancer patient for potential future use. Even in breast cancer patients, most would not be candidates for oocyte or embryo freezing due to concerns that high estrogen levels might have detrimental effects on the primary tumor. Additionally, not all patients have partners with whom they can create embryos for cryopreservation.

Therefore, most female cancer patients of reproductive age do not have the option of utilizing established assisted reproductive technologies to safeguard their fertility so far.

For women facing upcoming cancer therapies, cryopreservation of ovarian tissue and oocytes is a technology that holds promise for banking reproductive potential for the future.

Also, oocytes freezing offers future "social choice" in single woman, for ethical or religious problems or for governmental regulation. Non-human primates serve as research models for humans in a wide variety of fields, things work the other way around when it comes to female germplasm cryopreservation (Almondin et al., 2010; Cranfield et al., 1992). Industry needs pushed frozen-thawed ET in the cattle industry to commercial levels (Abe & Hoshi, 2003; Armstrong et al., 1995). According to a recent report by the International ET Society, over 300 000 frozen-thawed bovine embryos were transferred in 2008 worldwide. In this species, oocyte cryopreservation is very successful, and it has led to develop other correlates methods, such as superovulation techniques, and ovum pick up and *In Vitro* Embryo Production (IVEP) with no surgical methods.

The domestic buffalo (Bubalus bubalis) is a multipurpose livestock species in many countries of the world, particularly in South Asia, the Mediterranean region of Europe and South America, and is an indispensable source of employment to the marginal farmers and landless labourers. Recent advances in reproductive techniques, including superovulation, ovum pick-up and cryopreservation of oocytes offer numerous possibilities for the wider exploitation and dissemination of superior buffalo genotypes. Although the horse was probably the first animal to experience and benefit from artificial insemination, it trailed the field somewhat with regard to the application of embryo transfer and other oocyte and embryo-related modern breeding technologies.

In wild animals, especially with endangered species, it is very rare to collected the embryo but the collection of oocytes or ovary is possible, eventually also post mortem. For example the cryopreservation of female germoplasm is an important tool in assisted reproduction programs of feline species. Gamete cryopreservation represents an important tool for the development of efficient ART, and oocyte cryopreservation could facilitate the preservation of genetic resources in domestic and wild animals. It has been demonstrated that the domestic cat oocytes can serve as a successful recipient of nuclear transfer from related non-domestic cats (Cocchia et al., 2010).

Maintenance of biodiversity has intrinsic value for the genetic preservation of valuable domestic cat breeds and an extrinsic value for conservation management of taxonomically related non-domestic feline species (Luvoni, 2006). These observations are valid in different wild species as carnivore or ungulate. However, while live offspring have been produced using cryopreserved oocytes in a number of species: man (Chen, 1986); mouse, cattle, horse (Maclellan et al., 2002). The oocytes collection before cryopreservation or *in vitro* embryo production can be performed at different stage. The oocytes at a very early stage of maturation or immature (GV stage) can be collected from birth or sexually immature animals from ovary or ovarian tissue collected by surgery or post mortem. The mature oocytes (MII stage) can be collected from woman and mammalian after puberty by hormonal stimulation and non-surgery ovum pick-up.

To be fertilized, an oocyte needs to reach the metaphase II (MII) stage of maturation, or otherwise the probability of fertilization is very low (Luvoni & Pellizzari 2000). Thus, an *in vitro* maturation (IVM) procedure should be in hand to handle immature oocytes, and this process is currently developed for only a handful of species and even for these success is often fairly limited (Krisher, 2004). Furthermore, collection of immature oocytes following chemical stimulation disrupts the natural maturation process and thus compromises the quality of oocytes even if they were later matured *in vitro* (Moor et al., 1998; Takagi et al., 2001). During oocyte maturation and follicular growth, oocytes accumulate large quantities of mRNA and proteins needed for continuation of meiosis, fertilization, and embryonic development (Krisher, 2004). In the absence of the entire supporting system during IVC, production of some needed components is hampered resulting in suboptimal oocytes

(Krisher, 2004). Despite numerous studies on the issue, to date, no morphological or other method is able to accurately predict which oocytes have optimal developmental potential (Coticchio et al. 2004). Even so, it is clear that oocyte quality is a major determining factor in the success of IVF, early embryonic survival, establishment and maintenance of pregnancy, fetal development, and even adult disease (Coticchio et al. 2004, Krisher 2004; Wolf et al., 1989). Once all these hurdles have been overcome and keeping in mind the importance of oocyte quality, the next major hurdle to overcome is oocyte cryopreservation (Allen, 2010).

7.2 Oocyte cryopreservation

7.2.1 Factors affecting oocyte freezing and resolution

Oocytes are very different from sperm or embryos with respect to cryopreservation. The volume of the mammalian oocyte is in the range of three to four orders of magnitude larger than that of the spermatozoa, thus substantially decreasing the surface-to-volume ratio and making them very sensitive to chilling and highly susceptible to intracellular ice formation (Ruffing et al., 1993, Arav et al., 1996).

This problem becomes even more pronounced in non-mammalian vertebrates (fish, birds, amphibians, and reptiles) whose oocytes are considerably larger than those of mammals (Guenther et al., 2006). Oocytes of amphibians, for example, are 20–25 times larger than human oocytes. Several parameters have been taken into account in oocyte cryopreservation: cell characteristics, permeability to the cryoprotectants, toxicity, temperature and time of exposure to the cryoprotectants. Chilling injury is the main obstacle to successful oocyte cryopreservation. It has been reported that chilling injury affects the membrane, the microtubule, the cytoskeletal organization and the zona pellucida. Chromosome abnormalities also were observed after cryopreservation of human and mouse oocytes. Most striking sample is the effects of freezing on the second meiotic spindle where microtubules are disrupted or disassembled because of tubulin depolimerization.

Several approaches have been used to overcome the damage caused by chilling injury. Significant improvements have been obtained with rapid cooling throughout the transition phase, or by the addition of substance known to stabilize the plasma membrane against the thermal effect of oocytes: such as proteins (linoleic acid–albumin), sugar (sucrose or trehalose) anti-oxidant (Butylated Hydroxytoluene). In addition, supplementation of choline and higher sucrose concentration in the freezing solution can promote the retention of an intact chromosome segregation apparatus comparable in incidence to freshly collected oocytes (Willadsen et al., 1974).

7.2.2 Effect of meiotic stage

The meiotic stage seems to influence the survival of oocytes after freezing. Differing sensitivity to the cooling procedures for the oocyte cryopreservation has been related to the cell cycle stage during meiosis. The metaphase-II (MII) oocyte is extremely fragile due to its large size, water content, and chromosomal arrangement. In the mature oocyte, the metaphase chromosomes are lined up by the meiotic spindle along the equatorial plate.

Increases in chromosomal aberrations in matured oocytes were observed upon cooling and cryopreservation due to the alteration to the meiotic spindle. MII oocytes are susceptible to cryopreservation damage because of disruption of the metaphase spindle microtubule integrity during slow cooling, which may result in aneuploidy after fertilization of thawed oocytes. The plasma membrane of oocytes at the MII stage has a low permeability coefficient, thus making the movement of CPs and water slower (Ruffing et al., 1993). They are surrounded by zona pellucida, which acts as an additional barrier to movement of water and CPs into and out of the oocyte. As a result of the freeze–thaw process, premature cortical granule exocytosis may take place, leading to zona pellucida hardening and making sperm penetration and fertilization impossible (Mavrides & Morroll, 2005), a process that can be overcome by the use of ICSI or subzonal sperm insertion. Oocytes also have high cytoplasmic lipid content that increases chilling sensitivity (Ruffing et al., 1993). They have less submembranous actin microtubules making their membrane less robust. Cryopreservation can cause cytoskeleton disorganization, and chromosome and DNA abnormalities (Luvoni, 2006). The meiotic spindle, which has been formed by the MII stage, is very sensitive to chilling and may be compromised as well (Ciotti et al., 2009). It does, however, tend to recover to some extent after thawing or warming and IVC, recovery that is faster following vitrification than following slow freezing (Ciotti et al., 2009). Oocytes are also more susceptible to damaging effects of reactive oxygen species (Gupta et al., 2010). Despite many advances in the field of cryopreservation, specifically with regards to oocytes (ovulated, mature or immature), their cryopreservation is still not considered an established procedure and thus its current label as experimental technique (Noyes et al., 2010).

An alternative to cryopreservation of mature oocyte is to freeze oocyte when they have reached full size and become meiotically competent, but before they resume maturation and proceed to MII. It has been showed that oocytes frozen at the germinal vesicle (GV) stage survive better than those frozen at the metaphase-II stage (Luvoni & Pellizzari, 2000). Additionally, oocytes frozen at the GV stage have lower rates of abnormalities in the resulting meiotic spindle than oocytes frozen at the MII stage. At this stage the oocyte does not present a chilling-sensitive microtubular or meiotic spindle. Several other reports, however, paradoxically showed that the immature oocytes are more sensitive to freezing than mature oocytes, probably due to lower cell membrane stability and a particular cytoskeletal formation. This sensitivity to cryopreservation also seems to be due to the damage or interruption of cumulus cell projections, which may control the intercellular communication between cumulus cells and oocytes during maturation. Even though GV oocytes have a superior thaw survival rate and a lower incidence of meiotic spindle damage, the continued inefficiency of *in vitro* maturation protocols results in a final yield of mature oocytes that is similar to that obtained with cryopreserved metaphase-II oocytes.

Immature oocytes seem to be less prone to damages caused by the chilling (at the nuclear level), freezing, and thawing procedures, and they, too, can be cryopreserved by controlled-rate freezing (Luvoni & Pellizzari, 2000) or vitrification (Arav et al., 1993). Preantral oocytes can be preserved inside the follicle, and about 10% seem to be physiologically active after thawing and 1 week of culture (Nayudu et al., 2003). However, culture conditions that allow these oocytes to grow and reach full maturation are still largely unknown despite attempts in several species. The only species in which live young were produced from fresh (Eppig & O'Brien, 1996) or frozen–thawed (Carroll et al., 1990) primary follicles is the mouse. Some very limited success was also reported in cats, where following vitrification in 40% EG, 3.7% of the *in vitro* matured oocytes were able to develop to the blastocyst stage following IVF (Murakami et al., 2004).

The problems associated with maturation of early-stage oocytes *in vitro* are the need to develop the complex endocrine system that supports the development at different stages, other culture conditions that will ensure survival (oxygen pressure for example) and, in many species, the duration of time required to keep the follicles in culture. Another option for isolated oocyte freezing is freezing individual primordial follicles and later transplanting them to the ovarian bursa, where they can mature and eventually produce young offspring following natural mating as was shown in mice. Alternatively, ovarian cortex tissue or the entire ovary can be frozen or vitrified and then, after thawing/warming, transplanted to allow maturation *in vivo* (Candy et al. 1995), or else the oocytes can be fertilized and the resulting embryos can then be cryopreserved.

7.3 Female germplasm cryopreservation techniques

Cryopreservation holds tissues at temperatures between -140^0 and -200^{0}C, at which no biological activity can occur, producing a state of "suspended animation" of tissues that can be maintained indefinitely. It is the process of cooling and warming, not long-term cryo-storage, that harms cells or tissue. The success of these approaches depends upon the tissue, the cryoprotectant, and the freezing vessel used.

In the intervening years, variation to oocytes cryopreservation methods including changes in sucrose and sodium concentration in slow freezing media, along with the first report of successful oocyte vitrification and the development of novel cryotools have combined to provide consistently improved survival and pregnancy rate for oocyte cryopreservation. Two basic techniques have currently been used in the field of female germplasm cryopreservation, that is, slow freezing technique (Whittingham, 1977, Whittingham et al., 1972, Wilmut, 1972, Willadsen et al., 1976; 1978) and vitrification. Slow freezing method is a standard operating procedure in most IVF centers, but it is a time consuming procedure. In the slow freezing technique germplasm is gradually exposed to relatively low concentration of permeating cryoprotectants (CPs). These are usually glycerol or DMSO in the range of 1.0–1.5 M, which are added to the culture medium. Other cryoprotectants are widely used, alone or in various combinations. These include permeating CPs such as ethylene glycol (EG) and propylene glycol (e.g. Chen, 1986) and non-permeating ones such as sucrose, glucose, or fructose. The germplasm is then loaded in small volumes into straws and cooled to −7°C at −1 to −2°C/min, seeded at −7°C, and further cooled to −30°C to −35°C at −0.3°C/min, then free falling to −50°C before plunging into liquid nitrogen. This process often takes about 3 h. To date, there is no enough evidence to show that such slow cooling is necessary.

Another important method to improve the survivial of cryopreserved oocytes is vitrification. The vitrification is an ultra rapid freezing method and requires three important factors: high cooling rate, high viscosity of the medium and small volume. (Arav, 1992, Arav et al., 2002). Cooling rate is achieved by directly putting sample into liquid nitrogen. The sample is plunged into liquid nitrogen resulting in cooling rates of hundreds to tens of thousands degrees Celsius per min, depending on the container, the volume, the thermal conductivity, the solution composition, etc.. For enhancing the cooling rate, liquid nitrogen slush is employed instead of liquid nitrogen. Nitrogen slush can be produced from liquid nitrogen by using vacuum. To achieve liquid nitrogen slush, the liquid nitrogen needs to be cooled close to its freezing point (-210 °C). Slush is generated by the VitMaster (IMT Ltd,

Ness Ziona, Israel), a device that reduces the temperature of the LN to between -205 and -210° C. Oocytes or embryos are suspended in the viscous medium. This is defined by the concentration and behavior of various CPs and other additives during vitrification. The higher the concentration of CPs, the higher the glass transition temperature (Tg), thus lowering the chance of ice nucleation and crystallization. Different CPs and other additives have different toxicity, penetration rate, and Tg. The combination of different CPs is often used to increase viscosity and Tg, and reduce the level of toxicity. In the cattle industry, to avoid handling of the post-warmed embryos and to allow direct embryo transfer, EG is often used as the permeating CP because of its high penetration rate (Saha et al., 1996).

Recently, the less concentrated solution consisting of 15% (v/v) EG, 15% (v/v) DMSO or PROH and 0,5M sucrose with minimum volume can be used for human oocyte vitrification. This strategy further reduces solution toxicity. Another strategy to reduce toxic effects is the stepwise equilibration of cryoprotectants with 0.25 mL conventional straw. The cooling rate was around 2,500°C/minute and the warming rate was 1,300°C/minute. Using minimum volume method, a higher cooling rate can facilitate vitrification. Many techniques have been developed to reduce sample volume in the last decade. These techniques can generally be divided into two categories, surface technique and tubing technique.

The surface techniques include EM grid, minimum drop size, MDS (Arav 1992; Arav & Zeron, 1997), Cryotop, Cryoloop, Hemi-straw, solid surface, nylon mesh, Cryoleaf, direct cover vitrification, fiber plug, vitrification spatula, Cryo-E, plastic blade, and Vitri-Inga. The tubing techniques include the plastic straw, OPS, closed pulled straw (CPS), flexipet-denuding pipette, superfine OPS, CryoTip, pipette tip, high-security vitrification device, sealed pulled straw, Cryopette, Rapid-i and JY Straw. Each of these two groups has its specific advantages. In the surface methods, small drop (less 0.1ml) can achieve high cooling/warming rate because these systems are open. The tubing systems also may achieve high cooling rate in closed system and make samples untouched liquid nitrogen for safer and easier handle. Decreasing vitrified volume and increasing cooling rate allow a moderate decrease in CP concentration so as to minimize its toxic and osmotic hazardous effects (Barcelo-Fimbres & Seidel, 2007). The cryotop technique has been also modified by using a hermetically sealed container for storage to eliminate potential dangers of disease transmission.

7.4 Ovarian tissue cryopreservation

Another source of oocytes for gamete preservation is ovarian tissue removed for ovarian tissue cryopreservation. Large follicles 1 mm can easily be seen on the ovarian cortex and follicles greater than 5 mm may be aspirated to obtain immature cumulus-oocyte complexes.

As the ovarian tissue is processed, smaller antral follicles rupture releasing oocytes that fall to the bottom of the dish ranging in size and quality from incompetent denuded oocytes to larger cumulus enclosed oocytes. Oocytes are collected from the bottom of every dish used and matured *in vitro* up to 40 h. By 24 h in culture the cumulus granulosa, surrounding the oocyte, begins to mucify resulting in cumulus cell differentiation and expansion. By 40 h, oocytes are stripped of cumulus cells and are examined for meiotic stage; the resulting MII oocytes are vitrified for potential future use. Although there are numerous reports about pregnancies with *in vivo* matured cryopreserved oocytes, only a very few of pregnancies have been obtained using vitrified *in vitro* matured oocytes and no pregnancies with slow freezing *in vitro* matured oocytes by ovarian tissue cryopreservation. As mentioned previously, the cortex of a normal ovary is filled with arrested, immature, primordial follicles and hundreds of primordial follicles in a 1 mm^3 piece of tissue. Unlike freezing embryos and mature oocytes, the primordial follicles in cortical tissue contain small oocytes that easily survive after freezing process when the tissue is cut into small strips of 1-2 mm × 1-2 mm × 10 mm.

The common ovarian tissue slow freezing protocol is as follows: after incubation in 1.5 M ethylene glycol and 0.1 M sucrose for 20–30 min, cryovials with ovarian tissue pieces are cooled to −7°C at −2°C/min, seeded, and further cooled to −40°C at −0.3°C/min, then free falling to −100°C before storage in liquid nitrogen. Vials are thawed in a 37°C water bath, and tissue pieces are washed through progressively lower concentrations of cryoprotectant media (1.5, 1.0, 0.5,0) Methylene glycol.

Ovarian tissue transplant following tissue cryopreservation was first successfully completed in mouse and has since been successful in sheep and primates, whose ovaries more resemble those of humans. In the last few years, more than 30 cases have described the transplantation of cryopreserved or vitrified tissue to heterotopic sites such as the forearm, as well orthotopic sites such as the abdomen or back to the residual ovary. It was found, on average, that hormone ciclycity resumed within 3 and 5 months of the ovarian tissue transplant, which represents the time it takes for follicle recruitment and subsequent growth. Ovarian tissue transplantation has resulted in the birth of six children to date. As cortical tissue is isolated from the ovary, it can be cut into thin strips and cryopreserved as mentioned above; however, due to their increased oocyte size, primary and secondary follicles fail to survive the in situ freezing process. It is hypothesized that individual follicle isolation allows for better penetration of cryoprotectants, thus helping to stabilize physical connections between the follicle cells and the oocyte. Therefore, a portion of cortical tissue can be cut into smaller pieces (2 mm^3) and treated with enzymes such as liberase or collagenase that will break down stromal tissue to aid in the release of small follicles, which then can be cryopreserved for later use. Successful slow rate cryopreservation of small secondary follicles has been shown in mice, as well as in non-human primates and humans. After thawing, individual follicles can be encapsulated into a 3D matrix such as alginate, a hydrogel made from seaweed, which supports free passage of amino acids and secreted hormones and also serves as a scaffold for follicular development. It has been shown that fresh isolated follicles from prepubescent mice are capable of follicle growth from 150 to 350 μm within 8 days of culture in alginate.

8. Conclusion

The widespread introduction of assisted reproductive technology over the past 20 years has seen a simultaneous increase in the development and utilization of cryopreservation technology. Cryopreservation is now considered an essential adjunction to modern reproductive treatments. It is now possible cryopreserve both gametes and embryos at a variety of different maturational stage to offer patients a significant range of options to suit their individual fertility problem. In addition to an improvement of modalities for the treatment of human infertility, the progress in cryopreservation of reproductive cells and tissues is enabling better management of livestock and laboratory animal species and better conservation of biodiversity.

As with assisted reproduction in general, cryopreservation technology has led to the development of a number of moral and ethical issue surrounding its use. A number of these are unresolved and will continue to generate considerable debate.

9. References

Abe, H. & Hoshi, H. (2003). Evaluation of bovine embryos produced in high performance serum-free media, *Journal of Reproduction and Development* Vol.49:193–202.

Abe, Y., Suwa, Y., Asano, T., Ueta, Y.Y., Kobayashi, N., Ohshima, N., Shirasuna, S., Abdel-Ghani, M.A., Oi, M., Kobayashi, Y. et al. (2011). Cryopreservation of canine embryos, *Biology of Reproduction* [in press].

Abir, R., Nitke, S., Ben-Haroush, A., & Fisch, B. (2006). In vitro maturation of human primordial ovarian follicles: clinical significance, progress in mammals, and methods for growth evaluation, *Histol Histopathol* Vol.21(No. 8):887-898.

Aisen, E.G., Alvarez, H.L., Venturino, A. & Garde, J.J. (2000). Effect of trehalose and EDTA on cryoprotective action of ram semen diluents, *Theriogenology* Vol.53:1053–1061.

Ali, J .& Shelton, J.N. (1993). Design of vitrification solutions for the cryopreservation of embryos., *J Reprod Fertil* Vol. 99(No.2):471-477.

Allen, W.R. (2010). Sex, science and satisfaction: a heady brew, *Animal Reproduction Science* Vol. 121:262–278.

Aller, J.F., Rebuffi, G.E., Cancino, A.K. & Alberio, R.H. (2002). Successful transfer of vitrified llama (Lama glama) embryos, *Animal Reproduction Science* Vol.73:121–127.

Almodin, C.G., Minguetti-Camara, V.C., Paixao, C.L., & Pereira, P.C. (2010). Embryo development and gestation using fresh and vitrified oocytes, *Human Reproduction* Vol.25:1192–1198.

Amann, R.P. (1999) Cryopreservation of sperm, In: Knobil E, Neill JD (eds) *Encyclopedia of reproduction,* Academic Press, Burlington, MA, pp 773–783.

Andrabi, S., & Maxwell, W. (2007). A review on reproductive biotechnologies for conservation of endangered mammalian species, *Anim Reprod Sci* Vol.99:223–243.

Arav, A. (1992). Vitrification of oocytes and embryos, In A Lauria & F Gandolfi (eds) *New Trends in Embryo Transfer*,Cambridge: Portland Press, pp 255–264.

Arav, A. & Zeron, Y. (1997). Vitrification of bovine oocytes using modified minimum drop size technique (MDS) is effected by the composition and the concentration of the vitrification solution and by the cooling conditions, *Theriogenology* Vol.47:341.

Arav, A., Shehu, D. & Mattioli, M. (1993). Osmotic and cytotoxic study of vitrification of immature bovine oocytes, *Journal of Reproduction and Fertility* Vol.99:353–358.

Arav, A., Zeron, Y., Leslie, S.B., Behboodi, E., Anderson, G.B. & Crowe, J.H. (1996) Phase transition temperature and chilling sensitivity of bovine oocytes. *Cryobiology* Vol.33:589–599.

Arav, A., Yavin, S., Zeron, Y., Natan, D., Dekel, I., & Gacitua, H. (2002). New trends in gamete's cryopreservation, *Molecular and Cellular Endocrinology* Vol.187:77–81.

Armstrong, D.L., Looney, C.R., Lindsey, B.R., Gonseth, C.L., Johnson, D.L., Williams, K.R., Simmons, L.G. & Loskutoff, N.M. (1995). Transvaginal egg retrieval and in-vitro embryo production in gaur (Bos gaurus) with establishment of interspecies pregnancy, *Theriogenology* Vol.43:162.

Bailey, J.L., Bilodeau, J.F. & Cormier, N. (2000). Sperm cryopreservation in domestic animals: a damaging and capacitating phenomenon,,*J Androl* Vol.21:1-7.

Barbas, J.P., & Mascarenhas R.D. (2009). Cryopreservation of domestic animal sperm cells, *Cell Tissue Bank* Vol.10:49-62.

Barcelo-Fimbres, M. & Seidel, G.E. Jr. (2007). Effects of fetal calf serum, phenazine ethosulfate and either glucose or fructose during in vitro culture of bovine embryos on embryonic development after cryopreservation, *Molecular Reproduction and Development* Vol.74:1395–1405.

Barrett, S.L. &Woodruff, T.K. (2010). Gamete preservation *Carcer Treat Res* Vol.156:25-39.

Berg, van den L. (1959). The effect of addition of sodium and potassium chloride to the reciprocal system: KH2, P04-Na2, HPO4-H20 on pH and composition during freezing, *Arch Biochem*, Vol.84, 305-315.

Berg, van den, L. & Rose, D. (1959). Effect of freezing on the pH and composition of sodium and potassium phosphate solutions: the reciprocal system KH2PO4-Na2, HPO4-H20, *Arch Biochem* Vol.81, 319-329.

Bilton, R.J. & Moore, N.W. (1976). In vitro culture, storage and transfer of goat embryos, *Australian Journal of Biological Sciences* Vol.29:125–129.

Breed, W.G., Taggart, D.A., Bradtke, V., Leigh, C.M., Gameau, L. & Carroll, J. (1994). Effect of cryopreservation on development and ultrastructure of preimplantation embryos from the dasyurid marsupial Sminthopsis crassicaudata, *Journal of Reproduction and Fertility* Vol.100:429–438.

Bunge, R.G. & Sherman, J.K. (1953).. Fertilizing capacity of frozen human spermatozoa, *Nature* Vol.172:767-768.

Candy, C.J., Wood, M.J. & Whittingham, D.G. (1995). Follicular development in cryopreserved marmoset ovarian tissue after transplantation. Hum Reprod Vol.10(No.9):2334-2338.

Carroll, J., Depypere, H., Matthews, C.D. (1990). Freeze-thaw-induced changes of the zona pellucida explains decreased rates of fertilization in frozen-thawed mouse oocytes, *J Reprod Fertil* Vol.90(No.2):547-553.

Chen, C. (1986). Pregnancy after human oocyte cryopreservation, *Lancet* Vol.1:884–886.

Ciani, F., Cocchia, N., Rizzo, M., Ponzio, P., Tortora, G., Avallone, L. & Lorizio, R. (2008). Sex determining of cat embryo and some feline species, Zygote, Vol.16(No.2):169-177.

Ciotti, P.M., Porcu, E., Notarangelo, L., Magrini, O., Bazzocchi, A. & Venturoli, S. (2009). Meiotic spindle recovery is faster in vitrification of human oocytes compared to slow freezing, *Fertility and Sterility* Vol.91:2399–2407.

Cocchia, N., Ciani, F., El-Rass, R., Russo, M., Borzacchiello, G., Esposito, V., Montagnaro, S., Avallone, L., Tortora, G. & Lorizio, R. (2009). Cryopreservation of feline epididymal spermatozoa from dead and alive animals and its use in assisted reproduction, Zygote Vol.18(No.1):1-8.

Cocchia, N., Ciani, F., Russo, M., El Rass, R., Rosapane, I., Avallone, L., Tortora, G. & Lorizio, R, (2010) Immature cat oocyte vitrification in open pulled straws (OPSs) using a cryoprotectant mixture, *Cryobiology* Vol.60(No.2):229-34.

Comizzoli, P., Mermillod, P. & Mauget, R. (2000). Reproductive biotechnologies for endangered mammalian specie, *Reprod Nutr Dev.* Vol40(No.5):493-504.

Coticchio, G., Sereni, E., Serrao, L., Mazzone, S., Iadarola, I. & Borini, A. (2004). What criteria for the definition of oocyte quality? *Annals of the New York Academy of Sciences* Vol.1034:132–144.

Cranfield, M.R., Berger, N.G., Kempske, S., Bavister, B.D., Boatman, D.E. & Ialeggio, D.M. (1992). Macaque monkey birth following transfer of in vitro fertilized, frozen–thawed embryos to a surrogate mother, *Theriogenology* Vol.37:197.

Donnelly, E.T., Steele, E.K., McClure, N. & Lewis, S.E. (2001). Assessment of DNA integrity and morphology of ejaculated spermatozoa from fertile and infertile men before and after cryopreservation, *Hum. Reprod.* Vol.16:1191–1199.

Dresser, B.L., Gelwicks, E.J., Wachs, K.B. & Keller, G.L. (1988). First successful transfer of cryopreserved feline (Felis catus) embryos resulting in live offspring, *J Exp Zool* Vol.246(No.2):180-186.

Edwards, R.G., Bavister, B.D. & Steptoe, P.C. (1969). Early Stages of Fertilization in vitro of Human Oocytes Matured in vitro, *Nature* Vol.221, 632-635.

Eppig, J.J., O'Brien, M., Wigglesworth, K. (1996). Mammalian oocyte growth and development in vitro, *Mol Reprod Dev* Vol.44(No.2):260-273.

Fabbri, R. (2006). Cryopreservation of human oocytes and ovarian tissue, *Cell Tissue Bank* Vol.7(No.2):113-122.

Fabbri, R., Pasquinelli, G., Braconer, G., Orrico, C., Di Tommaso, B. & Venturoli, S. (2006). Cryopreservation of human ovarian tissue, *Cell Tissue Bank* Vol.7(No.2): 123-133.

Farrant, J., Walter, C., Lee, H. & McGann, L. (1977). Use of two-step cooling procedures to examine factors influencing cell survival following freezing and thawing, *Cryobiology* Vol.14:273-286.

Fuller, B. & Paynter, S. (2004). Fundamentals of cryobiology in reproductive medicine, *Reprod Biomed Online* Vol.9(No.6):680-691.

Fuller, B. & Paynter, S. (2007). Cryopreservation of mammalian embryos, *Methods Mol Biol* Vol.368:325-339.

Gao, D.Y., Mazur, P. & Critser, J.K. (1997). Fundamental cryobiology of mammalian spermatozoa, In: Karow AM, Critser JK (eds) *Reproductive tissue banking*, Academic press, San Diego pp 263–327.

Guenther, J.F., Seki, S., Kleinhans, F.W., Edashige, K., Roberts, D.M. & Mazur, P. (2006). Extra- and intra-cellular ice formation in stage I and II Xenopus laevis oocytes, *Cryobiology* Vol.52:401–416.

Gupta, M.K., Uhm, S.J. & Lee, H.T. (2010). Effect of vitrification and betamercaptoethanol on reactive oxygen species activity and in vitro development of oocytes vitrified before or after in vitro fertilization, *Fertility and Sterility* Vol93:2602–2607.

Herrero, L., Martinez, M. & Garcia-Velasco, J.A. (2011). Current status of human oocyte and embryo cryopreservation, *Curr Op Obstetr Gynecol* Vol.23(No.4):245-250.

Holt, W.V. (1997). Alternative strategies for long-term preservation, *Reprod Fertil Dev* Vol.9:309–319.

Holt, W.V. (2000). Basic aspects of frozen storage semen, *Anim Reprod Sci* Vol.62:3–22.

Isachenko, E. (2003). Vitrification of mammalian spermatozoa in the absence of cryoprotectants: from past practical difficulties to present success, *Reprod Biomed Online* Vol.6(No.2):191–200.

Isachenko, E., Isachenko, V., Katkov, I.I., Rahimi, G., Schöndorf, T., Mallmann, P., Dessole, S. & Nawroth, F. (2004a). DNA integrity and motility of human spermatozoa after standard slow freezing versus cryoprotectant-free vitrification, *Hum Reprod* Vol.19:932–93.

Isachenko, V., Isachenko, E., Katkov, I.I., Montag, M., Dessole, S., Nawroth, F. & Van Der Ven, H. (2004b). Cryoprotectant-free cryopreservation of human spermatozoa by vitrification and freezing in vapor: effect on motility, DNA integrity, and fertilization ability, *Biol Reprod* Vol.71:1167–1173.

Jensen, J.R., Morbeck, D.E. & Coddington, C.C. 3rd. (2011). Fertility preservation, *Mayo Clin Proc* Vol.86(No.1):45-49.

Kelly, S.M., Buckett, W.M., Abdul-Jalil, A.K. & Tan S.L. (2003). The cryobiology of assisted reproduction, *Minerva Ginecol* Vol.55(No.5):389-398.Krisher, R.L. (2004). The effect of oocyte quality on development, *Journal of Animal Science* Vol.82:E14–E23.

Krisher, R.L. (2004). The effect of oocyte quality on development, *Journal of Animal Science* Vol.82: E14–E23.

Kuczyński, W., Dhont, M., Grygoruk, C., Grochowski, D., Wołczyński, S. & Szamatowicz, M. (2001) The outcome of intracytoplasmic injection of fresh and cryopreserved ejaculated spermatozoa—a prospective randomized study, *Hum. Reprod.* Vol.16: 2109–2113.

Kuleshova, L., Gianaroli, L., Magli, C., Ferraretti, A. & Trounson, A. (1999). Birth following vitrification of a small number of human oocytes: case report, Hum Reprod Vol.14:3077–3079.

Kundu, C.N., Chakraborty, J., Dutta, P., Bhattacharyya, D., Ghosh, A. &, Majumder, G.C. (2002). Effects of dextrans on cryopreservation of goat cauda epididymal spermatozoa using a chemically defined medium, *Reproduction* Vol.123:907–913.

Law, P., Sprott, D., Lepock, J. & Kruuv, J. (1980) Post-thaw lysing and osmotic reactivation of frozen-thawed cell, *Cryo Lett* Vol.1:173-180.

Leaf, A. (1959). Maintenance of concentration gradients and regulation of cell volume, *Ann. N. Y. Acad. Sci.* Vol.72:396-404.

Leibo, S.P., McGrath, J.J., Cravalho, E.G. (1978). Microscopic observation of intracellular ice formation in unfertilized mouse ova as a function of cooling rate, *Cryobiology* Vol.15(No.3):257–71.

Liebermann, J., Nawroth, F., Isachenko, V., Isachenko, E., Rahimi, G. & Tucker, M.J. (2002). Potential importance of vitrification in reproductive medicine, *Biol Reprod* Vol.67:1671–1680.

Liebermann, J., Tucker, M.J., Sills, E.S. (2003). Cryoloop vitrification in assisted reproduction: analysis of survival rates in >1000 human oocytes after ultra-rapid cooling with polymer augmented cryoprotectants,. *Clin Exp Obstet Gynecol* Vol.30:125–129.

Loskutoff, N.M., Bartels, P., Meintjes, M., Godke, R.A. & Schiewe, M.C. (1995). Assisted reproductive technology in nondomestic ungulates: a model approach to preserving and managing genetic diversity, *Theriogenology* Vol.43: 3–12.

Luvoni, G.C. & Pellizzari, P. (2000). Embryo development in vitro of cat oocytes cryopreserved at different maturation stages, *Theriogenology* Vol.53:1529–1540.

Lovelock, J.E. (1955). The physical instability of human red blood cells, *Biochem J* Vol.60(No.4):692-6.

Luvoni, G.C. (2006). Gamete cryopreservation in ther domestic cat. *Theriogenology* Vol.66(No.1):101-111.Luvoni, G.C. & Pellizzari, P. (2000). Embryo development in vitro of cat oocytes cryopreserved at different maturation stages, *Theriogenology* Vol.53:1529–1540.

Loskutoff, N.M., Bartels, P., Meintjes, M., Godke, R.A. & Schiewe, M.C. (1995). Assisted reproductive technology in nondomestic ungulates: a model approach to preserving and managing genetic diversity, *Theriogenology* Vol.43:3–12

Lyons, J. M. (1972). Phase transitions and control of cellular metabolism at low temperatures, *Crvobiology* Vol.9: 341-350.

Maclellan, L.J., Carnevale, E.M., Coutinho da Silva, M.A., Scoggin, C.F., Bruemmer, J.E. & Squires, E.L. (2002). Pregnancies from vitrified equine oocytes collected from super-stimulated and non-stimulated mares,. *Theriogenology*Vol. 58(No.5):911-919.

Mavrides, A. & Morroll, D. (2005). Bypassing the effect of zona pellucida changes on embryo formation following cryopreservation of bovine oocytes, *Eur J Obstet Gynecol Reprod Biol* Vol.118(No.1):66-70.

Mazur, P. (1963). Kinetics of water loss from cells at subzero temperatures and the likelihood of intracellular freezing *J Gen Physiol*. Vol.47:347-369.

Mazur, P. (1977). Slow-freezing injury in mammalian cells, *Ciba Found Symp* Vol.52:19-48.

Mazur, P., Leibo, S.P. & Chu, E.H.Y. (1972). A two factor hypothesis of freezing injury, *Exp Cell Res* Vol.71:345-355.

Mazur, P. & Schmidt, J. (1968). Interactions of cooling velocity, temperature, and warming velocity on the survival of frozen and thawed yeast, *Cryobiology* Vol.5:1-17.

Mazur, P. & Schneider, U. (1986). Osmotic responses of preimplantation mouse and bovine embryos and their cryobiological implication, *Cell Biophys* Vol.8:259-285.

McGann, L. & Farrant J. (1976). Survival of tissue culture cells frozen by a two-step procedure to -196° C. II. Warming rate and concentration of dimethylsulfoxide, *Cryobiology* Vol.13:269-273.

Medeiros, C.M., Forell, F., Oliveira, A.T. & Rodriguez, J.L. (2002). Current status of sperm cryopreservation: why isn't better? *Theriogenology* Vol.57:327-344.

Meistrich, M.L., Wilson, G., Ye, W.S., Thrash, C. & Huhtaniemi, I. (1996). Relationship among hormonal treatments, suppression of spermatogenesis, and testicular protection from chemotherapy-induced damage, *Endocrinology* Vol.137: 3823–3831.

Moor, R.M., Dai, Y., Lee, C., Fulka, J. Jr. (1998). Oocyte maturation and embryonic failure, *Human Reproduction Update* Vol.4:223–226.

Morris, G.J., Acton, E, & Avery, A. (1999).A novel approach to sperm cryopreservation, *Hum Reprod* Vol.14:1013-1021.

Muldrew, K. & McGann, L.E. (1990). Mechanisms of intracellular ice formation, *Biophys J Biophysical Society* Vol.57:525-532.

Mullen, S.F. & Critser, J.K. (2007). The science of cryobiology, in Woodruff T.K. & Snyder K.A. (eds) *Oncofertility: fertility preservation for cancer survivors*, New York: Springer pp. 83-103.

Murakami, M., Otoi, T., Karja, N.W., Wongsrikeao, P., Agung, B. & Suzuki, T. (2004). Blastocysts derived from in vitro-fertilized cat oocytes after vitrification and dilution with sucrose, *Cryobiology* Vol-48:341–348.

Nayudu, P., Wu, J. & Michelmann, H. (2003). In vitro development of marmoset monkey oocytes by pre-antral follicle culture, *Reproduction in Domestic Animals* Vol.38:90–96.

Nawroth, F., Rahimi, G., Isachenko, E., Isachenko, V., Lieberman, M., Tucker, M.J. & Lieberman, J. (2005). Cryopreservation I Assisted Reproductive Technology: New Trends, *Seminars Reprod Med* Vol.23(No.4):325-335.

Noyes, N., Boldt, J. & Nagy, Z.P. (2010). Oocyte cryopreservation: is it time to remove its experimental label? *Journal of Assisted Reproduction and Genetics* Vol.27:69-74.

Palermo, G., Devroey, P., Van Steirteghem, A.C. & Joris, H. (1992). Pregnancies after intracytoplasmic injection of single spermatozoon into an oocyte, *Lancet* Vol.340:17-18.

Pegg, D. (1976). Long-term preservation of cells and tissues: a review, *J cli. Path* Vol.29: 271-285.

Pegg, D.E. (2007). Principles of cryopreservation, *Methods Mol Biol* Vol.368:39-57.

Polge, C., Smith, A.Y. & Parkes, A.S. (1949). Revival of spermatozoa after vitrification and dehydration at low temperature, *Nature* Vol.164:666.

Pope, C.E. (2000). Embryo technology in conservation efforts for endangered felids, *Theriogenology* Vol.53:163-174.

Pope, C.E., Pope, V.Z. & Beck, L.R. (1984). Live birth following cryopreservation and transfer of a baboon embryo, *Fertility and Sterility* Vol.42:143-145.

Ptak, G., Clinton, M., Barboni, B., Muzzeddu, M., Cappai, P., Tischner, M. & Loi, P. (2002). Preservation of the wild European mouflon: the first example of genetic management using a complete program of reproductive biotechnologies *Biology of Reproduction* Vol.66:796-801.

Purdy, P.H. (2006). A review on goat sperm cryopreservation, *Small Rum Res* Vol.6:215-225.

Rall, W.F. & Fahy, G.M. (1985). Ice-free cryopreservation of mouse embryos at -196°C by vitrification, *Nature* Vol.313:573-575.

Roth, T.L., Armstrong, D.L., Barrie, M.T. & Wildt, D.E. (1997). Seasonal effects on ovarian responsiveness to exogenous gonadotrophins and successful artificial insemination in the snow leopard (Uncia uncia) *Reprod Fertil Dev* Vol.9(No.3):285-295.

Ruffing, N.A., Steponkus, P.L., Pitt, R.E. & Parks, J.E. (1993):.Osmometric behavior, hydraulic conductivity, and incidence of intracellular ice formation in bovine oocytes at different developmental stages, *Cryobiology* Vol.30(No.6):562-80.

Saha, S., Otoi, T., Takagi, M., Boediono, A., Sumantri, C. & Suzuki, T. (1996). Normal calves obtained after direct transfer of vitrified bovine embryos using ethylene glycol, trehalose, and polyvinylpyrrolidone, *Cryobiology* Vol.33:291-299.

Salamon, S. & Maxwell, W.M. (2006). Storage of ram semen, *Anim Reprod Sci* Vol.62:77-111.

Saragusty, J.J. & Arav, A. (2011). Current progress in oocyte and embryo cryopreservation by slow freezing and vitrification, *Reproduction* Vol141:1-19.

Siimes, M.A. & Rautonen, J. (1990). Small testicles with impaired production of sperm in adult male survivors of childhood malignancies, *Cancer* Vol.65:1303-1306.

Shaw, J.M. (2000). Cryopreservation of oocytes and embryos. In Trounson AO; Gardner DK (eds) *Handbook of in vitro fertilization*. 2. Boca Raton: CRC Press LLC, p.373-368.

Sherman, J.K. (1964). Low temperature research on spermatozoa and eggs, *Cryobiology* Vol.1(No.2): 103-129.

Sherman, JK (1973). Synopsis of the use of frozen human semen since 1964: state of the art of human semen banking, *Fertil. Steril.* Vol.24:397-412.

Song, Y., Sharp, R., Lu, F. & Hassan, M. (2010). The future potential of cryopreservation for assisted reproduction, *Cryobiology* Vol.60:S60-S65.

Takagi, M., Kim, I.H., Izadyar, F., Hyttel, P., Bevers, M.M., Dieleman, S.J., Hendriksen, P.J. & Vos. P.L. (2001). Impaired final follicular maturation in heifers after superovulation with recombinant human FSH, *Reproduction* Vol.121:941-951.

Thomson, B., Campbell, A.J., Irvine, D.C., Anderson, A.R., Kelnar, C.J. & Wallace, W.H. (2002). Semen quality and spermatozoal DNA integrity in survivors of childwood cancer: a case-control study, *Lancet* Vol.360:361-367.

Thurston, L.M., Siggins, A., Mileham, P.F., Watson, P.F. & Holt, W.V. (2002). Identification of amplified restriction fragment length polymorphism markers linked to genes controlling boar sperm viability following cryopreservation, *Biol Reprod* Vol.66:545–554.

Vajta, G. & Nagy, Z.P. (2006). Are programmable freezers still needed in the embryo laboratory? Review on vitrificatio, *Reprod Biomed Online* Vol.12:779–96.

Whittingham, D.G. (1977). Fertilization in vitro and development to term of unfertilized mouse oocytes previously stored at K196 8C, *Journal of Reproduction and Fertility* Vol.49:89–94.

Whittingham, D.G. & Adams, C.E. (1974). Low temperature preservation of rabbit embryos, *Cryobiology* Vol.11:560–561.

Whittingham, D.G., Leibo, S.P. & Mazur, P. (1972). Survival of mouse embryos frozen to K196 8C and K269 8C, *Science* Vol.178 411–414.

Willadsen, S.M., Polge, C., Rowson, L.E.A. & Moor, R.M. (1974). Preservation of sheep embryos in liquid nitrogen, *Cryobiology* Vol11:560.

Willadsen, S.M., Polge, C., Rowson, L.E.A. & Moor, R.M.. (1976). Deep freezing of sheep embryos, *Journal of Reproduction and Fertility* Vol.46:151–154.

Willadsen, S., Polge, C. & Rowson, L.E.A. (1978). The viability of deep-frozen cow embryos. *Journal of Reproduction and Fertility* Vol.52:391–393.

Wilmut, I. (1972). The effect of cooling rate, warming rate, cryoprotective agent and stage of development of survival of mouse embryos during freezing and thawing, *Life Sciences* Vol.11:1071–1079.

Wilmut, I. & Rowson, L.E. (1973). Experiments on the low-temperature preservation of cow embryos, *Veterinary Record* Vol.92:686–690.

Wolf, D.P., Vandevoort, C.A., Meyer-Haas, G.R., Zelinski-Wooten, M.B., Hess, D.L., Baughman, W.L. & Stouffer, R.L. (1989). In vitro fertilization and embryo transfer in the rhesus monkey, *Biology of Reproduction* Vol.41:335–346.

Woods, E.J., Benson, J.D., Agca, Y. & Crister, J.K. (2004). Fundamental cryobiology of reproductive cells and tissue, *Cryobiology* Vol.48:146-156.